MW01627357

The Complete Seven Rays of Healing System

The Complete Seven Rays of Healing System

ISBN 978-1-63625-393-0
Printed in the United States of America

Published by
Fifth World Wisdom Press

Other books by Mark Amaru Pinkham
THE RETURN OF THE SERPENTS OF WISDOM
CONVERSATIONS WITH THE GREAT GODDESS
FROM THE GREEN MAN TO JESUS: THE ORIGIN AND EVOLUTION OF THE CHRIST MYTH
GUARDIANS OF THE HOLY GRAIL
WORLD GNOSIS: THE COMING GNOSTIC CIVILIZATION
SEDONA: CITY OF THE STAR PEOPLE
SACRED GEOMETRY THE CREATION OF THE UNIVERSE
AN INITIATE'S GUIDE TO THE PATH OF THE DRAGON

TABLE OF CONTENTS

Introduction: The Origin of Seven Ray Healing............................pg.1

Chapter 1: The Theory of the Seven Rays...................................pg.14

Chapter 2: The Characteristics, Abilities & Destinies
of People born under each of the the Seven Rays.......................pg.43

Chapter 3: Seven Rays Color and Sound Healing...................... pg.74

Chapter 4: The Inner Organs: Diagnosis and Treatment.............pg.98

Chapter 5: The Dragon Body of Meridians & Chakras.................pg.119

Chapter 6: Seven Ray Reiki and Polarity Therapy.......................pg.171

Chapter 7:Creating a Seven Ray Healing Temple.......................pg.184

Chapter 8:Giving a Seven Ray Balancing Treatment.................pg.200

Chapter 9:Advanced Diagnosis Techniques and

Treatment of the Inner Organs..pg.223

Appendix 1: Additional Seven Rays of Healing Modalities........pg.243

Appendix 2: The Dragon Body Activation Technique..............pg.245

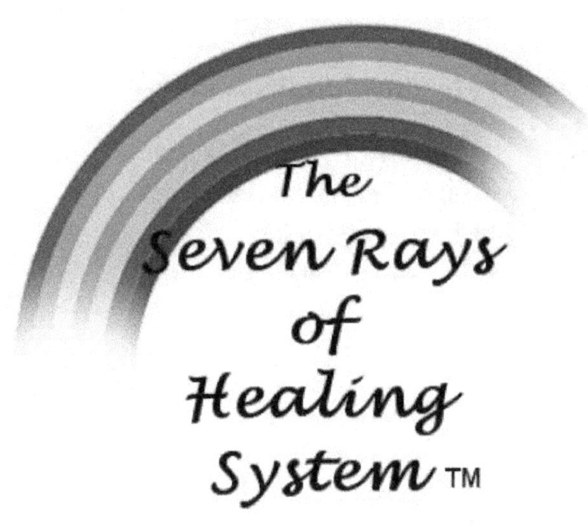

Introduction: The Origin of Seven Ray Healing

The Origin of the Seven Rays of Healing System

The Seven Rays of Healing was first taught on the ancient Pacific continent of Lemuria many thousands of years ago. The system emerged within the Order of the Seven Rays, which was founded by the Lord of the Seven Rays, Sanat Kumara or Karttikeya, the "Son of the Pleiades." Karttikeya was sent to Earth by his Mother, Sophia, the Lady of the Seven Rays and Goddess of the Pleiades, when She decided that Her "children" on Earth should realize their spiritual greatness.

Sanat Kumara brought to Earth the Gnostic-Alchemical tradition or "Siddha Marga," the Path to Human Perfection, that consisted of practices designed to awaken the dormant alchemical force of Kundalini in the human body and transform each person into a fully enlightened, God-Realized soul. A God-Realized adept is one that knows he or she is "God," the Infinite Spirit, that created the universe and has existed for eternity.

The Order of the Seven Rays was founded to preserve and teach the Gnostic-Alchemical Path. Within it emerged the Seven Rays of Healing System. The Seven Ray Order and Healing System became a mystical branch of the primal nature religion of the Goddess & Her Son that once covered Lemuria.

When most of Lemuria eventually sank to the bottom of the Pacific Ocean, waves of missionaries took both the Order of the Seven Rays and the Seven Rays of Healing System to fledgling Atlantis on the opposite side of the planet, and to the Pan-Pacific countries that surrounded MU, including India, China and Peru. It was from these lands that the Seven Ray Order and Healing System were then taken to other parts of the globe. Many years later the Order of the Seven Rays became known as the Great White Brotherhood and the Seven Rays of Healing re-emerged as a complete natural healing system.

The Seven Pleiades: Home of the Seven Rays

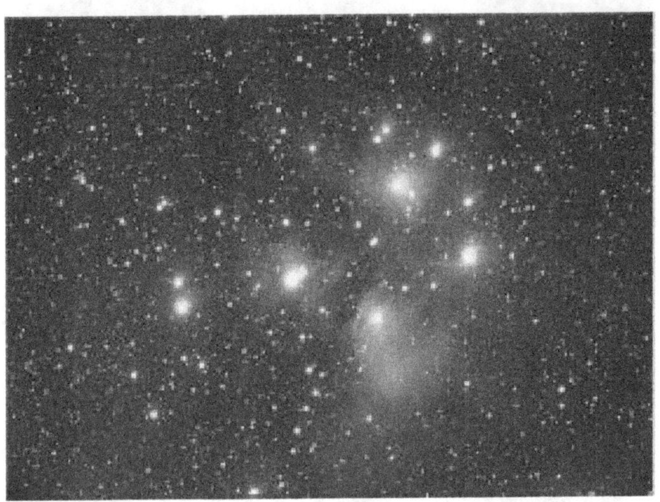

Collectively the Pleiades are

Sophia: The Lady of the Seven Rays

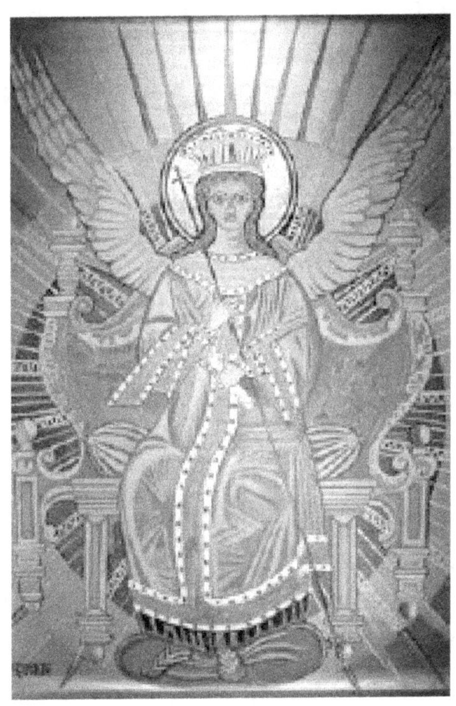

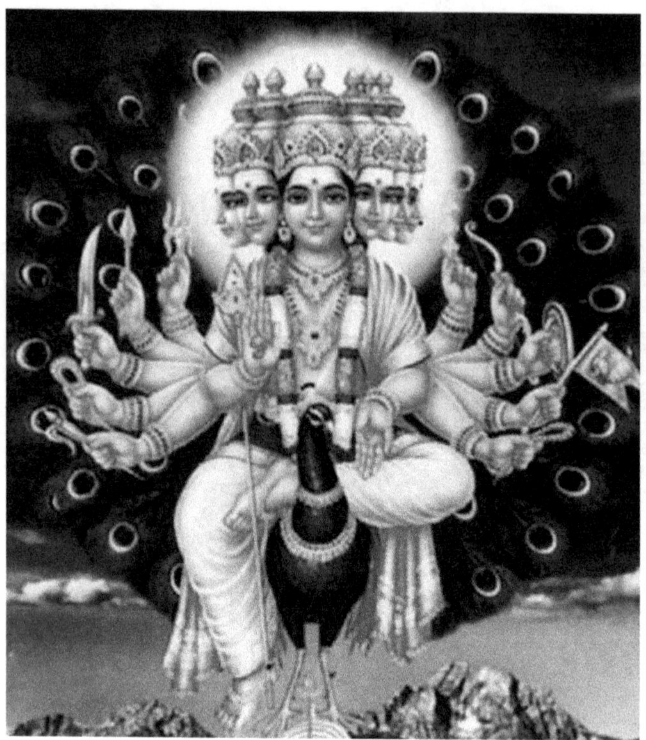

Lord of the Seven Rays
The Son of Goddess Sophia
The Founder of Seven Rays Healing

The Divine Son, Sanat Kumara as Karttikeya: "Son of the Pleiades."
Sent to Earth by Sophia from the Seven Sisters
He founded the Order of the Seven Rays
aka the Great White Brotherhood.
Together, his Seven Heads
(One is invisible)
Denote the
7 Rays

Invoke Sanat Kumara when you begin to practice Seven Ray Healing
use the Sanscrit mantra "Om Namo Skandaya Namaha"
Skanda is Sanat Kumara's "Serpent" or Energy Name
Kan or Can is the universal name of the Serpent

Among the Yezidis of northern Iraq, the Lord of the Seven Rays became known as the Peacock Angel

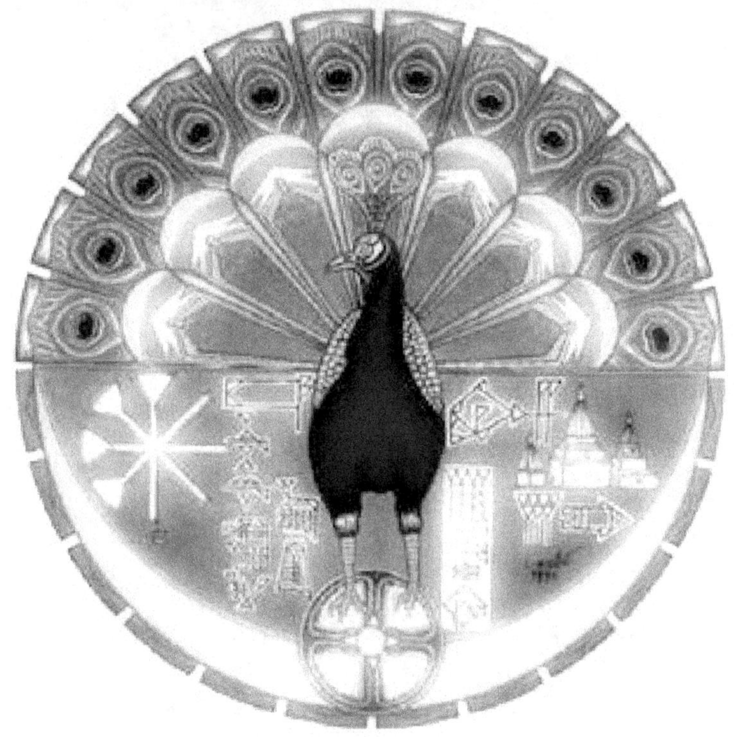

The Peacock Angel

The Lord and Embodiment of the Seven Rays

The Peacock Angel brought the Seven Rays to Earth .Notice the three feathers on his head. They represent the first Three Rays. And the seven red feathers just behind them represent all the Seven Rays.

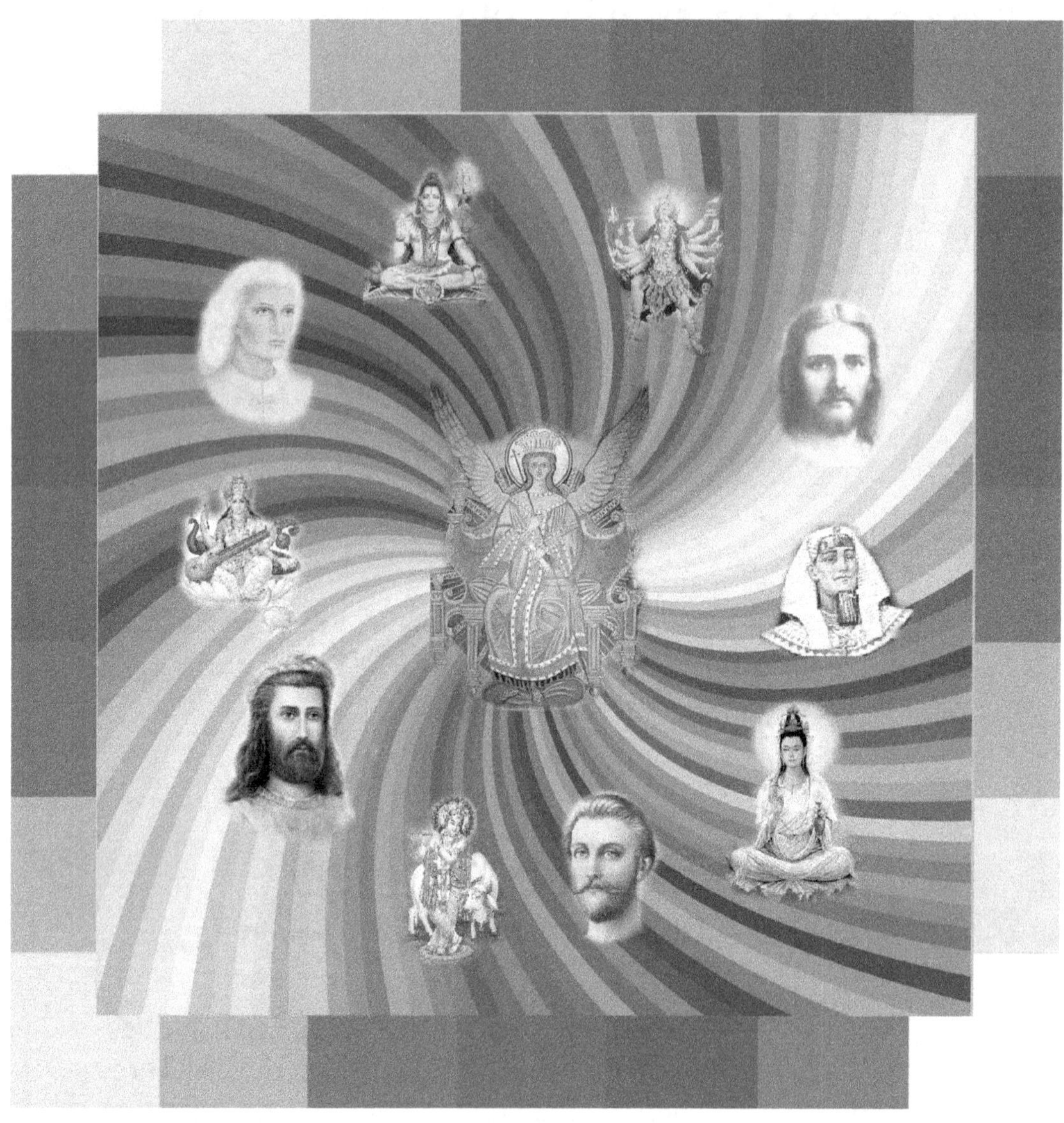

Sophia, Lady of the Seven Rays, and Her "Sons" and "Daughters," the Lords and Ladies of the individual Rays

The Seven Rays of Healing System in India, China and Peru

The Seven Rays of Healing in India

Before arriving in India the Seven Rays of Healing System was practiced in the Pandyan Kingdom, which once existed on the landmass that united India with Lemuria. The principal teacher of the Pandyan Kingdom was the Siddha Agastya, a direct disciple of Sanat Kumara. When his homeland sank below the waves of the Indian Ocean, Agastya took the teachings of the Siddha Marga north into South India and made the Pothigai Hills his new home and headquarters. Agastya then trained many new Siddhas and instructed them to take the teachings of the Siddha Marga around the Indian sub-continent and found schools of yoga. Foremost among the Siddha disciples and missionaries of Agastya was Siddha Goraknath, the founder of the school of Hatha Yoga, Bogarnath, the founder of the alchemical school of Rasayana, and the Siddha Babaji, founder of Kriya Yoga.

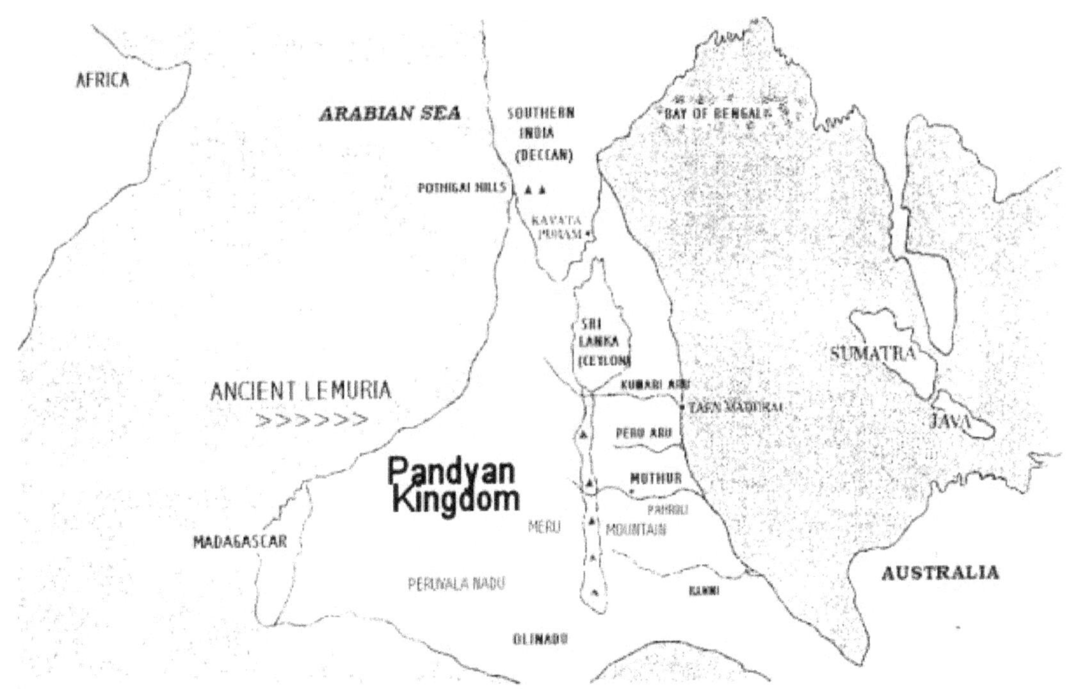

In India, Seven Ray Healing became part of the spiritual/healing traditions of the Vedas, Tantras and Siddha Medicine. Perhaps the best surviving example of the Seven Rays and their correspondences can be found within the science of Jyotish, the "Science of Light," which is know in the west as Hindu or Vedic Astrology. Vedic Astrology is based upon both the Solar Zodiac of twelve astrological signs, as well as the Lunar Zodiac of twenty-seven Lunar Mansions (approximately one lunar sign per day of a lunar month). It recognizes the Moon (symbol of the female principle) as the most important astrological "planet," and is, therefore, more closely aligned with the ancient Goddess Tradition than the astrology of the west which pivots around the movement of the Sun and the male principle it represents.

The esoteric texts of Jyotish maintain that the one primal life force divides into seven Rays or spirits, and each of these move through the seven "planets," the Sun, Moon, Mercury, Venus, Mars, Jupiter, and Saturn, before arriving on Earth and influencing the existence of every life form. The science of Jyotish makes correspondences between the Seven Rays and the seven astrological "planets" (Saturn, Jupiter, Mars, Venus, Mercury, Sun and Moon), as well as the seven color frequencies, and the seven sound frequencies.

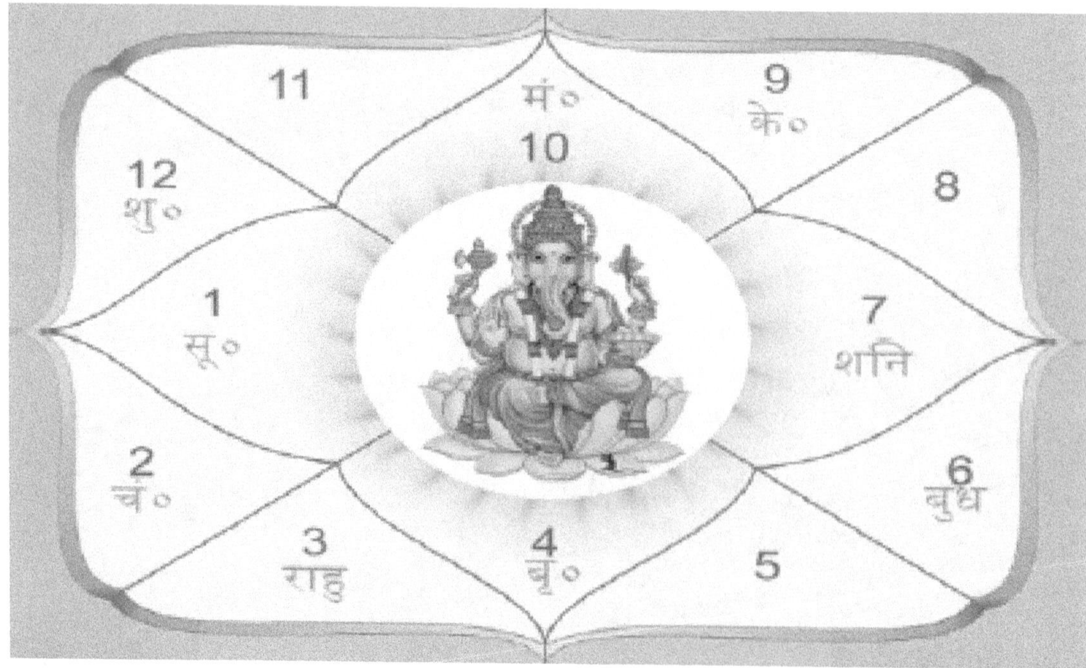

The Seven Rays of Healing in China

China was also initially united with Lemuria. When the two lands separated emissaries of the Order of the Seven Rays landed on the coast of China and moved inland. Some arrived from the Islands of the Immortals and the Gulf of Chihli, and then fanned out along the Yellow River. These missionaries and their descendants built sacred temple cities, the remains of which include the compound of 16 pyramids in Xian province that were originally painted in the colors of the Seven Rays.

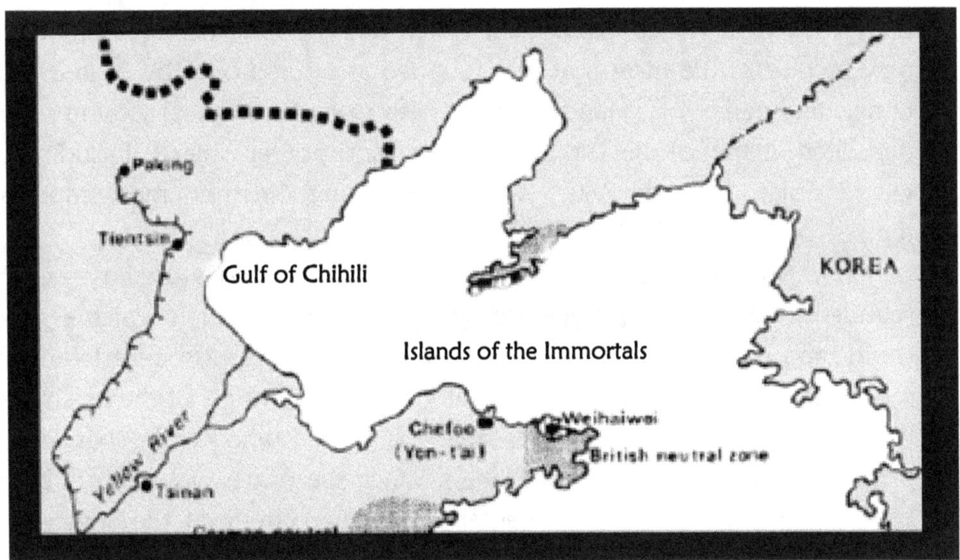

As part of its Taoist healing tradition, the Chinese made detailed correspondences between the Seven Rays, the 14 Major Meridians (2x7) and their Acu-Points, as well as the 7 Yin and 7 Yang inner organs they connect with. These correspondences will be elaborated upon in Chapter 5.

The Seven Rays of Healing in Peru

Legend has it that the Lemurian Order of the Seven Rays dispatched one of its leading members, Aramu Muru, to the Andes with the teachings and power objects of the order during the time of the continent's fateful destruction approximately 12,000 years ago. Aramu Muru first built the Monastery of the Seven Rays deep within the Andes to serve as a headquarters for the Order of the Seven Rays and a reliquary for its sacred objects and records. When the time was right, however, Aramu Muru left the monastery and met other missionaries from Lemuria known as the Kapac Kuna at Lake Titicaca. Together they traveled throughout the Andes while building megalithic temple cities.

When they reached a special Andean valley the Kapac Kuna built the megalithic city of Cuzco, which then became headquarters of the new empire of the Incas that was founded and ruled over by Aramu Muru under the name of Manco Kapac. It was here that Aramu Muru deposited many of his Lemurian records and power objects, including the sacred Solar Disc of Mu, which he hung in the most important temple of Cuzco, the Coricancha, the "Temple of Gold."

In his new Incan empire Aramu Muru flew the Seven Ray flag and founded a branch of the Order of the Seven Rays through which a seeker could progress through seven levels, each of which was associated with one of the Seven Rays. Many of those that graduated through all the levels were Illiac Umas, those with "heads full of light," who wore bands and ornaments decorated with Seven Rays. When the Andes was overrun by the Spanish Conquistadors the Order and Healing System of the Seven Rays became circumspect and forced "underground." Today the teachings and practices of the Order of the Seven Rays and Seven Ray Healing System are principally known of by the Andean Shamans, certain Andean esoteric societies such as the Brotherhood of the Sun, and solitary groups of Incas, including the Qeros, who have survived by living deep within the Andes and upon the mountains' highest elevations.

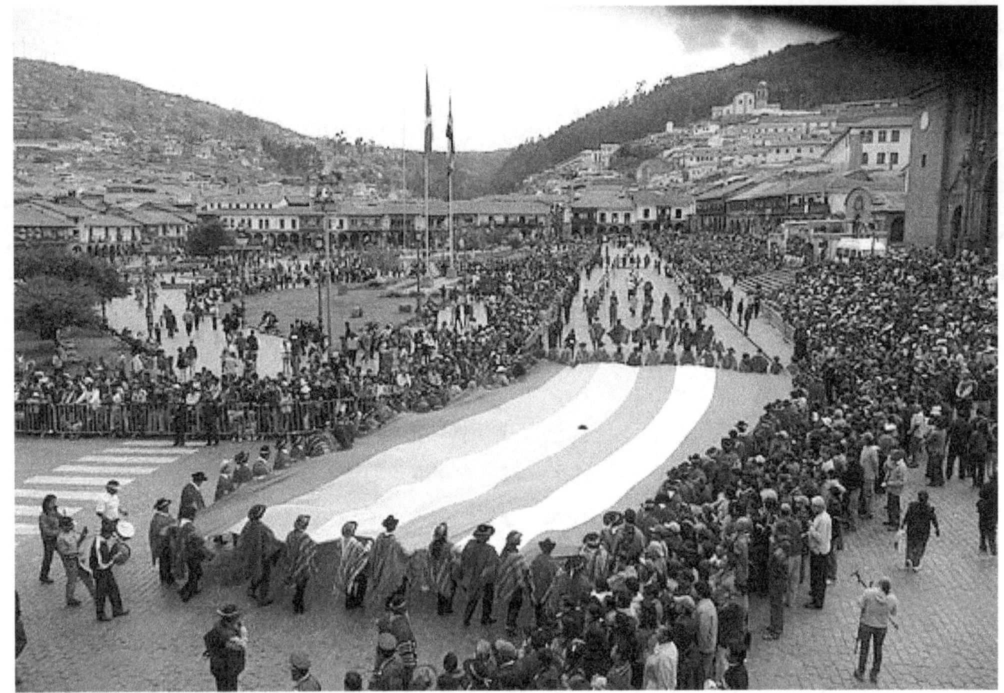

The Inca Seven Ray Flag

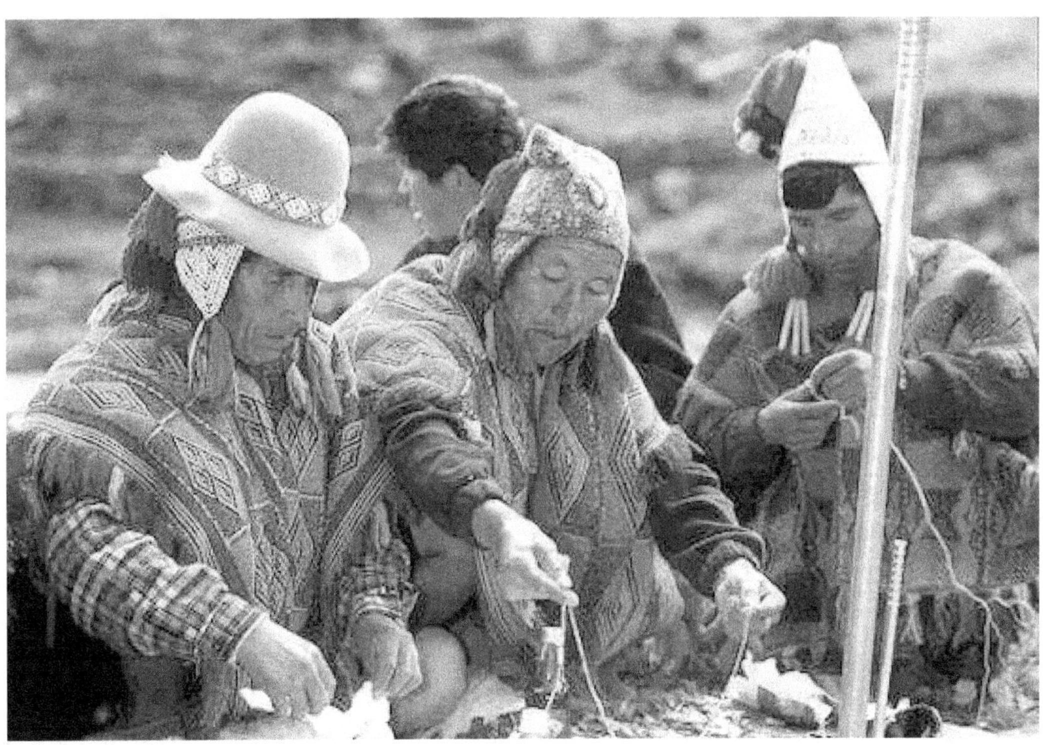

Peruvian Qeros wear shawls and hats covered with the colors of the Seven Rays

Another group of Lemurian missionaries settled in a part of Peru that was much closer to the Pacific coast. At an elevation of 10,000 feet in the Andes they built a pyramidal temple city that is today known as Chavin de Hauntar. One of the temples of the city was more feminine than the rest and designed specifically for Goddess rites. It was circular in shape and used solely for ceremony that involved imbibing a liquid made from Wachuma (San Pedro cactus) that the missionaries had used on Lemuria and brought with them to the Andes. Through the psychoactive effects of this plant each participant of a Wachuma ceremony acquired the ability to behold their beloved Goddess with Her "coat of crystals and seven rays of color." Wachuma was one of the principal plants on Lemuria that had been used to commune with both the Goddess and Her Son.

It is believed that the Masters of Chavin achieved enlightenment solely through the consumption of the sacred Wachuma. In doing so they acquired the three powers of the Goddess, which are associated with Her first three rays: creation, preservation and destruction. These three powers, which were acquired one after the other by each initiate, were associated with the three sacred animals of the Andes: the condor, the puma and the snake. In order to reveal that they had acquired mastery of all these three animals, their powers, and the three worlds associated with them (Heaven, Earth, Underworld), the builders of Chavin left behind carved stone heads of themselves that combined the features of all three sacred animals. Many of the heads also feature top knots, representing that the Chavin Masters also had fully awakened and active Crown Chakras

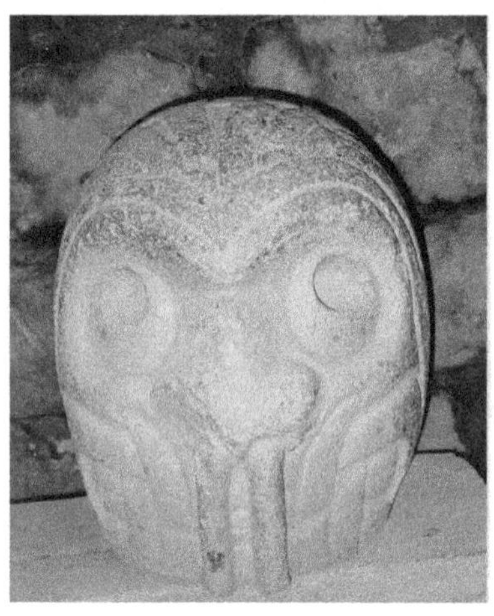 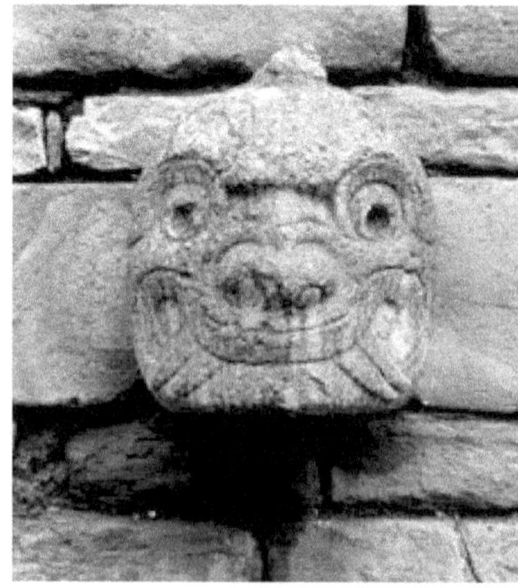 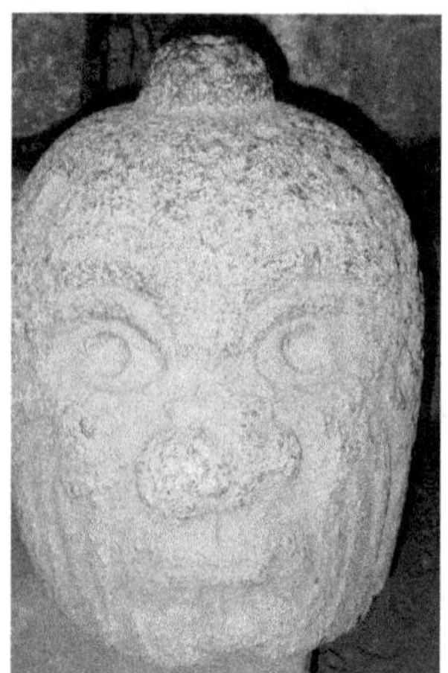

The Revival of Seven Ray Healing

Leading up to the coming new era is the re-introduction of all components of the Goddess tradition, including Seven Ray Healing. This science, which was brought to Earth with the Kumara Sons of God/Goddess, is important for today because it is not only a healing system but can also activate the evolutionary power and thereby lead to the goal of humankind, God-Realization. The re-introduction of Seven Ray Healing began in the last century with the work of Alice Bailey, a channel for a Tibetan master of the Great White Brotherhood known as Djwhal Khul, who presented to the world the esoteric philosophy of the Seven Rays. Djwhal Khul, who normally introduced himself to Ms. Bailey simply as "the Tibetan," also expounded upon the Kumaras, their history, and their intimate association with the Seven Rays. Ms. Bailey apparently came to realize the true connection between Sanat Kumara and Lucifer and named her publishing company Lucifer Publishing, a title she was eventually forced to change to Lucis Publishing because of the acrimonious Christian indignation directed against her.

Ms. Bailey eventually published an extensive series of books on the ancient Goddess mysteries. The most important in regards to the Seven Rays are ***Initiation, Human and Solar*** and ***The Rays and the Initiations.*** Although some of the correspondences in Bailey's books are becoming a little too abstruse and outdated for the contemporary world, her books are still a good resource for the study of the philosophy of the Seven Rays.

Another messenger of the Great White Brotherhood who has played an important role in re-popularizing the Seven Rays is Elizabeth Clare Prophet, director of the Church Universal and Triumphant in Montana. Ms. Prophet, whose organization until recently was known as the Summit Lighthouse, was founded in conjunction with her late husband, Mark Prophet, after the couple met the Great White Brotherhood adept Master Morya in Washington D.C. in the 1950s. Master Morya became the sponsor and patron of the original Summit Lighthouse and guided the Prophets in their mission of channeling the wisdom of various masters of the Great White Brotherhood for the benefit of the world. Part of the information the Prophets channeled is related to the Lords of the Seven Rays and was published as ***Lords of the Seven Rays: Mirror of Consciousness.*** Within this text the Lords of each of the Rays are presented, along with the physical embodiments they have taken throughout the course of history. Although it is difficult to prove or disprove the Prophets' information, the text is a good introduction to the Ray Lords and their functions.

The Prophets' were greatly influenced by the tradition of Theosophy founded by Madame Blavatsky in the nineteenth century, as well as the I AM Church established by Godfrey Ray King in the early twentieth century. In the late 1800s Blavatsky brought forth channeled information from members of the Great White Brotherhood, including Master Morya, Master Kuthumi and Saint Germain. These were the invisible patrons of her organization, the Theosophical Society, which was initially headquartered in Chennai, the city patronized by Sanat Kumara as peacock-riding Murugan in south India. In the books written by Blavatsky and her students there is an abundance of information regarding the earlier epochs of the world, such as the Lemurian and Atlantean Ages, as well as a few treatises on the Seven Rays. Her most famous tome, ***The Secret Doctrine,*** is one of the best texts on Earth's esoteric history ever published. Godfrey Ray King, the author of some classic texts recounting his training with Saint Germain, including ***Unveiled Mysteries*** and ***The Magic Presence,*** also helped infuse the wisdom of the existence of the Great White Brotherhood into the public domain. His I AM Church has published some manuscripts and teachings regarding the Seven Rays and their Lords, although the organization is particularly dedicated to the introduction of Saint Germain and his function as Lord of the Seventh Ray. According to the I AM Church, as the Earth moves to a higher octave of vibration it passes through the Seventh Ray, which is why Saint Germain is so important to these times. He is the guiding presence of our current world transformation. And since the United States is playing such an important role in the planetary transformation, Saint Germain is the special patron and guide of the US.

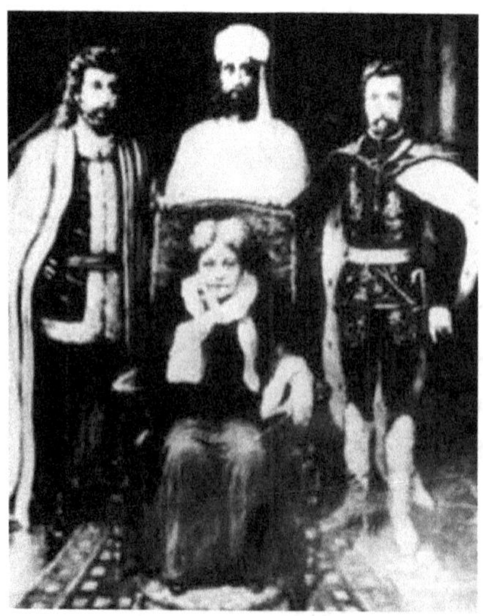

Kuthumi, Master Morya, Saint Germain, Madam Blavatsky (seated)

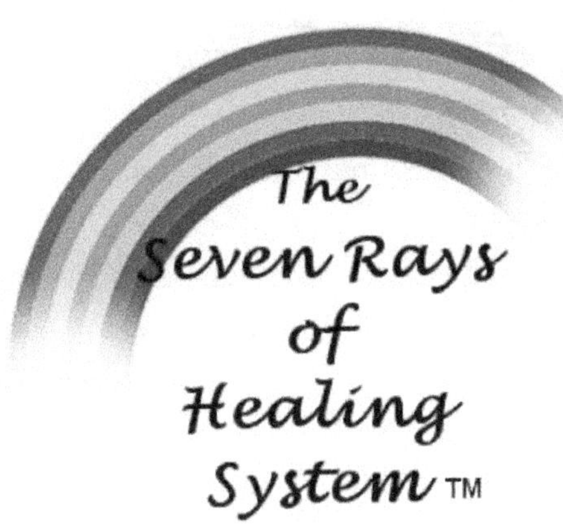

Chapter 1

The Theory of the Seven Rays

The Creation of the Seven Rays

The Seven Ray Primal Serpent

The creation of the Seven Rays begins with the Primal Serpent who emerged from the Cosmic Ocean of Consciousness at the beginning of time and became the vehicle for the Infinite Spirit to create the universe. The Primal Serpent was pure, high frequency life force that moved in a serpentine spiral and possessed seven component parts. These are the Seven Rays. As the the Primal Serpent created the universe out of its own body it endowed every object and life form with the characteristics of the Seven Rays.

In order to reveal the Seven Rays of the Primal Serpent it was often portrayed iconically with seven heads, seven tails and/or seven curves to its torturous body. Such septenary images of the Primal Serpent can be found all over the globe.

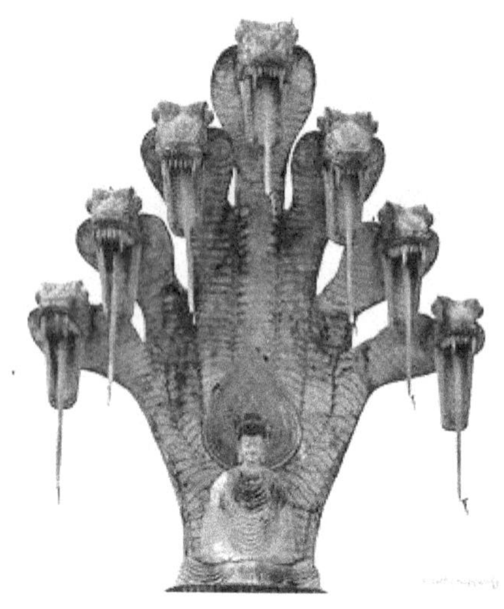

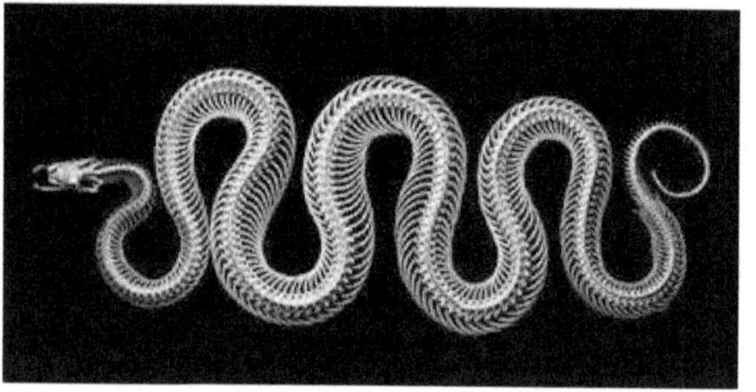

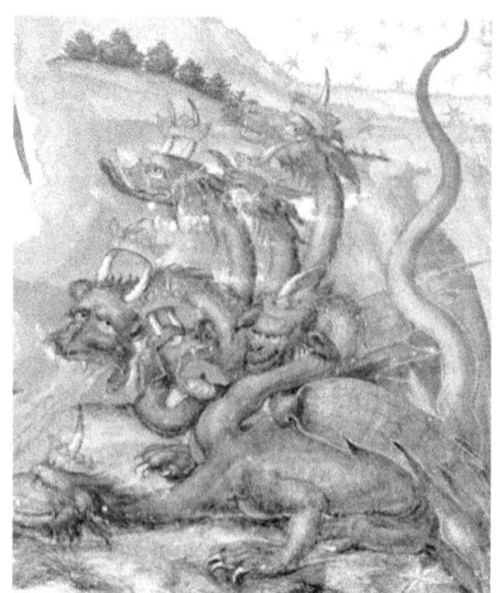

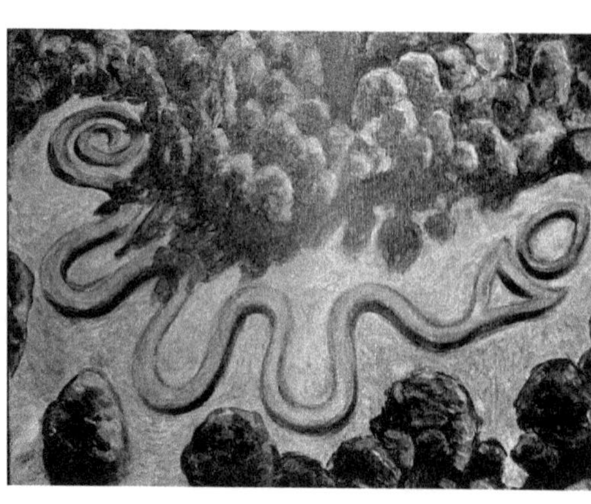

The Seven Ray Serpent Goddess

Many of the ancient cosmologists identified the Primal Serpent as the Goddess which had emanated out of the Infinite Spirit. She was the female counterpart of the "male" Spirit and embodied its power and wisdom.

In Her manifestation as the serpentine life force and Primal Serpent the Goddess has been represented in iconography worldwide as slithering snakes that emanate from a "male" God. In Hindu iconography She is the Goddess Shakti who is often depicted as snakes coiled around the anthropomorphic body of Shiva, the "male" Infinite Spirit. In the ancient Persian tradition of Zervanism, which later evolved into Mithraism, the Goddess was worshiped as a huge snake coiled around a lion-headed man that represented the "male" Infinite Spirit.

Throughout the Middle East the serpentine nature of the Goddess was always depicted in iconography as either a snake or as a woman in possession of a snake. Her serpentine images as Ishtar/Inanna (Mespotamia), Cybel (Phrygia), Isis and Sekhmet (Egypt), and Athene (Greece) bear this out.

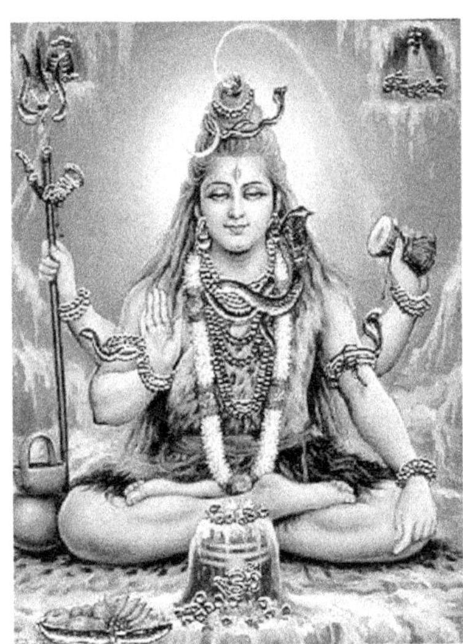

Shiva with Goddess Shakti as dangling snakes.

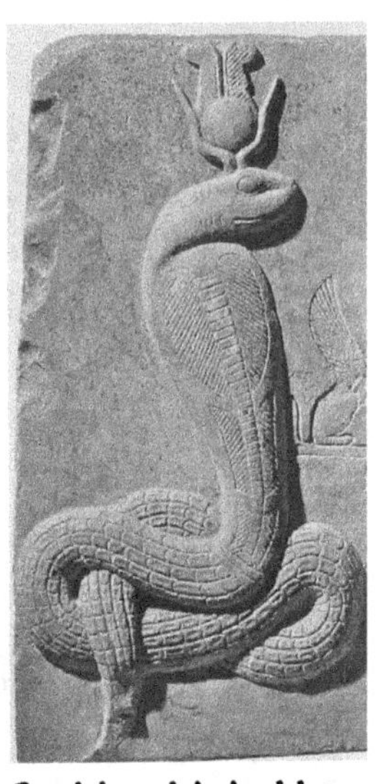

Goddess Isis in Her serpent form as Isiopolis

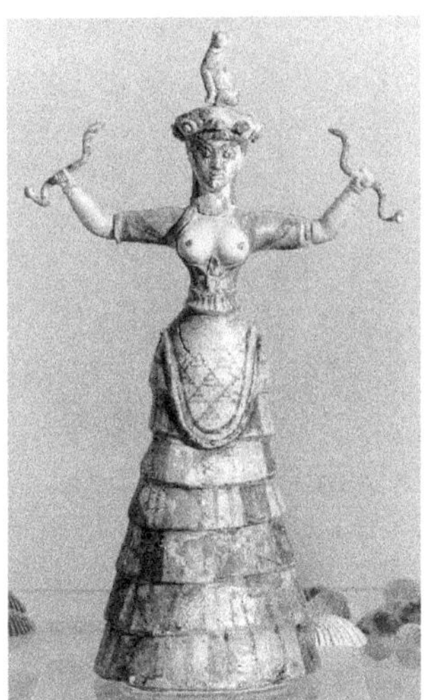

Cretan Snake Goddess

The Goddess's First Son: The First Ray

In Her form of the Primal Serpent the Goddess eventually divided herself into two, three and then Seven Rays. These Rays are referred to as the seven parts of the Goddess as well as Her Seven Sons.

When the Goddess gave birth to Her First Son his features completely mirrored those of his mother. Like her he was also the synthesis of the Seven Rays and possessed a serpentine body. He became Lord of the Seven Rays and She became Lady of the Seven Rays.

Since the First Son was the embodiment of the First Blue Ray all the other six rays descended from him. Thus, like his mother he was also recognized as the creator or parent of all the Seven Rays.

So even though the Son descends from the Goddess, both Goddess and Son have individually been referred to by different cultures worldwide as *the* Primal Serpent that created the universe. The Sumerians were unique, however, in referring to both the Goddess and Her Son, whom they knew as Inanna and Dammuzi, as "the serpent [of energy] that emanated from the Heaven God Anu [the Infinite Spirit]."

Because of the Son's association with the Primal Serpent he, like his mother, has also been represented globally by serpent icons. Dammuzi/Tammuz and other Sons of the Goddess were always portrayed as snakes, including Sanat Kumara/ Murugan, Dionysus, Osiris, Adonis, and Attis. And since he was also the synthesis of the Seven Rays, the Son has additionally been depicted as a snake with seven heads or as a seven-headed boy. This is his image as Karttikeya/Sanat Kumara, who has seven heads, although one is associated with the invisible Spirit and hidden.

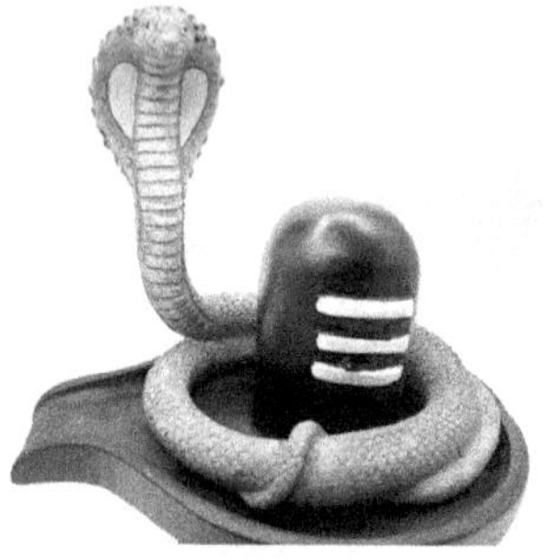

A Snake encoils a Shiva Lingam; A form of Murugan/Sanat Kumara

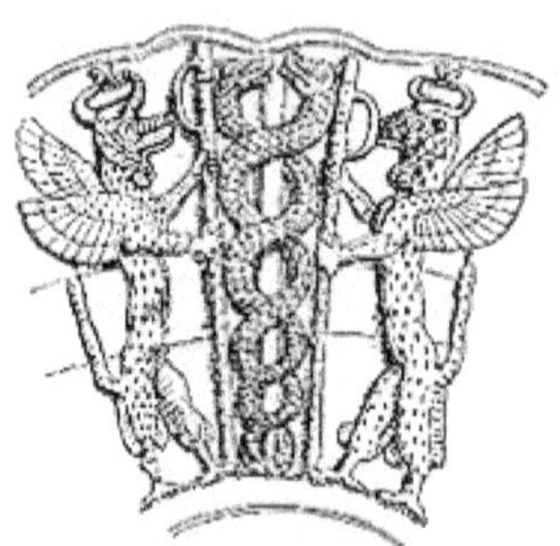

Intertwined snakes: A form of Dammuzi/Tammuz

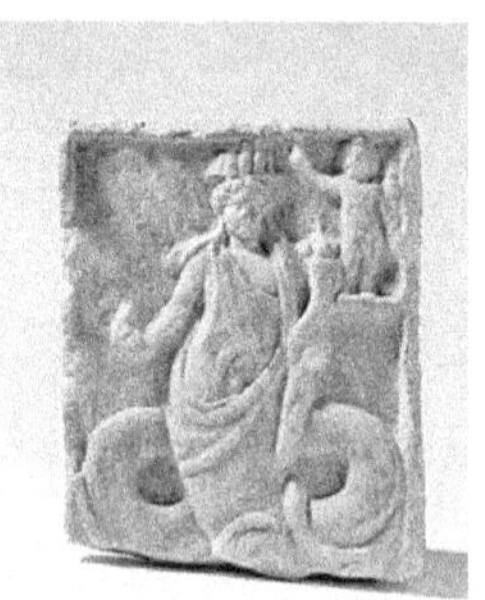

Dionysus with snake body

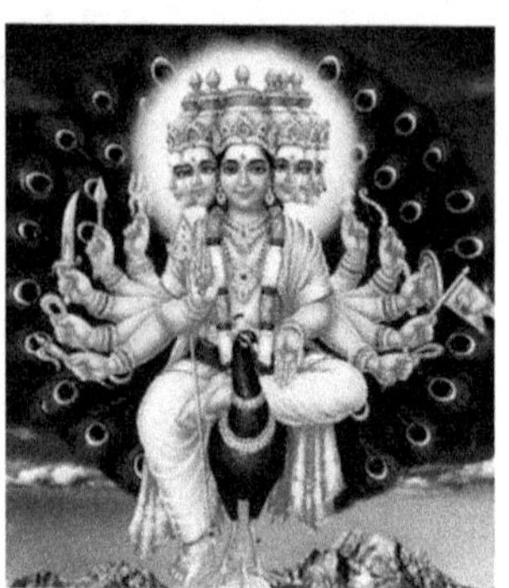

The "Seven" Headed Karttikeya

One iconic image of the Goddess or Son as the Primal Serpent is the Serpent on the Tree in the Garden of Eden. The "Tree" that the Goddess or Son spirals around is the Universal Tree that unites all the dimensions. It slithers down the tree from the highest dimension of the Infinite Spirit before arriving in Eden.

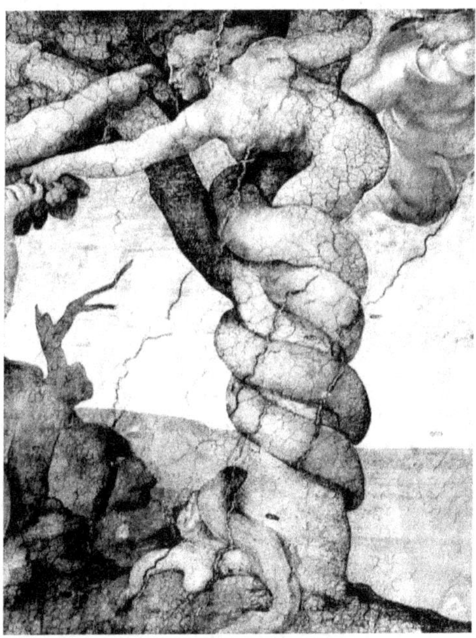

The Eden Serpent as the Goddess in the Sistine Chapel

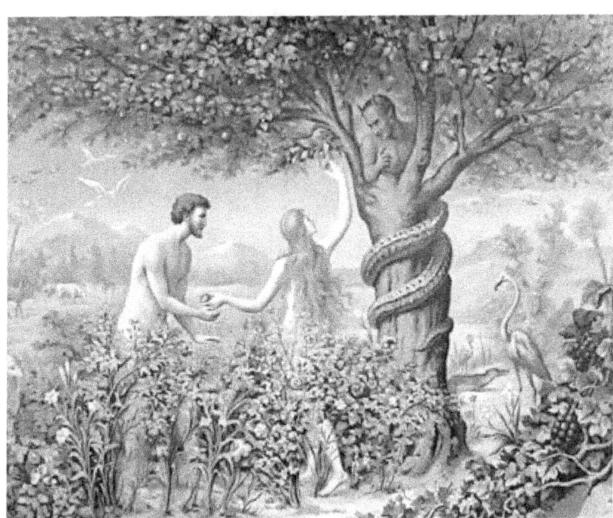

The Eden Serpent as the Son

The Goddess/Son Becomes the Twins: The First 2 Rays

As the Primal Serpent, whose body was neutral or "androgynous" energy, the Goddess and Her Son in their incipient serpentine forms were androgynous. Their dual nature is explicitly portrayed in their anthropomorphic iconography. In Sumeria, the dual Goddess Ishtar/Inanna was the goddess of the polar opposites of love and war, and in Syria She was Aphrodite with a beard. One iconic form of the androgynous Egyptian Goddess Hathor possessed two heads, one for each polarity. The androgyny of the Son has also been implicit. It is revealed by the androgynous pre-pubescent images of the Hindu Sanat Kumara/Murugan and the Egyptian Horus, as well as by the overtly bisexual Dionysus of Greece.

As the Primal Serpent, the Goddess or Son split during the creation of the universe into their their positive/negative, male/female polarity. This split was necessary in order to keep the universe in a state of balance and harmony. These dual parts of the Primal Serpent are the first Two Rays of the Goddess/Son.

The polar opposite aspects of the Goddess have been portrayed worldwide as both Twin Serpents as well as anthropomorphic Twin Boys, known variously as Sananda and Sanat Kumara, the Ashwin Twins (India), the Dioscouri Twins (Greece), the Kaberoi Twins (Egypt, Greece, Asia Minor), Hunapu and Xbalenque (Maya), the Poyangs (Hopis), the Ahayutas (the Zunis), and Monster Slayer and Child of the Waters (the Navajos). These Sons of the Goddess are said to have assisted in the creation of the Earth and wielded their mother's power of creation (the Twin of Light) and destruction (the Twin of Darkness). In later patriarchal religions these twins became known as Christ and Lucifer.

The Twins are alternately said to be the two halves of the Son. From this perspective, the First Son, who is Lord of all the Seven Rays, "divides" to become himself, Lord of the First Ray, and his Twin, Lord of the Second Ray. Thus, Sanat Kumara divides to become himself, Sanat Kumara, and his Twin, Sananda Kumara.

Iconic images of the Goddess or Her Son as Twin Serpents include the Caduceus of Mercury and the motif of twin snakes or dragon wrapped around identical pillars. Both motifs are an evolution of the Serpent on the Tree in the Garden of Eden, which has been portrayed both as the Goddess and Her Son.

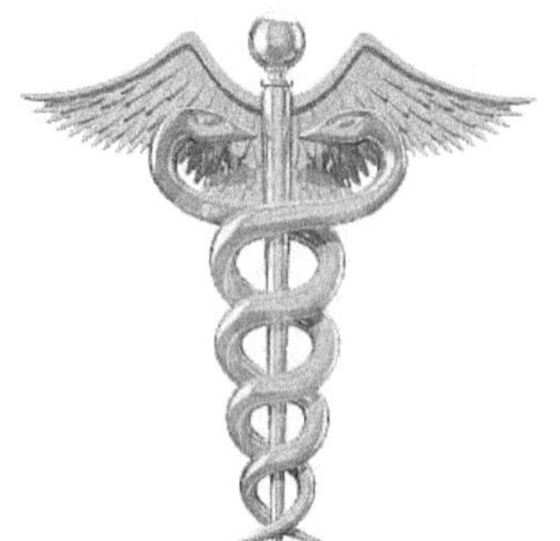

Caduceus of Mercury

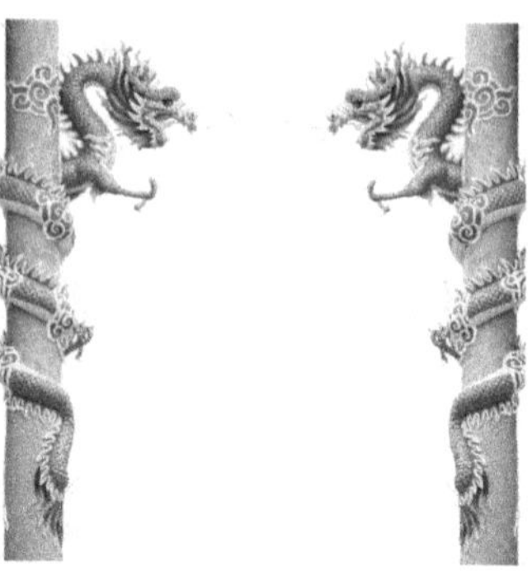

Twin Dragons wrapped around identical pillars

Manifestations of the Twin Sons of the Goddess

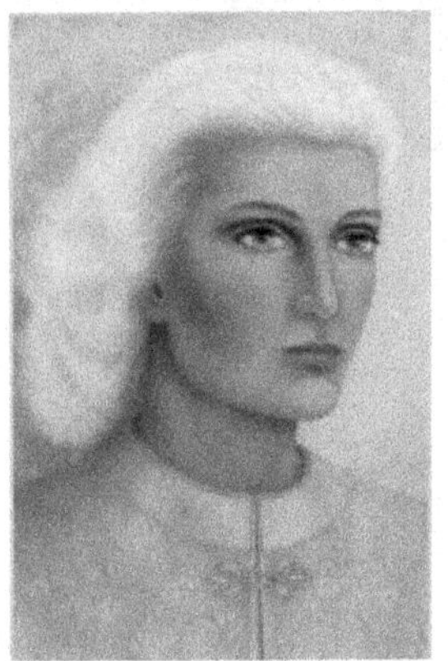

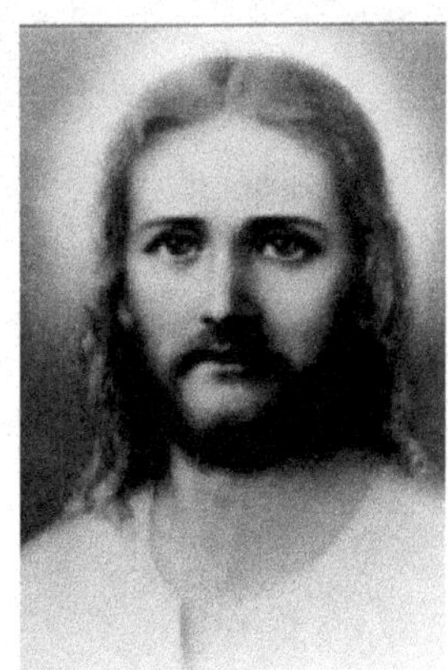

Sanat and Sananda Kumara

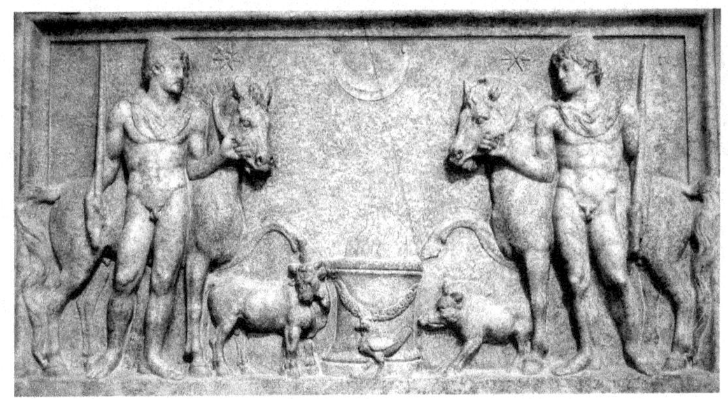

The Dioscouri Twins

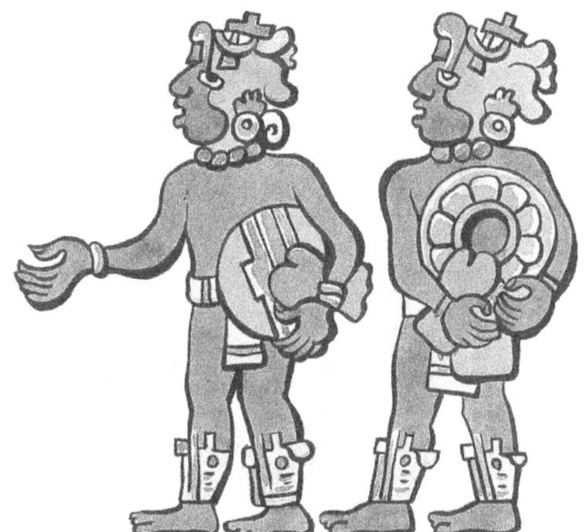

Hunapu and Xbalenque

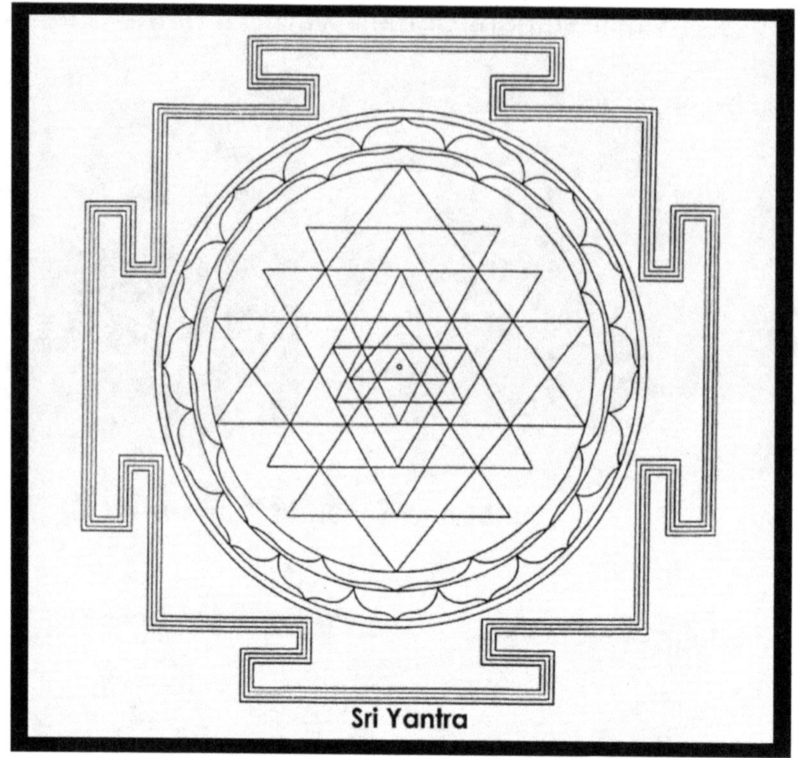

Sri Yantra

The two dual parts of the Goddess or Son are reflected in the Sri Yantra and Star of David, which are the Sacred Geometrical forms of the Universal Goddess and Her Son. The Twins are manifest in the Sri Yantra and Star of David as the upward and downward interlocking triangles.

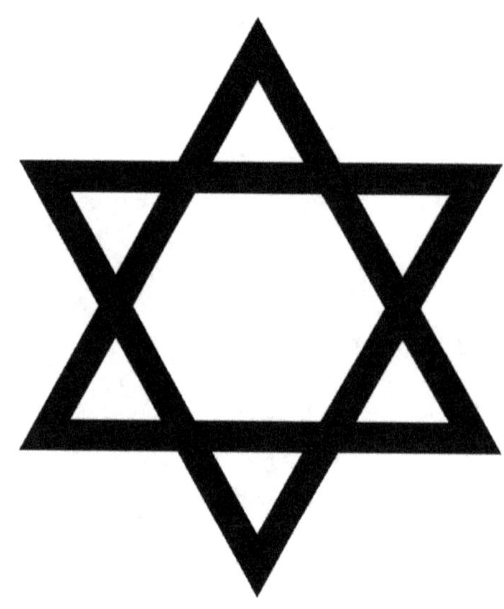

The Three-Fold Goddess: The First 3 Rays

The First Two Rays of the Goddess embodied Her polarity of light/dark, male/female as well as Her Twin Powers of Creation and Destruction. Her Third Son and Third Ray was then born to embody Her third power of Preservation. Now the Goddess had three Sons.

In India, the three Sons of the Goddess are known as Brahma, Vishnu, and Shiva. Brahma and Shiva embody the Goddess' powers of creation and destruction, and Vishnu personifies Her power of preservation which is arises through the harmonious balance of the powers of creation and destruction and their union.

Because of Her three powers and Sons, the Goddess is often referred to as the Triune, Triple or Three-fold Goddess. In Her Triple Goddess manifestation the three parts of the Goddess have been portrayed as three female figures: the maid, mother, and crone. As the Three-fold Goddess of the Hindus, She is known as Tripura Sundari, the Goddess of three parts.

The three powers of the Goddess are intrinsic to the life force. The Goddess as the life force creates the universe out of Her own etheric substance, She then nurtures and sustains the universe by giving all crystallized physical life forms the requisite amount of life force to survive, and She finally destroys the universe by returning all physical forms back into pure energy or life force.

The three powers of the Goddess as the life force are reflected in the iconic images of three-headed serpents, the trident, and Her sound/name of AUM. This is the mantra of three letters that correspond to the three powers of creation, preservation, and destruction. AUM is known as the "Pranava" because its vibration generates life force or prana. It is because the AUM reverberated at the beginning of time that the life force came into being; and life force can be created anytime through the intonation of AUM or its variations, such as Amen. Prayers typically begin and/or end with AUM or Amen in order to create the life force needed to manifest the prayers.

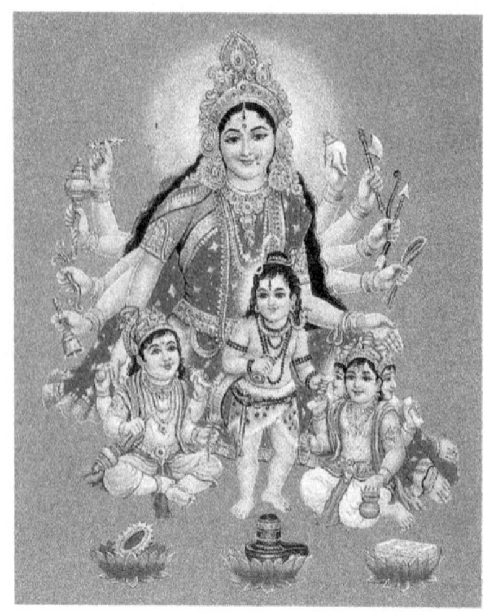

Tripura Sundari and Her 3 Powers as 3 "Sons"

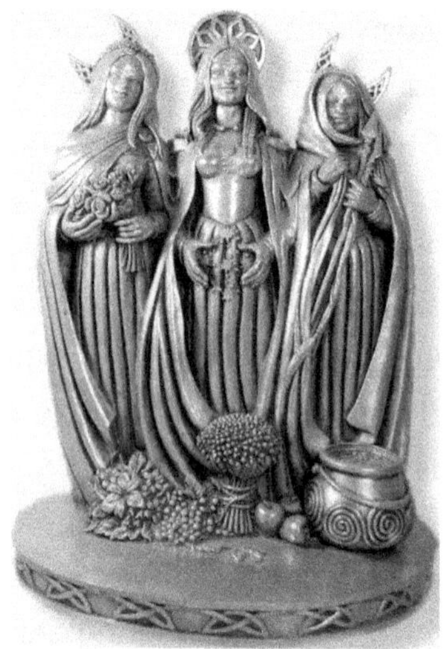

Triple Goddess as Maid, Mother, & Crone

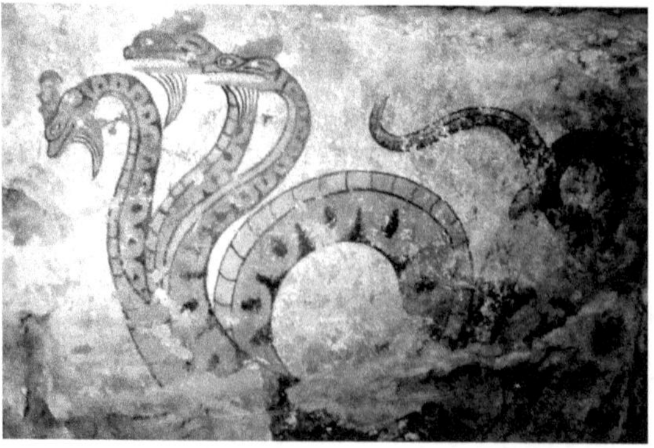

Ancient Etruscan image of the 3-headed Primal Serpent

In India, the Goddess Shakti, whose name denotes "Power," divides Herself into three sub-shaktis or sub-powers: Iccha Shakti, Jnana Shakti, and Kriya Shakti. These sub-shaktis are alternate names for the three Sons of Tripura Sundari. Brahma personifies the Goddess's Iccha Shakti, Her creative power; Vishnu personifies the Goddess's Jnana Shakti, Her preserving power; and Shiva (or Rudra, Shiva's alternate name, because Shiva is commonly used as the name of the Infinite Spirit) personifies the Goddess's Kriya Shakti, Her power of action and destruction.

In the West, the Goddess and Her three powers evolved into Father, Mother, and Son, and later into Father, Son and Holy Ghost. The Father, who is the Creator of the Universe, personifies the Goddess's power of creation; the Mother is mater or matter that is governed by time that breaks down through entropy and destroys/transforms, so She personifies the Goddess's power of destruction; and the Son, who is the union of Father and Mother, personifies the Goddess's power of preservation by occasionally being sent to sent to Earth to preserve the world and humanity.

Since the creation phase of the universe has been completed, it is the preserving power of the life force that most immediately affects us now on Earth. In its preserving manifestation it is the life force that helps to synthesize and nourish new buds and seedlings each spring, and it is the preserving life force in the human body that fuels and accomplishes all our bodily processes. In India, it is said that to accomplish this task the Goddess as the life force divides up into five different pranas in the body, each of which has a specific task. As "Prana" the Goddess moves air into the lungs through inhalation, as "Apana" She moves air out of the body through exhalation, and as Apana She moves waste down and out of the body. As "Samana" She digests our food; as "Vyana," the Goddess moves blood and energy throughout the body; and as "Udyana" She moves energy upwards in the body and thereby keeps the body upright. The Chinese have a similar perspective. They divide chi into "Ancestral Chi", the chi that energizes the heart; "Source Chi," the chi that nourishes the kidneys; "Food Chi", the chi that moves through the body to nourish it, as well as numerous other sub-categories of chi.

The Trident and the Trinity

One of the pre-eminent symbols of the first the three powers of the Primal Dragon as either the Goddess or Son is the trident. The trident image below perfectly reveals that the inner prong of the Son and his power of preservation is the union of the two outer prongs of Father and Mother and their powers of creation and preservation. When separated from the trident the middle prong is a pre-eminent symbol of the Son and represents the Vel or spear of Sanat Kumara (see following page).

Within certain religious sects the trident does not represent three powers, but solely the power of destruction. This is often the case when the trident becomes the identifiable "weapon" of the third Son and who embodies the Goddess's power of destruction. Thus, it has been the outstanding symbol of the Goddess's Sons who are the Lords of Fire and Destruction, including Rudra/Shiva in the Hindu pantheon, and Lucifer or the Devil of the Christian faith. But the "fire" the trident represents is not dense physical fire but high frequency Cosmic Fire, the prana or life force that manifested at the beginning of time and wielded all three powers of creation, preservation and destruction. This truth is reflected in the ancient Sanscrit AUM symbol, which when turned vertically is the trident. The AUM symbol represents Cosmic Fire or high frequency prana and its associated three powers of creation, preservation, and destruction.

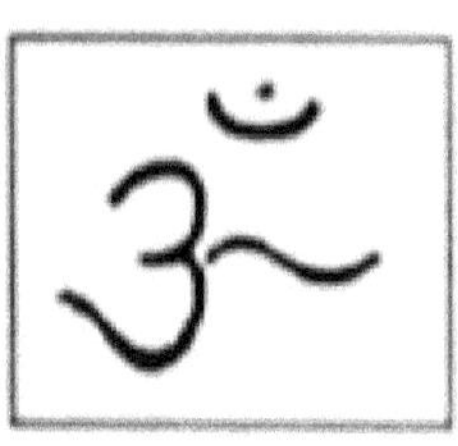

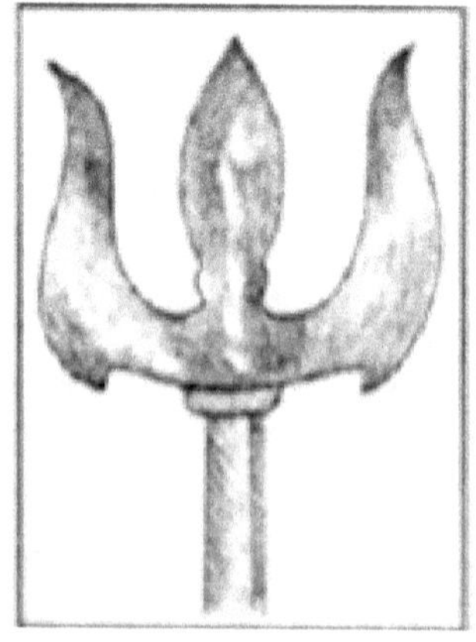

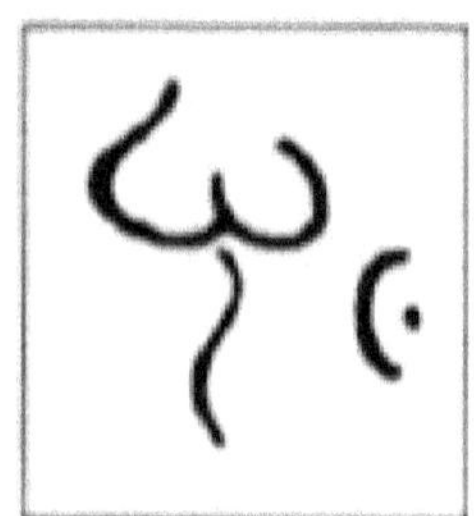

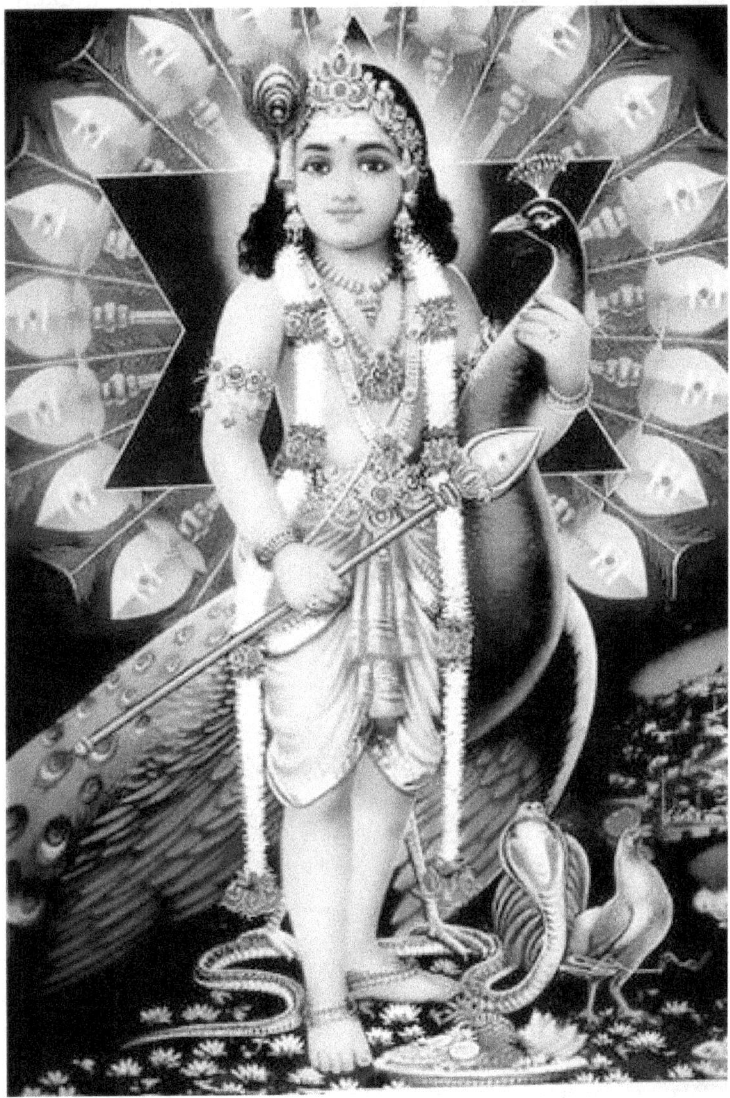

The Divine Son, Sanat Kumara as Murugan, with his sacred Vel spear. The Vel is associated with the middle prong of the trident and is the symbol of both the Son and Jnana, "Wisdom."

The Trinity in the Kabbala

Another symbolic representation of the Three Rays can be found in the Jewish secret tradition known as the Kabbala. Below is a diagram taken from the Sepher Yetzirah, the Kabbala "Book of Creation," which represents the creation of the universe from sound. The inner triangle represents the first Three Rays as three primal sounds (which are collectively the primal AUM). These first three sounds are represented by the three "Mother Letters" of the Hebrew alphabet, Resh, Mem, and Shen, and correspond both to the elements of air, fire, and water, as well as Iccha, Jnana and Kriya Shaktis. As you can see, the Hebrew letter for fire, Shen, is written as a trident. Another Kabbalic diagram, the Tree of Life (below right), similarly represents of the first three Rays. The first three Rays are represented in this format as the first three Sephiroth (there are ten in total) at the top of the tree, Kether, Chockmah, and Binah, which also correspond to air, fire, and water. The first three Rays are also manifest as the three pillars of the Tree of Life.

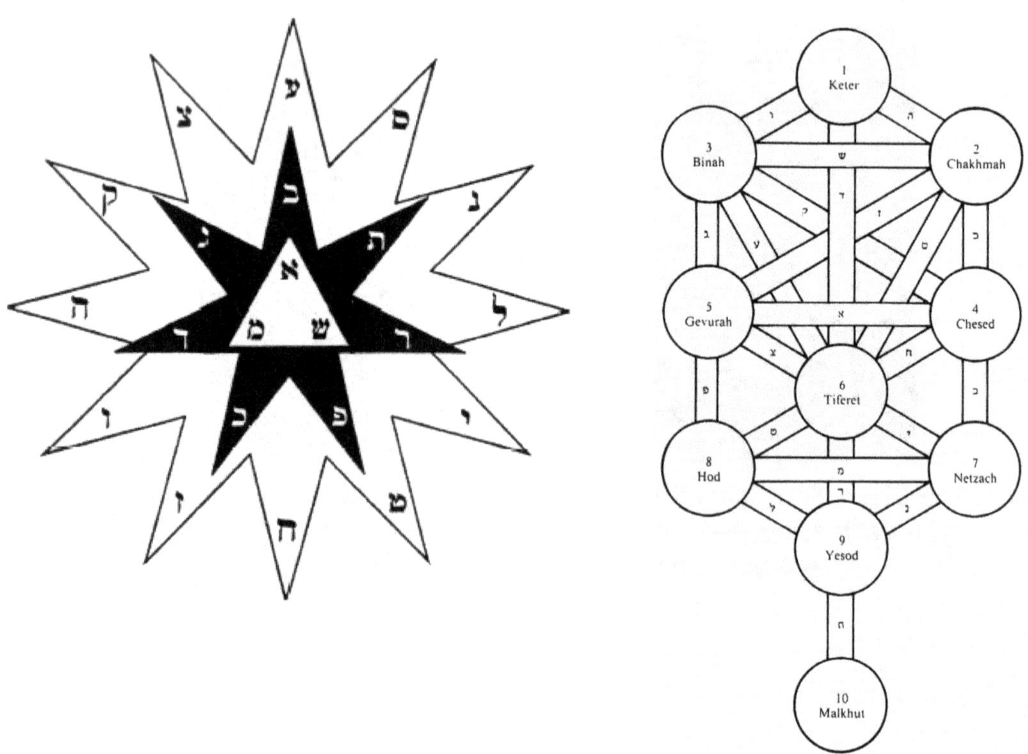

TheTrinityoftheThree Sacred AnimalsoftheAndes

The three powers of the Goddess are also associated with the three sacred animals of Andean Shamanism. In Her form as the Primal Dragon, the Goddess is the synthesis of these three animals – the condor, puma and serpent (amaru). form. When She divided Herself into three parts She placed one of these animals at three of the four directions as its guardian and sentinel. The condor embodies the Goddess's power of creation (and beginnings) and rules the east direction, where the Sun begins its march across the sky each day. The puma rules the Goddess's power of preservation and governs the west, the direction from which the modern technology that preserves the world comes from. And the serpent rules the Goddess's power of destruction and the north, the direction of darkness and bitter cold. The Dragoness Goddess, whose body is pure life force, rules the south, the direction where the life force is most prolific and gives rise to the lush vegetation of the jungles. By knowing the deities, animals, and the powers that are associated with the four directions, you can consciously choose which deity to commune with by facing its corresponding direction. If, for example, you want to create something in you life you will want to summon the power of creation and its animal, the condor-eagle, by facing the east. If you want to you want to destroy something in your life you will connect with the serpent, the power of death and the underworld, and face the north. And if your desire is to commune with and absorb the powers of preservation you would face the west, the direction of the puma-jaguar.

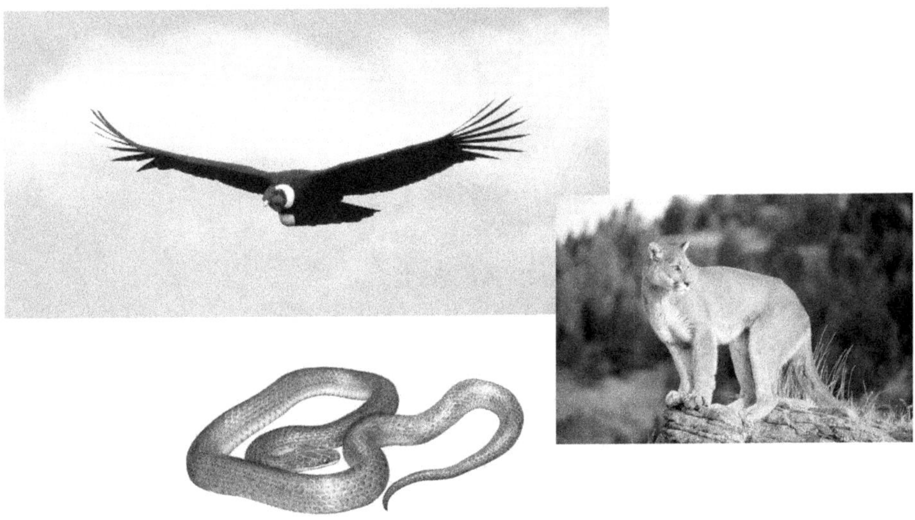

The Four Directions

South

Season: Summer
Activity
Deity: The Goddess, Dragoness, Shakti
All 3 animals & all 3 powers of the Life Force
Color: Red

Spring
Creation
Dawn

East

Sananda
Condor
Spiritual
Wisdom
Morning Star
Gold

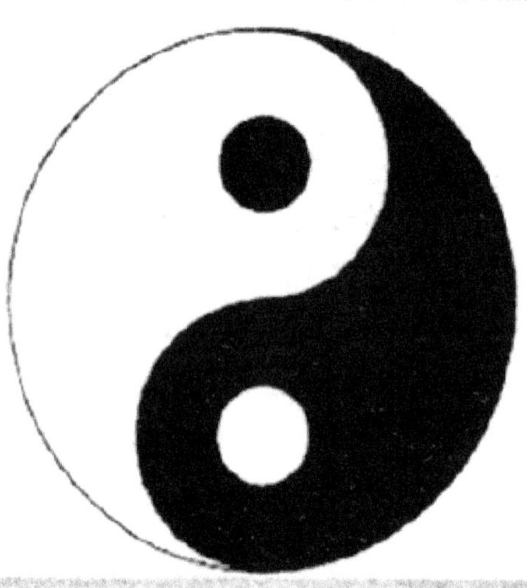

Autumn
Destruction
Dusk

West

Sanat Kumara
Puma
Materialism
Rulership
Evening Star
Blue

North

Season: Winter
Inaction, Solidity
The God, Lord Shiva
Animal: Amaru
The Underworld, Inner Reflection
Color: White

Sanat and Sananda Kumara are also associated with the with the east and west directions respectively. As you will discover in Chapter 2, Sananda is Lord of the 2nd Ray of Wisdom and especially connected to the east, the direction of divine wisdom. And Sanat, who is the Lord of the 1st Ray of Will and Power, is especially associated with the west because from the west have emerged the conquerors who have ruled the world. As pictured, Shiva and Shakti also occupy the north and south directions. Shiva is the dark nothingness of the Infinite Spirit that emanates from itself Shakti, the life force.

The Trinity in the Antahkarana

One more representation of the first three Rays is the symbol known as the Antahkarana that can be found decorating the walls of Tibetan temples and monasteries. **According to the tradition of Johrei Reiki , which uses the symbol for healing, the Antakarana was anciently used by Tibetan monks during special initiations.** Since it is a symbol of the three Rays or powers of the life force, represented by the three inner chevrons and the three concentric circles, it appears that the symbol had the effect of activating the inner fire, the Kundalini, within a Tibetan monk and thus initiating him or her on the path of alchemical transmutation. You can also use this symbol for the same purpose. I would recommend placing it, or copies of it, in your meditation and/ or healing temple in order to fill it with both healing and transformative energy that you can use during your treatments. See Chapter 7.

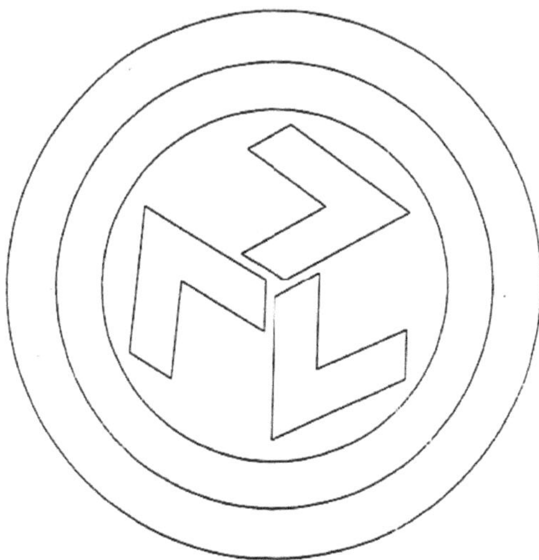

The Antahkarana

The Three-Fold Goddess

On the following page is a chart that combines numerous correspondences of the Trinity and three powers of the Goddess they embody. These correspondences should help you deepen your understanding of the first Three Rays and the three intrinsic powers of the life force. For example, Iccha Shakti, the power of creation, corresponds to the creative power associated with the element of air (or prana), while Jnana Shakti corresponds to the nurturing power of water, and Kriya Shakti corresponds to the destructive nature of fire. The creative Kundalini also corresponds to Iccha Shakti, while the Ida and Pingala Nadis, the subtle pathways traveled by the essences of water and fire in the human body, correspond to the Jnana and Kriya Shaktis and their powers of preservation and destruction. Iccha, which is the Sanscrit word for "will" corresponds to the will to create; Jnana, which is the Sanscrit term for "wisdom," corresponds to the wisdom needed by humankind to preserve itself, and Kriya, meaning "action," corresponds to the destruction which often accompanies intense or excess activity.

The chart also includes color and deity correspondences. The color corresponding to Iccha Shakti is the color of "creative" Heaven, blue; the color of Jnana Shakti is gold/yellow, the color of "preserving" wisdom; and red, the color of movement, passion, activity, and ultimately destruction, is the color that corresponds to Kriya Shakti. In terms of deities, besides Brahma, Vishnu and Shiva/ Rudra, there are other deities and Sons of the Goddess that personify and rule each of the three powers of the life force. Sanat Kumara, the First Son of the Goddess who transmitted his spirit into the Earth and became the Will of our planet, the Planetary Logos, is the deity that personifies Iccha Shakti; he is the Father whose Will reigns supreme. Sananda Kumara, the Second Son of the Goddess, is the personification of spiritual wisdom and the ruler of Jnana Shakti; and the Third Son, Satan/Lucifer, is the deity that personifies and rules the unbridled and destructive activity associated with Kriya Shakti. Since the three primal Sons are also identified as divisions of the First Son, Sanat Kumara, they are sometimes referred to as Sanat Kumara, Sanat/Sananda, and Sanat/Lucifer.

The Three-Fold Goddess

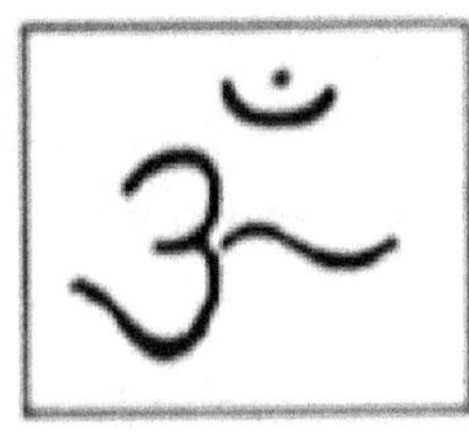

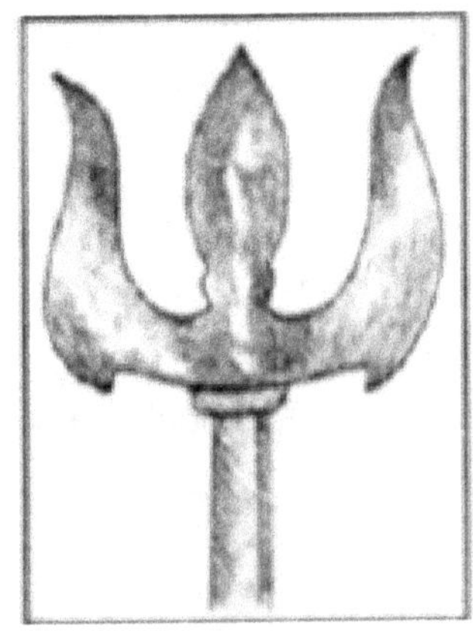

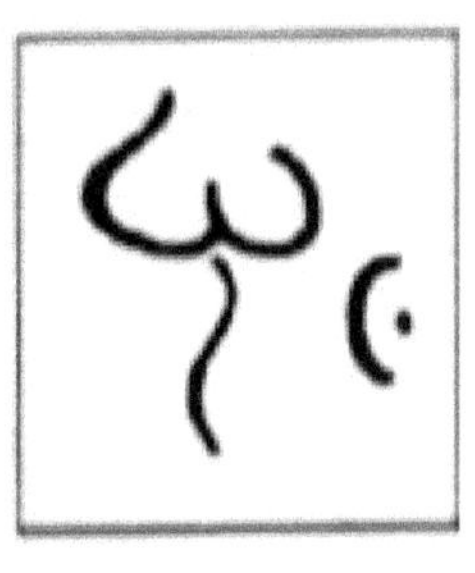

Iccha Shakti	Jnana Shakti	Kriya Shakti
Brahma	Vishnu	Shiva/Rudra
Will	Wisdom	Action
Creation	Preservation	Destruction
Father	Son	Mother/Holy Spirit
Air	Water	Fire
Blue	Yellow/Gold	Red/Orange
Sanat Kumara	Sanat-Sananda	Sanat-Lucifer

The Septenary Goddess or Son

Eventually the Goddess or Son as the Primal Serpent became fully divided into its seven component parts, which collectively are the Seven Rays. Also known as the Seven Sons of the Goddess or Son, as well as the Seven Great Angels and Seven Archangels, the Seven Rays worked together to create the myriad objects and life forms of the physical universe, including Earth humans, that reflect and are governed by one or more of the Seven Rays. The Seven Rays also became the spirits of the Seven Astrological planets (Saturn, Jupiter, Mars, Venus, Mercury, Sun and Moon) and the 12 Zodiacal signs they govern.

The Star of Creation from the Kabbala (below) reveals the separation of the primal sound into the Trinity, the Seven Rays, and the 12 signs. The same sequential separation can be seen in the sequential division feathers of the Peacock Angel, a form of the Primal Dragon venerated by the Yezidis of northern Iraq. According to the Yezidis, the Peacock Angel is the form taken by the First Son and leader of the Seven Great Angels who joined together to create the universe.

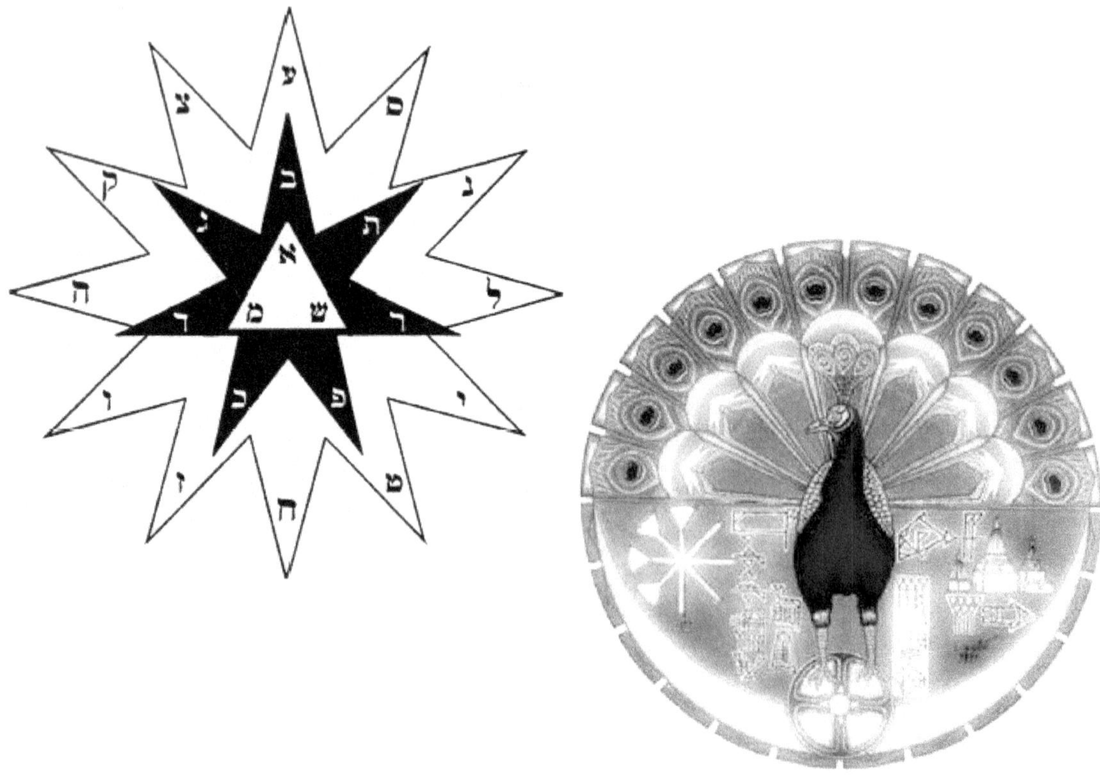

The Seven Rays and the Stages of Creation

As the Seven Rays created the universe each one was responsible for one level and one of the seven successive stages that unfold during the creation of the universe.

The 1st Ray of Iccha Shakti, the Will of God, was the first emanation from Spirit that preceded the manifestation of any physical form in the universe. Before anything can be created there must be the will to create. Once the will became strong, the 2nd Ray of Wisdom manifested.

The 2nd Ray of Jnana Shakti is associated with the Divine Mind of God, within which the Creator formulated a blueprint for the ensuing universe.

The 3rd Ray of Kriya Shakti corresponds to the stage of creation when subtle or Cosmic Fire becomes physical fire, such as during the Big Bang. This is the first phase in the creation of physical matter. This Ray is ruled by Sanat-Lucifer and the fire lords of the Hindu and Judeo-Christian pantheons. During the stage associated with the 3rd Ray, volatile streams of fire shoot through the universe and begin the process of making stars.

Following the 3rd Ray is the 4th Ray of love, harmony and beauty. During the period associated with this Ray the universe cools down and comes to a place of harmony, love, and beauty. Without the balance fostered by the 4th Ray the universe would eventually burn itself out.

Once harmony is established in the cosmos, the new inhabitants of the universe are faced with the practical questions of how to survive on a daily basis. **The 5th Ray, the Ray of Healing and Technology** then manifests to assist them in this pursuit. Then, during **the 6th Ray of Devotion and Mysticism,** the universal citizens understand that they need to align their technology with universal principles or risk destroying themselves. They also develop the desire to unite with the Creator in order to fully know Him or Her.

Finally, during the 7th Ray of Alchemy and Transformation, the citizens in the universe decide they want more than to just understand the Creator, they want to BECOME THE CREATOR. They then move into the 7th Ray of Alchemy and Transformation and thus complete the evolution of the universe which was created so that God could know Himself through the human body.

Understanding the Division of the Seven Rays

The Male and Female Rays

To encapsulate what has been already stated regarding the sequential creation and powers of the Seven Rays:

The First and Second Rays correspond to the polarity of the Primal Dragon and its division at the beginning of time. **The two primary male/female Rays of the Primal Serpent are personified as the first two Sons of the Goddess, Sanat and Sananda Kumara.** Sanat Kumara is the male polarity of the Primal Serpent and Sananda is its female polarity.

Sanat Kumara rules over the 1st Ray of Will and Power. He embodies Iccha Shakti, the Will of God, which is active and masculine. **Sananda, the Christ, is the embodiment of the female principle and rules over the 2nd Ray of Jnana Shakti, the Ray of Wisdom.**

The first two Rays are the most important of the Seven Rays because each Ray is predominantly masculine or feminine in nature and therefore a nuance of the 1st or 2nd Ray. **The odd numbered Rays are masculine and associated with Sanat Kumara, and the even numbered Rays are feminine and associated with Sananda.** The masculine Rays are active and intellectual and the female Rays are emotional and intuitive.

After the first two Rays the 3rd Ray is the most important. The 3rd Ray is the Ray of Kriya Shakti, the Ray of Activity. Because of its nature to be generate explosive and raucous activity, this is also the Ray of Destruction.

The Three Rays of Essence

Collectively, the first three Rays are known as Rays of Essence because all the other Rays partake of their nature. Each of the other four Rays partakes of the essence of the first Three Rays by expressing a nature that is predominantly creative, preserving, or destructive.

The Four Rays of Aspect and Activity

Just as the three primary colors give rise to the four secondary colors, so do the first three Rays give rise to the four secondary Rays. In fact, there is a close correspondence between the colors and the Rays. The first three Rays rule over the three primary colors and the four secondary Rays govern the four secondary colors.

The four Secondary Rays are known as the Rays of Aspect and Activity. They incorporate one or more of the Essence Rays, and they are often referred to as sub-Rays of the 3rd Ray. This is because the 3rd Ray is associated with the creation of the physical universe and they are all related to activity in the third dimensional plane.

The Seven Ray Lords and Ladies

The Lords and Ladies of the Rays consist of deities and spiritual masters aligned with and governing each Ray. The Gnostics claimed that the original Lords of the Seven Rays were the Sons of the Goddess, but it can also be said that they are the seven parts or Seven Sons of Sanat Kumara, the First Son who is the synthesis of all the Seven Rays. In this regard, they have been called the Seven Kumaras.

Sanat and Sananda Kumara initially became the Lords of the 1st and 2nd Rays, while other Kumaras assumed lordship over the other five Rays. Since all persons are governed by one or two Rays, over millennium some have ascended along their Ray and become Ascended Masters of their Ray. They then became additional lords of their associated Ray.

Because the world is moving into a new cycle known as the Fifth World, the Lords and Ladies of the 7th Ray are especially active right now. This includes Goddess Kali and Saint Germain.

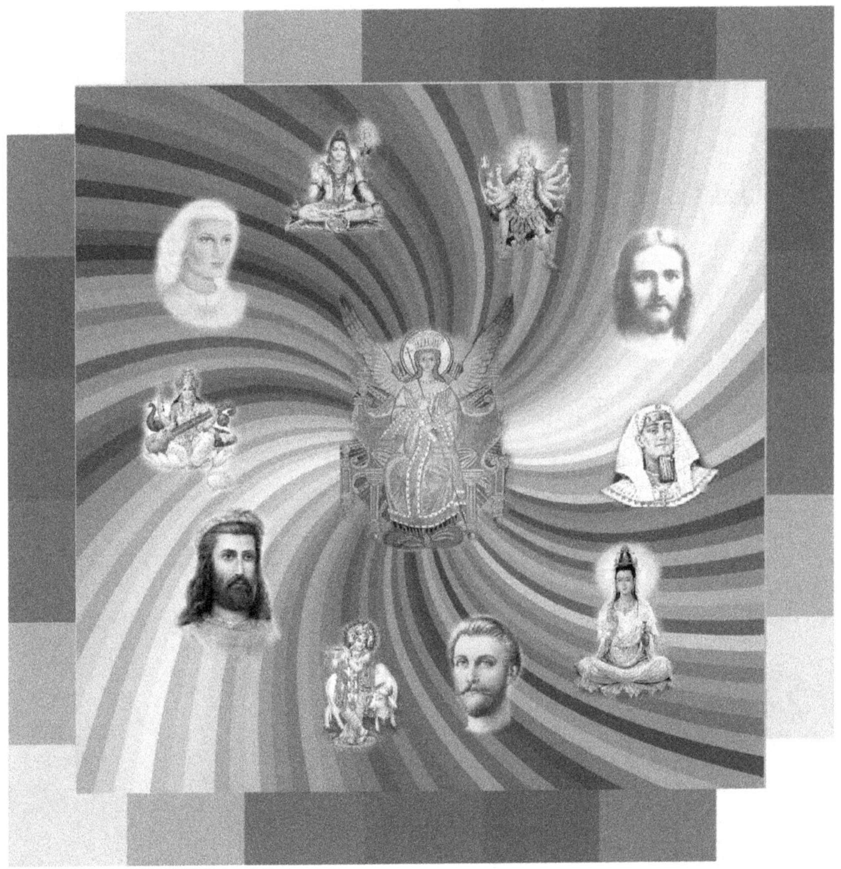

The Seven Rays and the Planets

One important vehicle the Seven Rays have used to govern Earth and all its life forms are the Astrological Planets: the Sun, the Moon, Mercury, Venus, Mars, Jupiter, Saturn, Uranus, Neptune, and Pluto. A basic approach to understanding the planet-ray link is to think of the planet Saturn as embodying the spirit of the 1st Ray and the planets between it and the Sun as embodying the spirits of the successive rays. This continues until the 6th and 7th Rays which are embodied by Neptune and Pluto. Saturn corresponds to the 1st Ray because the planet and its ray are both associated with form. They both denote the first form and color of the Infinite Spirit as it initially comes into physical manifestation. Neptune and Pluto's association with the 6th and 7th Rays occurs because the two planets and their rays both denote the transcendence, breakup and transformation of the physical plane. This is how the planets and rays line up.

Planet	Ray
Saturn	1st Ray
Jupiter	2nd Ray
Mars	3rd Ray
Venus	4th Ray
Mercury	5th Ray
Neptune	6th Ray
Pluto	7th Ray

Now, look at the association chart below. You will find the 3rd, 4th and 5th Rays are each associated with two planets. Saturn, the planet of organization and power governs the 1st Ray of Will and Power; Jupiter, the planet of religion and philosophy, governs the 2nd Ray of Wisdom; Mars, the planet of activity, governs the 3rd Ray of Activity; Venus and the Moon, two "planets" involved with peaceful relationship, govern the 4th Ray of Harmony; Uranus and Mercury, planets of scientific intelligence, govern the 5th Ray of Technology; Neptune, the planet of transcendental experience, governs the 6th Ray of Devotion; and Pluto, the planet of transformation, channels the 7th Ray of Alchemy.

Planet	Ray
Saturn	1st Ray
Jupiter	2nd Ray
Mars	3rd Ray
Venus, Moon	4th Ray
Mercury, Uranus	5th Ray
Neptune	6th Ray
Pluto	7th Ray

Determining a Person's Birth Ray

Thus, every life form governed by a Ray is ruled over by one or more Ray Lords and one or more planets. In order to determine which Ray or Rays govern a person's current incarnation, you will need to determine their Ruling Planet, which is the planet or planets that govern the Rising Sign in their astrological Natal (Birth) Chart. The Rising Sign, which is the astrological sign at the beginning of the First House in a chart, represents a person's theme for the current incarnation. It rules what they are meant to accomplish and learn in the world, as well as their body type and personality. You can determine which planets and Rays are governing a person's life by learning what planet(s) rule their Rising Sign. If the person is born with a Sagittarius Rising, for example, they are ruled by Jupiter because Jupiter rules the sign Sagittarius. And since they are ruled by Jupiter, their Ray is the 2nd Ray. If the person is born with Scorpio Rising, a sign governed by both Mars and Pluto, they are ruled by both the 3rd and 7th Rays. It will be a help to you to learn what planets govern which signs in order to more easily determine a person Ray or Rays.

This is important! The Rising Sign you use to determine a person's Ray is the Rising Sign of their Vedic or Hindu Astrology Chart, not their Western Chart. Don't let this scare you. You can easily find an online website offering free Vedic Astrology Natal Charts and simply type in a person's date time and place of birth to the form provided. The website does all the calculation. Or you can find an online website offering free Western Astrology Natal Charts. If you go that route you will have to determine the person's Vedic Rising Sign through subtracting 23 ½ degrees from their Western Rising Sign. This is also quite easy to do.

Steps to determine a person's Vedic Rising Sign via their Western Rising Sign

1. Find out the degree of the person's Western Rising Sign. Each sign has 30 degrees, so the degree will be between 0-and 30.

2. Now subtract 23 ½ degrees from the Western Rising Sign degree.

3. If after subtracting the degrees from the person's Western Rising Sign the resulting degree is still in the same sign, then the person's Vedic Rising Sign is the same as their Western Rising Sign. But if after subtracting the degrees from the Western Rising Sign the result is a degree in the previous sign, then that is the person's Vedic Rising Sign.

4. If, for example, the person's Rising Sign in the Western System is 26 degrees of Sagittarius, you simply subtract 23½ degrees and get 2½ degrees Sagittarius. Therefore, the person's Vedic Rising Sign is also Sagittarius. But If the person's Western Rising Sign is 5 degrees of Sagittarius and you subtract 23½ degrees from it you will get 11½ degrees of Scorpio. Therefore the Vedic Rising Sign is Scorpio.

5. When you subtract 23½ degrees from 5 degrees of Sagittarius you first subtract 5 degrees to get to the beginning of the sign, which is 0 degrees of Sagittarius; then you subtract the remaining 18½ degrees and get 11 ½ degrees of Scorpio.

6. On the following page are the Vedic and Western Natal Charts of John F. Kennedy. The Western Chart at the top of the page shows a Rising Sign degree of 20 degrees of Libra while the Vedic Chart at the bottom has the Rising Sign at 27 degrees of Virgo (The Vedic Rising Sign is the house with the diagonal line across it). Thus, JFK"s Vedic Rising Sign is approximately a 23 degree behind his Western Rising Sign. This is approximately the degree difference between the Western and Vedic Systems when JFK was born. Now it is 23 ½ degrees.

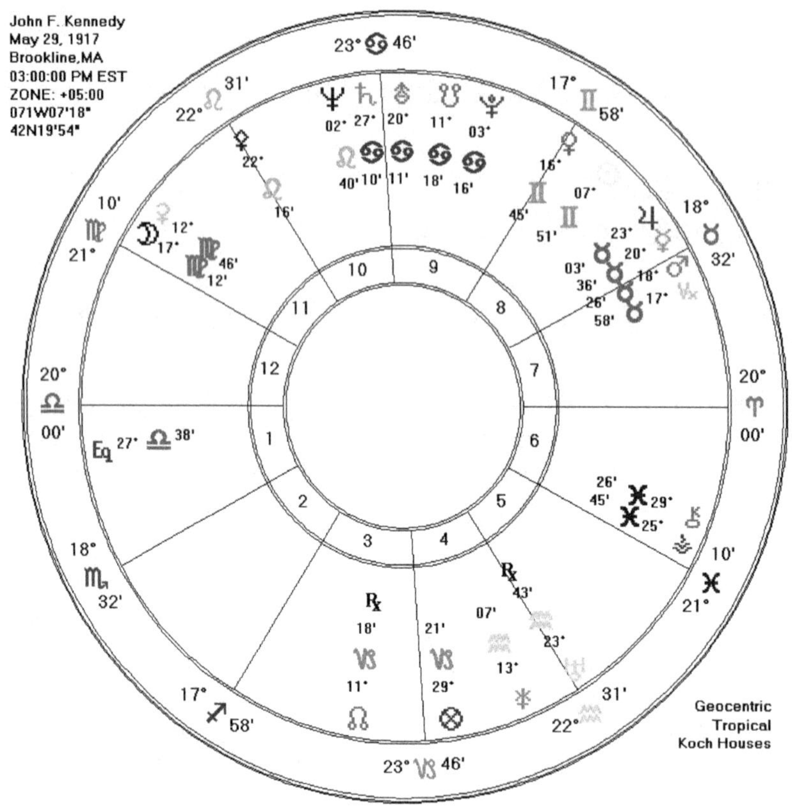

♓	♈ ♂ 25° 45′ ☿D 27° 53′	♉ ♃ 00° 21′ ☉ 15° 09′ ♀ 24° 04′	♊ ☋ 19° 46′
♒	**RASI**		♋ ♄ 04° 28′
♑			♌ ☽ 24° 30′
♐ ☊ 19° 46	♏	♎	♍ 27° 10′

Determining a Person's Ray of their Current Planetary Cycle

Although it is not necessary for a Seven Rays of Healing evaluation of a person's birth Ray, determining a person's Dasas, their Vedic Planetary Cycles, can also supply helpful information regarding what additional and current Ray influences they may be under.

The Vedic Planetary Cycles and their Rays

When a person is born their life is divided into Dasas, planetary cycles, that together total 120 years. Although most people will not reach 120 years of age, during their lives they will progress through the majority of their cycles. Since each cycle is governed by a planet and each planet is associated with one or two of the Seven Rays, determining what cycle a person is currently moving through is a good way to pin-point another Ray(s) influence (besides their natal life Ray) affecting their lives. This information can be very valuable when diagnosing and administering a Seven Rays of Healing treatment.

A person's Dasas are determined when their Vedic Chart is drawn up. Through erecting an online Vedic Astrology Chart on a free Vedic Astrology website, or by acquiring your own Vedic Astrology program, you can easily discover what Dasa a person is currently moving through and the Ray currently governing them.

The Dasa a person begins and ends their life with will be different for each person, but the sequence of Dasas will be the same for everyone. Every person's Mars cycle will last seven years, for example, and their Sun Cycle will always unfold at the end of their Mars Cycle. The length of each planetary cycle and their sequence is shown below.

Sun Cycle -- 6 Years
Moon Cycle -- 10 years
Mars Cycle -- 7 Years
Rahu Cycle-- 18 Years
Jupiter Cycle -- 16 Years
Saturn Cycle -- 1 years
Mercury Cycle - 17 Years
Ketu Cycle -- 7 Years
Venus Cycle -- 20 Years

If a person is currently moving through their Sun Cycle then they have the Sun prominently affecting their life. Since the Sun is associated with the 3rd Ray, the 3rd Ray is operating as a secondary influence after their Birth Ray. This should be taken into account when diagnosing a person. More on this in a future chapter.

Rahu and Ketu are the Vedic counterparts of Neptune and Pluto and should be interpreted similarly. Rahu is also associated with the 7th Ray and Ketu with the 6th Ray.

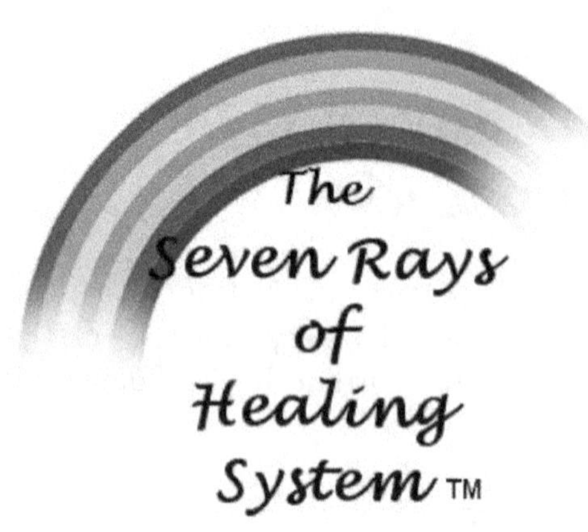

CHAPTER 2

The Characteristics, Abilities and Destinies of People born under the Seven Rays

This chapter will cover all the Seven Rays and the people who are aligned with each Ray At the end of this chapter you will be able to determine a person's Ray as well as know their life path, character traits, potential health issues, protective gems, Spirit Animals and Ascended Guides.

Please read this chapter over many times in order to begin to fully grasp the nature of each Ray and what it rules over. And at the same time practice determining peoples' Rays according to the directions at the end of Chapter 1 and then explaining to them the characteristics of their Ray. Begin by memorizing the Zodiacal signs and the planets that rule them listed below. It will also assist you to do your own astrological overview of the nature of the different planets and signs.

Sign	***Ruled by...***
Aries	**Mars**
Taurus	**Venus**
Gemini	**Mercury**
Cancer	**Moon**
Leo	**Sun**
Virgo	**Mercury**
Libra	**Venus**
Scorpio	**Mars & Pluto**
Sagittarius	**Jupiter**
Capricorn	**Saturn**
Aquarius	**Saturn & Uranus**
Pisces	**Jupiter & Neptune**

Now, memorize which planet (or planets) is associated with what ray or rays

Planet	Ray
Mars	3rd Ray
Venus	4th Ray
Mercury	5th Ray
The Moon	4th Ray
The Sun	3rd Ray
Jupiter	2nd Ray
Saturn	1st Ray
Uranus	5th Ray
Neptune	6th Ray
Pluto	7th Ray

Now, memorize what colored gem stones are associated with each planet.

Planet	Color of Gem
Mars	Orange
Venus	Clear, transparent
Mercury	Green
The Moon	Milky white
The Sun	Red
Jupiter	Yellow-gold
Saturn	Blue
Uranus	Silvery
Neptune	Purple, Violet
Pluto	Black, Red, Violet

The Three Rays of Essence

The 1st Ray of Will and Power

1st Ray Goddess Power: Of the Goddess's three powers of Creation, Preservation, and Destruction, the 1st Ray is associated with the power of Creation.

1st Ray in Trinity: The 1st Ray is associated with Brahma, the Lord of Creation in the Hindu Trinity, and with the first "person" or Father of the Christian Trinity.

The 1st Ray Colors: The color of this ray is dark blue, the color of the upper heavens, and of Spirit.

Note on the Colors : In general, the first three rays are associated with the Primary Colors of blue, yellow, and red, while the other four rays are associated with the Secondary Colors.

The 1st Ray Realm and Stage in the Creation of the Universe: The 1st Ray was the first ray to emanate out of the Infinite Spirit and is inclusive of all the Seven Rays. From dark blue all the colors of the other rays descend. The 1st Ray is both the Divine Will and Divine Power. The "Will" of the 1st Ray begins the creative process even though it precedes the actual manifestation of physical forms in the universe that occurs via the 3rd Ray. The 1st Ray corresponds to the First Day of *Genesis*, when "the Spirit of God moved upon the face of the waters. And darkness was upon the face of the deep."

Note on the Realms : As previously mentioned each ray is associated both with a level of the multi-leveled universe and/or one of the seven stages in the process of universal creation. The multi-layered model of the universe used in this book is based upon the ancient cosmological systems developed by the sages of the East and the Gnostics and Neo-Platonists of the West.

1st Ray Lords and Ladies: The Lords and Ladies of the 1st Ray include those deities which are the synthesis of all the Seven Rays and a manifestation of the Primal Dragon, the first material form of the Infinite Spirit, Shiva. This includes Sophia, the Lady of the Seven Rays, as well as Her Son, Sanat Kumara, the Lord of the Seven Rays. Sanat Kumara is known in the West as St. Michael, as well as the Peacock Angel among the Yezidis and Enki of the Sumerians. So these are also Lords of the 1st Ray. Brahma of the Hindu Trinity and Master Morya of the Ascended Masters tradition are additionally Lords of the 1st Ray.

1st Ray People: These people are the rulers, leaders, and authority figures in the world. Their wills reign supreme. Some become titled authority figures, such as CEOs, senators, commanders, presidents and prime ministers, whereas others are simply rulers of their own "nest" or household, or they may simply function in the role of organizer. 1st Ray people are good managers, supervisors, and have good organizational skills. They serve with greater or lesser worldly authority and power under the etheric King of the World, the ray lord Sanat Kumara. **Negatively**, these people can be over authoritarian, bossy, dictatorial, rigid, and both self-serving and self-glorifying. **Positively**, they can be well organized, self-abnegating and rule in accordance with Divine Will solely for the greater good. They can also be warriors for righteousness and fairness, and in this regard they reflect their ray lord St. Michael.

1st Ray Urges and Desires: 1st Ray persons often have the desire to lead and rule others. They also have a need to organize a situation, persons, places and/or things in their environment.

1st Ray Mental Tendencies: Being aligned with a male ray, 1st Ray persons tend to be intellectual. They separate and categorize events and objects in their lives, which is what makes them such good organizers. The more highly evolved 1st Ray natives are also philosophical as well as intuitive.

1st Ray Emotional Tendencies: The 1st Ray people ruled by Saturn (see 1st Ray Planets and Zodiacal Signs) can tend towards cultivating a realistic approach to life, but also one that can lead to negativity, anger, fear, and depression. Because of all the responsibilities they often need to shoulder, life can often feel heavy and burdensome.

1st Ray Spirit Animal: The Puma, Lion, or the wildcat in general, is the spirit animal of 1st Ray people. Just as the Lion is King of the Beasts, the 1st Ray person is king within his own domain. The Puma is the Andean sacred animal that rules the middle plane, Earth, the plane once ruled by kings and queens. It is the balance of the other two worlds and their corresponding animals – the upper world ruled by the Condor, and the lower world ruled by the snake or serpent. The cat teaches us how to move in balance in this world while uniting the higher self and the Divine Will of the upper world (the Condor) with the lower world of the ego (the snake). The direction of the Puma is west; so 1st Ray people can assimilate the nature and wisdom of the Puma by facing west during meditation and/or while observing spiritual practices.

The 1st Ray Chakras: 1st Ray persons consistently function out of many chakras. They operate out of the 1st and 2nd chakras, which are associated specifically with will and power, as well as the 5th chakra, an upper chakra that is also associated with the power of the spoken word. They also have an active 6th chakra, especially in its role of controlling the Master Gland, the Pituitary Gland. The more evolved 1st Ray persons also have the higher functions of the 6th chakra active and can clearly intuit the Divine Will.

The 1st Ray Planets and Zodiacal Signs: 1st Ray persons are born with their Vedic Ascendants in the sign of Capricorn. Their ruling planet is Saturn, the planet of organization, ambition, control and authority.

The 1st Ray Gems: In order to align with their ray, 1st Ray persons can wear blue stones. If they are born with Capricorn on the ascendant they would seek to align with the planet Saturn through wearing on their bodies dark blue stones, such as Blue Sapphire, Blue Topaz, and Lapis Lazuli. The blue stones should be set in a gold setting – preferably with the stone touching the skin, and worn either as a pendant or ring. In a ring, the blue stone is worn over the middle finger, Saturn's finger.

Note on Gems : In general, all stones ruled by any of the rays that are worn or set into a ring or pendant should ideally be able to touch the skin. They should be two carats in size or larger, and of good quality. In generals, the stones associated with the male rays, i.e., the odd number rays, are set into the "male" metal, gold, and those associated with the female rays, i.e., are set into the "female" metal, silver.

1st Ray Mantras: The 1st Ray mantras are the mantras of Saturn, which is known as Sani in the Vedic System of Astrology. the mantra for Saturn is Om Sanischarya Namaha, "Salutations to Saturn." By repeating this mantras during times of worship, at least 108 times and 1-2x a day, a 1st Ray person can more fully align with the 1st Ray and thereby better fulfill his or her destiny.

Note on Mantras : Mantras for any of the rays are the names of the planets the rays move through. Planetary mantras are used to help align one with his or her ray, as well as to neutralize the potential bad influences coming from such planets. It is good to repeat the mantra a sacred number of times, such as 7, 9, 13, 33, 52, or 108. Repeating it 108 times will give the best result.

When pronouncing Sanscrit mantras, e is pronounced as a long a, i is pronounced as a long e, and a is pronounced as a short a.

1st Ray Organs and Body Parts: The body organs ruled by the 1st Ray include the pituitary gland, the kidneys and adrenals, as well as the heart. The pituitary gland is the first and "Master Gland" that regulates all the other glands, especially the thyroid and adrenal glands. The kidney/adrenals, which are regarded as one organ in Chinese medicine since the adrenals sit right on top of the kidneys, are a person's source of will and power. When the kidney/adrenals become weakened through malfunctioning thyroid gland and/or stress and overwork, a common 1st Ray syndrome, a person can lose his or her power and will to succeed, or to even do anything in life. The kidneys govern the lower back, and back trouble is also a common symptom of 1st Ray people who try to carry the world on their backs.

The Kidneys are also the source of the "watery essence" or what the Chinese refer to as Jing. When Jing is strong it transports a portion of itself to the head to help form up the brain – which is the Blue Ray organ that controls the body. A person with deficient Jing will have weak knees (a symptom of not being able to move forward with their ambitions, as well as vertigo, spacey-ness and difficulty making decisions and leading others.

Every organ rules over an emotion; for the kidney/adrenals that emotion is fear. 1st Ray persons experience fear because of their tendency to separate and perceive differences. This keeps them from feeling connected and supported by others or by a higher power. When their fear becomes profound enough, what happens? They involuntarily urinate. This demonstrates how the kidneys and the organ connected to them, the bladder, are linked to the emotion of fear.

Of all possible heath conditions, First Ray persons are the most likely to suffer from kidney/adrenal problems. They are also subject to problems with teeth, bones and skin. These are parts of the body ruled over by Saturn, the planet that governs the hardest and densest matter, including solid rocks. Saturn rules over skin because it is the planet governing boundaries, and our skin is the boundary between our bodies and the outer world.

1st Ray Treatment

1st Ray Counseling: One way 1st Ray persons can suffer from the above mentioned emotional and physical disharmonies is by not being aligned with their ray. Such persons will have difficulty fulfilling their destinies, and the energy circulating through the bodies of such persons can become easily blocked and stuck. When that happens, certain organs and parts of the body are not able to receive the nourishment they need and physical disease symptoms are soon to follow. Besides physical illness, such persons will also suffer from a lack emotional fulfillment and inner peace. By counseling 1st Ray persons and advising them how they can align with their rays (mantras, gems, etc. and what they could be doing in life to fulfill their destinies (organize, supervise, direct, be successful and achieve status in the world, etc., you can help assist them in regaining health on all levels.

1st Ray Color Therapy: Use the 1st Ray colors. This includes dark blue or indigo. The color should be dark blue to black, like deep within the ocean or the sky as it meets the darkness of space. The Kidneys are the seat of the watery "ocean" in the human body. They are the root of the other organs just as black and dark blue are the root of the seven colors and the blackness of space is the root of all life. Red is another 1st Ray color. It especifically nurtures the Adrenal Glands. When performing color therapy on someone with 1st Ray Kidney symptomology, either dark blue to black, or red, can be broadcast over the kidney/adrenal region at the lower back. Dark blue-black primarily nourishes the Kidneys themselves and red feeds the adrenals sitting upon them.

1st Ray Sound Therapy: When using the red color for kidney/adrenal disorders the musical note of G can be used in tandem. Use the musical note of D when broadcasting very dark blue to black on these organs. Bass drumming sounds can also be used with these colors. Classical music, which unites many instruments together in harmony, is helpful for 1st Ray people who function as organizers and directors.

A note on colors and sounds: For optimum results administer color therapy in conjunction with sound therapy for at least 30-45 minutes.

1st Ray Meridian Therapy: When working with 1st Ray conditions acupressure points along the Kidney and Du Meridians (a Meridian that runs up the center of the back can be used. Seven Ray Acupressure will be covered in its entirety in a later chapter.

1st Ray Yogas: The asanas of Hatha Yoga can be prescribed for any ray related illness because they benefit the entire physical body. In the case of 1st Ray people the asanas that stretch and strengthen the spine are very efficacious. Karma Yoga, the path of work, is a good yoga for busy 1st Ray natives to follow. Karma Yoga involves dedicating the fruits of one's labors to God. Work without desire for the fruits. The best scripture and handbook for those on the path of Karma Yoga is the *Bhagavad Gita.* The path of Jnana Yoga, the path of wisdom, is also good for 1st ray people who are by nature intellectual and philosophical. Jnana Yoga is the path of contemplation and study of God and the meaning and goal of existence. All scriptures and sacred books are part of the path of Jnana Yoga.

The 2nd Ray of Wisdom

2nd Ray Goddess Power: The 2nd Ray is associated with the Goddess's power of Preservation.

2nd Ray in Trinity: The 2nd Ray corresponds to the Son and Second "Person" of the Holy Trinity.

2nd Ray Color: The color of the 2nd Ray is yellow-gold, the color of high wisdom.

2nd Ray Realm and Stage in the Creation of the Universe: The 2nd Ray is associated with the Goddess, the embodiment of Love and Wisdom that emanates from the Blue Spirit of the 1st Ray. The 2nd Ray corresponds to the Mental or Causal Plane, i.e., the plane that is the cause of all the other planes of existence. Also known as the archetypal plane, it is where the Divine Mind resides and the archetypes and the blueprints of all eventual physical forms first manifest. This is the realm of perfection, because it is the realm where all form is in perfect alignment and harmony with the Divine Will. As such, it is also the realm of love, which is the emotion associated with balance and a harmonious relationship with the Divine Will.

2nd Ray Lords and Ladies: As the definitive "female" ray, one of the 2nd Ray Lords is Sophia, the Lady of the Seven Rays and Goddess of Wisdom or Gnosis. The Lords of this ray include Sananda Kumara and the Avatars of Lord Vishnu who out of love take a physical body on Earth in order to share their wisdom and save the world from destruction. These Avatars include Krishna, Rama, Buddha and Jesus. In the archangelic tradition Raphael is associated with the 2nd Ray, and in the Ascended Master tradition the 2nd Ray Lord is Kuthumi.

2nd Ray People: 2nd Ray people are here to participate in and become leaders of the world's spiritual traditions. They can be called "Priests after the Order of Melchizedek (a name for Sanat Kumara.") As shamans, gurus, spiritual teachers, philosophers, priests, priestesses, and enlightened adepts, they assist in the administration of established religious traditions or found new ones. Not all 2nd Ray persons are, however, destined to be spiritual leaders. Some contribute to the world's spirituality simply through leading spiritual lives and serving as a guide and example for others. **Negatively**, 2nd Ray persons can be dogmatic and controlling and/or arrogant with what wisdom they have acquired. **Positively**, 2nd Ray people project wisdom and love into their surroundings. They are compassionate towards the down trodden, whom they seek to serve. And they strive to live righteous lives, which serve as an example for others.

2nd Ray Urges and Desires: 2nd Ray people are normally drawn to align with some spiritual tradition and serve within it as priests, priestesses and teachers. They usually have an insatiable appetite to know and understand the universe and the meaning of life, and many have the desire to then teach or share these topics with others. The higher evolved 2nd Ray natives are also usually intensely interested in serving the world, sometimes to the point of self-abnegation.

2nd Ray Mental Tendencies: The principal 2nd Ray mental tendency is to be philosophical. 2nd Ray persons normally assimilate life's experiences through a philosophical filter. The lower evolved 2nd Ray are also intellectual and critical (or judgmental), while the higher evolved often have well-developed intuitions.

2nd Ray Emotional Tendencies: 2nd Ray persons can succumb to the emotions of anger and depression, two emotions ruled by the liver, which is one of the principal organs that these persons can have problems with. 2nd Ray people tend to be optimistic, but their downfall is that they can tend to be overly optimistic and not realistic enough at times.

2nd Ray Spirit Animal: The spirit animal of the 2nd Ray is the Condor (South America) or Eagle (North America), the high-flying bird of philosophy and spiritual wisdom that can see life from a broader and higher perspective than most any other creature. The Condor or Eagle is the pre-eminent bird of wisdom and justice. Its direction is the east, which is the direction of wisdom. 2nd Ray persons can sit facing the east for meditation and spiritual work in order to assimilate the wisdom of the Condor/Eagle.

2nd Ray Chakras: 2nd Ray people function principally out of the 3rd, 4th, 6th, and 7th chakras. Their desire to assimilate information and experiences – and take in all that life can give – requires an active third chakra. Their desire to serve with compassion leads them into their hearts and helps activate the fourth chakra. Their tendency to contemplate and philosophize stimulates the sixth chakra, and their desire for spiritual communion and oneness with God and all life activates the seventh chakra.

2nd Ray Planets and Zodiacal Signs: Those born with an alignment to the 2nd Ray have either the Zodiacal signs of Sagittarius or Pisces as their Vedic Ascendants or Rising Signs. Both Zodiacal signs are ruled by the planet Jupiter, the vehicle of the spirit of the 2nd Ray. Jupiter is called Guru in Vedic astrology, and those who are born under its influence embody the guru principle. They dispel darkness (gu) with light (ru) and give perfect wisdom.

2nd Ray Gems: The yellow-gold stones ruled by Jupiter help a 2nd Ray person align with their ray. The best of this group is Yellow Sapphire, and after that, the best is Yellow Topaz, followed by Citrine Quartz. Even though this is a feminine and even numbered ray, the Jupiter stones of the 2nd Ray should be set in gold, which with its yellow-gold color is the metal especially attuned to Jupiter. As a ring, these stones should be worn on the index finger, which is the Jupiter finger. They can be worn either as a pendant or as a ring.

2nd Ray Mantras: The mantras to align with the 2nd Ray are the names of Jupiter. Besides being known as Guru, it is also known as Brihaspati, the preceptor of the gods. Jupiter's mantra is Om Brihaspataye Namaha, meaning Om "Salutations to Jupiter." Repeat this mantra audibly or mentally at least 108 times and 1-2x a day.

2nd Ray Organs and Body Parts: The 2nd Ray and its color of golden yellow rules over the middle of the torso, home of the liver and stomach. Thus, 2nd Ray persons can have problems with both the liver and the stomach. Jupiter, the biggest planet in the Solar System and vehicle of the 2nd Ray, rules over the liver, the largest organ in the body. The liver is related to wisdom through being an organ that is involved with helping a person to make decisions about life. With a weak or malfunctioning liver it is hard for one to make decisions and feel that he or she has a firm direction in life. The liver also rules over the smooth flow of life force in the body. When the liver is congested the life force does not flow smoothly and a person's body feels tight and they are stressed out. Conversely, when we are not flowing with life and we become stressed, the life force gets blocked up and injures the liver. Life force congestion will eventually create fire (all stagnant energy eventually turns to fire) in the liver that will flare upwards and cause both anger and headaches. Since a diseased liver can also "attack" the stomach, 2nd Ray persons can also show symptoms of stomach disharmony, such a indigestion and belching.

2nd Ray Treatment

2nd Ray Counseling: When treating 2nd Ray persons you can first assess through counseling whether the person in question is aligning with their ray and fulfilling their destiny. They are likely to feel unfulfilled unless they are moving ahead spiritually and actively aligning with a spiritual tradition. They also need to serving others, and/or being a teacher, guide or guru for others. Look for signs of liver and stomach disharmony, such as anger, depression, headaches, and/or stomach discomfort and poor digestion to confirm a 2nd Ray imbalance.

2nd Ray Color Therapy: To treat 2nd Ray imbalances with color therapy, the color of yellow-gold can be broadcast over the entire body. For more specific treatment, yellow-gold can be broadcast across the middle of the torso or directly over the liver. Color therapy should be administered on the bare skin. If you do not get optimum results with yellow, green can also be used to heal the liver. Always administer color therapy for a minimum of 30 minutes. Yellow-gold can also enter the body as yellow-gold colored foods, such as bananas, yellow skinned vegetables, yellow-gold grains, pineapples, nuts, corn, yellow lentils, butter, etc.

2nd Ray Sound Therapy: The note of B along with the color yellow-gold will help alleviate liver and all 2nd Ray issues. When using Green light, play the note of C. Play these notes around the person or right over the liver area.

2nd Ray Meridian Therapy: The meridians associated with the 2nd Ray and the liver are: the Liver Channel, the Gall Bladder Channel (just as the kidney and adrenal are considered one organ system in Chinese Medicine, so are the liver and gall bladder one organ system), as well as the stomach and Ren Channel, the meridian in the center of the torso that moves up the front of the body. Certain points on these meridians are more efficacious in treating 2nd Ray and liver disharmonies. These will be discussed in a later lesson.

2nd Ray Yogas: All yogas are helpful to 2nd Ray persons, and some 2nd Ray natives will adopt many or all of them in their lifetime. A myriad of 2nd Ray persons will eventually teach one or more yoga path to others. Yoga is the "food" of the 2nd Ray and was first taught by 2nd Ray gurus. Yoga is the path of purification that one embarks upon in order to permanently unite with God.

The 3rd Ray of Action and Creativity

3rd Ray Goddess Power: The 3rd Ray embodies the Goddess's fiery Power of both Creativity and Destruction. Thus, this paradoxical ray is both creative and destructive. It is associated with the manifestation of physical fire, which can be creative if harnessed constructively but destructive if allowed to burn uncontrollably.

3rd Ray in the Trinity: The 3rd Ray is associated with the Third "Person" of the Trinity, the Holy Spirit.

3rd Ray Colors: The colors associated with the 3rd Ray are the "active" and "fiery" colors, red and orange.

3rd Ray Realm and Stage of the Universe: The 3rd Ray is associated with the third stage of the creation of the universe, when the archetypal forms of the Divine Mind begin to take shape physically. This comes under the guidance of the fiery Son and corresponds to the fire of the Big Bang, which is the raw material out of which all the physical forms of the universe will be composed. Initially this fire is volatile and destructive, but when it begins to cool and crystallize into the forms of the Divine Mind it becomes creative.

3rd Ray Lord and Ladies: The 3rd Ray Lords and Ladies include Shiva-Rudra, the deity of fire who is Lord of both Creation and Destruction (fire creates and destroys), as well as Kali, the Goddess of Destruction. It is also ruled by the third member of the archangelic trinity, Gabriel. Since it is an odd numbered and male ray, it is additionally governed by Sanat Kumara.

3rd Ray People: 3rd Ray people are usually the most active of all ray people. They are often athletic and sportsmen or sportswomen. They can be enterprising business people or they may be involved in physical professions, such as trainers and construction workers. They are generally fiery in nature. When their fire is used constructively they are creative, but when it is unharnessed and unbridled it can be destructive. 3rd Ray people sometimes direct their creativity into art projects and can eventually become renowned artists and musicians, but their downfall can be their big egos and their desire for fame and recognition. **Positively,** 3rd Ray people are creative, inventive, and possess good leadership abilities. **Negatively,** 3rd Ray people can be overly aggressive, destructive, raucous, egotistical, and excessively passionate. They may not use adequate discrimination when acting.

3rd Ray Urges and Desires: 3rd Ray persons desire to create, but they can also desire to harm and destroy. They have the desire to excel and shine in whatever they do. They also have the urge to be first in line and to lead others.

3rd Ray Mental Tendencies: Since theirs is an odd numbered and "male" ray, 3rd Ray persons tend to be intellectual and scientifically oriented.

3rd Ray Emotional Tendencies: 3rd Ray people usually have strong desires and can succumb to anger if their passions are not satisfied. It is often the un-realized desires of the 3rd Ray native that engenders his or her destructive tendencies. 3rd Ray people can also be defensive, as well as intensely excited and raucously enthusiastic.

3rd Ray Power Spirit Animal: The 3rd Ray people are aligned with the puma because they are naturally athletic and move well. They are warriors and often enjoy the role of leaders.

3rd Ray Chakras: 3rd Ray people function principally out of the lower three charkas. Their active energy and passion comes from the 1st and 2nd chakras, and their creativity comes from both the 2nd and 3rd chakras. The 3rd chakra is also the chakra of the ego and governs the desire for both power and personal recognition.

3rd Ray Planets and Zodiacal Signs: 3rd Ray people are governed by Mars and the Sun and the two fire signs they rule, Aries and Leo, as well as the sign of explosive energy, Scorpio. Third Ray persons with Aries on their Vedic Ascendant and ruled by Mars can be very active, passionate, competitive, and destructive. Those with Leo on the Ascendant and ruled by the Sun are both active and creative. They can also have an egotistical temperament and a very strong drive to be recognized and achieve fame. Those with Scorpio on the Ascendant and ruled by Mars are the most snake-like. They are secretive, intense, and can be explosive when threatened. They are, like Aries natives, also competitive, active, passionate, and sometimes destructive.

3rd Ray Gems: These are the red and orange stones ruled over by the Sun and Mars respectively. The red stones, which include Ruby and Garnet, should be set in gold and worn on the ring finger. The orange stones, which include Red Coral, Spondylus, and Carnelian, should also be set in gold. In a ring setting, the orange stones should be worn on the ring finger. 3rd Ray persons can also benefit by wearing Quartz Crystal, which has a naturally fiery vibration.

3rd Ray Mantras: 3rd Ray mantras are the names of Mars and the Sun, which are Kuja and Surya. If the person has Aries or Scorpio Ascendant, and are therefore ruled by Mars, their mantra should be Om Kujaya Namaha, Om "Salutations to Mars." If their Ascendant is Leo, their mantra should be Om Suryaya Namaha, Om "Salutations to the Sun." Repeat these mantras audibly or mentally at least 108 times and 1-2x a day.

3rd Ray Organs and Body Parts: The 3rd Ray of Activity governs both the lower part of the torso, especially the Adrenal Glands, as well as the Heart – the most active organ - in the upper part of the torso. 3rd Ray persons, especially those ruled by the Sun, can suffer from heart dis-harmonies, including palpitations and heart attacks. Those ruled by Mars can have afflictions to the charkas of physical movement and fiery passion, the lower two chakras and their corresponding organs. The organs specifically associated with these chakras are the kidney/adrenals, which control one's fight or flight reactions, and generally support the entire body with life force (more on this later), as well as the sexual organs. 3rd Ray persons, especially those ruled by Mars, can suffer from disharmonies with the kidney/adrenals (usually symptoms related to overuse) and the sexual organs. 3rd Ray natives can also have a dysfunctional liver, which can become afflicted with excess expressions of anger.

3rd Ray Treatment

3rd Ray Counseling: 3rd Ray people thrive best when they are active and creative and can feel unfulfilled when they are not. These people need to be making things happen in their lives; they need to be accomplishing. If a 3rd Ray person is living an inactive lifestyle and not able to live with zest and express and fulfill their passions, he or she is likely to suffer both physically and emotionally. A 3rd Ray person also needs to be able to lead others and feel special.

3rd Ray Color Therapy: Those 3rd Ray natives ruled by Mars can be bathed in orange light to help them realign with their ray, and the Sun ruled 3rd Ray persons can be bathed in red light for the same result. For kidney/adrenal or sexual organ related problems, bathe the lower part of the torso with both red and orange light. For heart problems, bathe the upper torso in red light. If a 3rd Ray native becomes too fiery, bathe him or her in blue light to bring them into balance. If the condition is Heart related, red can be broadcast over the heart region. Red feeds the heart, blue slows down an irregular rapid heartbeat. Red colored foods include red lentils, apples, strawberries, red peppers, rhubarb, cherries, red plums, as well as red beets, red cabbage, red meats, etc. Orange foods include oranges, papaya, cantaloupe, carrots, pumpkin, peaches, apricots, etc.

3rd Ray Sound Therapy: 3rd Ray kidney/adrenal and sexual organ problems respond to the note A as well as light drumming musical selections. Use note A for Orange lights and G for Red lights.

3rd Ray Meridian Therapy: For 3rd Ray kidney/adrenal or sexual organ problems use points along the Kidney Meridian. Points of the Du and Ren Channels can also be used, as well as points along the Heart, Liver and Gall Bladder Meridians (See Chapter 5).

3rd Ray Yoga Therapy: Since the 3rd Ray is an odd "male" ray, its natives are intellectual and so can benefit from the most intellectual form of yoga, Jnana Yoga. Since the are physical people, they can also benefit greatly from the most physical form of yoga, Hatha Yoga.

The Four Rays of Aspect

The 4th Ray of Love, Harmony and Beauty

4th Ray Colors: The 4th Ray rules over the softer, more balanced colors, such as pink and white. Since it is the middle ray, it is also associated with the middle color, green.

4th Ray Stage in the Creation of the Universe: The 4th Ray corresponds to the stage of creation when the volatile fire of the Big Bang moves into a state of equanimity. For life to thrive the universe must eventually come into a place of balance.

4th Ray Lords and Ladies: Since this is an even numbered "female" ray, it is ruled over by Sananda Kumara. It is also ruled over by all the Avatars who come to Earth to create harmony, as well as the Divine Mother in Her beneficent aspect as the nurturing and grace-bestowing life force. In the Ascended Masters tradition, Serapis Bey is Lord of the 4th Ray. Serapis Bey is especially associated with alchemy, the process that occurs when the polar opposite principles governing the universe (male/female, fire/water) come into a state of balance and then unite.

4th Ray People: 4th Ray people are here to help establish beauty and harmony on Earth. As relationship oriented and/or family persons they are constantly seeking to create harmony in their intimate relationships. Many 4th Ray persons study and read about the art of relationship and some go on to teach others this skill as counselors, therapists, and psychologists. Some use their relationship skills as diplomats and/or mediators.

4th Ray people often help to create harmony and beauty through an art medium. In this regard they can be painters, sculptors, musicians, interior decorators, and poets. 4th Ray persons also often contribute beauty to their environments by being physically attractive themselves.

Positively, 4th Ray persons are diplomatic, sociable, service oriented and nurturing to others. **Negatively**, they can be overly indulgent (they like the beautiful and "nicer things" of life), materialistic, excessively passionate (especially in relationship), and emotionally needy.

4th Ray Urges and Desires: 4th Ray persons possess the urge to create harmony and surround themselves with beauty. They desire to be in relationship with others and to give and receive love. Many 4th Ray persons also have a strong urge to nurture, counsel, and support others.

4th Ray Mental Tendencies: Since the 4th Ray is an even numbered and "female" ray, its natives tend to be less intellectual and more intuitive. These people also have the gift of "common sense."

4th Ray Emotional Tendencies: Being ruled by a female ray makes 4th Ray persons more emotional than those ruled by the male rays. They are given to worry and grief, and some are often moody and occasionally depressive.

4th Ray Power Spirit Animal: The 4th Ray power animal is the Dragon or Dragoness, which is the synthesis of the Puma, Condor, and Serpent, that come together in harmony, and its direction is south. The form of the Goddess, who is the principal deity of the 4th Ray, is often rendered as a dragoness. The Goddess's direction is south, in the warmer climates where the life force is the most concentrated and prolific.

4th Ray Chakras: The relationship oriented 4th Ray people live much of their lives through the heart chakra. More than any other ray, these natives can have emotionally injured hearts. Their passionate natures also give them active second chakras, and their need to relate to others makes their fifth chakras active.

4th Ray Planets and Zodiacal Signs: 4th Ray persons are born with the signs Libra, Taurus, or Cancer as their Vedic Ascendants. Libra and Taurus are ruled by Venus, the planet of relationship and beauty, and Cancer is ruled by the moon, the "planet" of home, family, the Goddess, and emotion. Libra and Taurus ruled people are usually more relationship oriented than are the Cancer ruled persons, but Cancerian types are more attached to home and family.

4th Ray Gems: Those with Taurus or Libra Ascendants should wear stones ruled by Venus. These are the clear stones, such as Diamond (the best and Clear Topaz, but they also do well wearing pink stones, such as Rose Quartz and Pink Tourmaline. Venus stones should be set in silver and worn on the ring finger. Those with Cancer Ascendants should wear milky white stones, such as Pearl and Moonstone. These stones are set in silver and worn as pendants or as rings on the ring finger. All 4th Ray persons can wear green stones, such as Emerald and Green Tourmaline. Watermelon Tourmaline, which unites Pink and Green Tourmaline, is an excellent 4th Ray stone. The green stones should be set in gold and worn as pendants or on the little finger, the Mercury finger.

4th Ray Mantras: These are the names of Venus and the Moon. Venus ruled persons should repeat Om Shukraya Namaha, Om "Salutations to Venus (Shukra)", and Moon ruled persons should repeat Om Chandraya Namaha, Om "Salutations to the Moon (Chandra)." Repeat these mantras audibly or mentally at least 108 times and 1-2x a day.

4th Ray Organs and Body Parts: The 4th Ray persons with Taurus Ascendants can have throat and lung problems, including Thyroid disharmonies, and those with Libra Ascendants can have kidney problems, since one of the functions of the kidneys is to create balance and harmony in the body of the male and female principles. When persons have an out-of-balance male principle (over or under assertive they can have difficulty with the right kidney, and when their female, receptive natures are not harmoniously expressed they can have problems with the left kidney. Those 4th Ray people with Cancer Ascendant can suffer from stomach problems because of too much worry. They can also have lymphatic problems because the Moon rules the fluids in the body.

4th Ray Treatment

4th Ray Counseling: Fourth Ray people can experience disharmonies and conflicts in their lives very acutely. They also can also have an extremely difficult time with the loss of a person(s or material security. Counseling for them often involves relationship counseling and learning good conflict resolution skills. Sometimes Fourth Ray people can give too much of themselves to others, so spending more time focusing on themselves can catalyze a healing for them.

4th Ray Color Therapy: For 4th Ray kidney disharmonies dark blue, black or red can be broadcast over the kidney area. Dark blue or black can help bring the left kidney back into alignment with the female principle, and red can similarly assist the right kidney with re-aligning the male principle. Yellow is good for 4th Ray stomach problems and white is good for lung problems. Blue can help the throat, unless the problem is low or inactive Thyroid functioning, in which case you would use a more stimulating color, such as orange. Green is an excellent color to be broadcast over the entire body. Yellow, blue, orange and red colored foods have been mentioned in association with the preceding rays.

4th Ray Sound Therapy: The note of C is beneficial when played to 4th Ray persons while using Green Lights. Play note D when using Blue light, G for Red lights and B for Yellow lights.

4th Ray Meridian Therapy: All depending on the problem, you would treat points on the following Meridians: the Heart, Kidney, Lung, Large Intestine (the Large Intestine Meridian moves through the throat), and Stomach and Spleen (the spleen is also associated with digestion – more on this later).

4th Ray Yoga Therapy: Since the 4th Ray is an even number "female" ray its natives respond more to devotional forms of yoga, such as Bhakti Yoga, the yoga of love and service. They reflect the female nature in wanting to merge with another person or deity, so Raja Yoga, the yoga of deep meditation is also sometimes attractive to 4th Ray persons.

The 5th Ray of Healing and Technology

5th Ray Color: The principal color of the 5th Ray is green, the color of healing.

5th Ray Stage in the Creation of the Universe: Once balance is created through the 4th Ray and life is then able to evolve, the inhabitants of the new universe need to consider practical issues, such as the scientific properties and uses of a planet's raw materials and how to heal from accidents and diseases. In the 5th Ray of Healing and Science the various facets of human culture become fully manifest.

5th Ray Lords and Ladies: Since the 5th Ray is an odd numbered and "male" ray, one of its deities is Sanat Kumara. It is also ruled over by Saraswati and Athene, the Hindu and Greek Goddesses of speech and learning. Among the Ascended Masters the ray is governed by Hilarion, the Ascended Master of Healing who once walked the planet as Saint Paul. Since the color of the 5th Ray is green, this ray is also associated with alchemy (green harmonizes and unites the polarity) and ruled over by Thoth-Hermes, the Lord of Alchemy, whose symbolic artifact is the Emerald Tablet. Just by being in proximity to the Emerald Tablet it is said that alchemy would be spontaneously initiated within a person.

5th Ray People: 5the Ray persons are usually involved with healing or science. They might be doctors, nurses, shamans, acupuncturists, massage therapists, etc, or they could be involved with one or more of the scientific fields as researchers, physicists, biologists, inventors, etc. They usually excel at technological trades. 5th Ray persons are the inventors and geniuses of the world. They are often the ones to introduce the new ideas and technologies that contribute to a developing civilization.

Positively, 5th Ray persons are desire to serve others with their healing skills and ingenuity. They have good powers of discrimination and a natural ability to diagnose and heal others.

Negatively, 5th Ray people can be arrogant, overly-critical, and skeptical of anything that is not scientific.

5th Ray Urge and Desires: Being people with practical and cutting-edge ideas, 5th Ray natives have the urge to communicate their ideas. They are academic and have the desire to understand a variety of ideas. They also have the urge to help heal and balance themselves and others.

5th Ray Mental Tendencies: 5th Ray people are intellectual and scientific. Some are geniuses in their fields.

5th Ray Emotional Tendencies: Possessing an over-active nervous system, 5th Ray persons can be chronically nervous. Otherwise, they can often tend to be detached and unemotional.

5th Ray Power Spirit Animal: The power animal or animals of the 5th Ray is the snake encoiled around the staff of the Greek god of Healing, Ascelpius, and the two snakes intertwined around the Caduceus of Mercury, the contemporary symbol of the medical profession. 5th Ray persons inherit the wisdom of the serpent that is specifically intellectual and categorical, as well as its power to heal. It is the serpentine life force that ultimately effectuates any cure.

5th Ray Chakras: 5th Ray people function out of the 5th chakra, the chakra of communication, as well as the 3rd chakra, the etheric wheel that rules over the assimilation of ideas, and the 6th charka, the chakra that becomes active in those who in moments of revelation receive new information. Among those 5th Ray persons who are healers, the heart or 4th chakra is also often active.

5th Ray Planets and Zodiacal Signs: 5th Ray persons are ruled by either Mercury or Uranus and have as their Ascendant one of Mercury's signs, Gemini or Virgo, or Uranus's sign of Aquarius. Thus, it will be seen that people with an Aquarius Ascendant are ruled by two planets, Saturn and Uranus, and they are aligned with two rays, the 1st and 5th. Both Mercury and Uranus are planets that influence the intellect. Mercury is the definitive planet of the intellect, and Uranus rules genius. Uranus is that component of the intellect that makes it assimilate and synthesize information very quickly, like a computer. Of the three signs associated with the 5th Ray, those born with Virgo Ascendant are the most likely to get involved with healing.

5th Ray Gems: 5th Ray stones are the green stones ruled over by Mercury. These include Emerald, Green Tourmaline, Moldavite and Malachite. The stones should be of good quality, approximately 2 carats of more in size, and set in gold. If worn as a ring, these stones should be worn on the little finger, the Mercury finger. Mercury stones will activate the intellect and communication skills, as well as open the heart and help promote healing. They also balance and unite the inner polarity, thus stimulating alchemy. Those 5th Ray persons who are on the path of alchemy can benefit by wearing a Mercury ball made of solid, detoxified Mercury. Such balls naturally stimulate the process of alchemy within the wearer.

Those 5th Ray persons born with Aquarius Rising and ruled by Uranus can wear green stones, especially Green Tourmaline, as well as stones with a silvery tint to them (the silver tint can be from silver inclusions within the stone. Uranus, which is rapid in action, rules Quicksilver. Stones that are rutilated (inclusions of Titanium Dioxide are highly electro-magnetic and also aligned with Uranus. Usually rutilated stones are of Clear Quartz.

5th Ray Mantras: These are the names of Mercury, which is known as Buddha in Vedic Astrology. The mantra of the 5th Ray is Om Budhaya Namaha, meaning Om "Salutations to Mercury." Repeat mantras audibly or mentally at least 108 times and 1-2x a day.

5th Ray Organs and Body Parts: All 5th Ray persons have sensitive nervous systems, which are often overtaxed from mental work. Those born with a Gemini Ascendant also can suffer from lung and arm problems, while those with a Virgo Ascendant can be prone to assimilation problems affecting the intestines, especially the large intestine. In Chinese Medicine the lung and large intestine are considered to be interconnected and part of the same system.

5th Ray Treatment

5th Ray Color Counseling: For 5th Ray persons to be happy and fulfilled they need to be actively using their intellects, their communication skills, their technical abilities, and/or their healing abilities. Their work is often incredibly important to them and they need to find a profession that they enjoy. Some 5th Ray persons suffer from work holism and need to spend more time relaxing and playing.

5th Ray Color Therapy: 5th Ray persons benefit from having their bodies bathed in green light as this will nurture and balance the nervous system. To treat Virgo Ascendants with intestinal problems, yellow light should be broadcast over the entire abdominal area. Lung related problems displayed by Gemini Ascendants respond to both green light and white light. Green colored foods have mentioned in association with the preceding rays.

5th Ray Sound Therapy: Soothing music helps to relax the overactive nervous system of a 5th Ray person. Broadcast note C when using Green colored light, D when using Blue, and B when using yellow lights.

5th Ray Meridian Therapy: To treat 5th Ray disharmonies use Lung, Large Intestine, Stomach, and Spleen Meridian points – all are good for digestive problems- as well as points along the heart meridian for relaxation and calming the mind.

5th Ray Yoga Therapy: The intellectual 5th Ray natives will benefit from Jnana Yoga, the Yoga of Wisdom, as well as Hatha Yoga. At least half of all Hatha Yoga postures work to stretch and nourish the spine, and the shoulder stand is excellent for any digestive problems. Pranayama, the controlled breathing patterns of Hatha Yoga, will strengthen and benefit both the digestion as well as the lungs.

The 6th Ray of Devotion and Mysticism

6th Ray Colors: 6th Ray colors include the high frequency colors of purple and violet, as well as the balancing colors of pink and green. These are yin or female colors and are aligned with this female and even numbered ray.

6th Ray Lords and Ladies: As a female ray the 6th Ray includes as one of its Lords Sananda Kumara. It is also governed by the etheric-natured Goddess Kwan Yin, and the Ascended Master Lady Nada. Avalokiteshwara, the Bodhisattva of Compassion, is also Lord of the 6th Ray.

6th Ray People: The persons of the 6th Ray are devoted to an ideal or deity and tend to be very idealistic about life. This trait can make it hard for 6th Ray persons to live on Earth, and it can promote escapism tendencies. 6th Ray persons are mystical, psychic, and sometimes work as clairvoyants and/or channels. They can be reclusive, preferring to meditate and merge with the Higher Self than participate in the mundane activities of the world. These persons would rather involve themselves in activities that assist them in completing their cycle of incarnations on the Earth plane, including meditation, spiritual practices, and service work. Their strong desire to merge into something greater than themselves can also attract them to a vocation in music, art, and shamanism.

Positively, 6th Ray persons are compassionate, devoted, and self-sacrificing towards others, while also seeking to cultivate, experience and share divine love. **Negatively**, they can be with withdrawn, prone to addictions and escapism, overly idealistic, overly sensitive, and ungrounded.

6th Ray Urges and Desires: 6th Ray people have the urge to worship and merge with something greater and/or transcend into perpetual communion with God. They have the desire to loose themselves in service work and/or sacrifice themselves for the greater good.

6th Ray Mental Tendencies: Of all the ray natives 6th Ray people are generally the most intuitive. They are on Earth to get their egos out of the way and channel wisdom and healing power from a higher source.

6th Ray Emotional Tendencies: 6th Ray people can tend to be confused and overwhelmed as they try to assimilate their experience with an intellect dominated by a developing intuition. They can also experience sadness and depression when the world does not live up to their idealism. Some can tend towards psychosis as they venture into the hidden and unseen dimensions of themselves or the universe while awakening their psychic vision.

6th Ray Spirit Animal: The 6th Ray power animal is the condor. The condor flies into the Heavens and takes a 6th Ray person to other worlds.

6th Ray Chakras: The principal 6th Ray chakra is the 6th Chakra, also known as the Ajna Chakra and 3rd Eye or Wisdom. They also receive energy from the 2nd chakra, the water chakra, which is also involved in psychic perception. Since 6th Ray persons are often ungrounded, they can suffer from an inactive or disharmonious 1st or Root Chakra, the Earth or "ground" chakra.

6th Ray Planets and Astrological Signs: 6th Ray persons have the sign of Pisces as their Ascendants. Pisces is ruled by both Jupiter and Neptune, so Pisces Ascendant persons are aligned with both the 2nd and 6th Rays. Neptune and Ketu are the astrological planets that rules over the 6th Ray. Ketu, which is known as the Dragon's Tail in Vedic Astrology and the South Node in Western Astrology, is not really a planet, but it is given the power and position of a planet in Hindu Astrology. Ketu is the polar opposite of Rahu, the Dragon's Head and the North Node of Western Astrology. Ketu is spiritual and Rahu is materialistic. You won't be using Ketu in your healing work unless you go deeper into Vedic Astrology and interpret a person's Dasas or Planetary Cycles. Even though each person is aligned with one or two primary rays they have a chance to experience and learn from all seven rays at different times of their life. When they will experience a specific ray is determined by their Dasas.

6th Ray Gems: The Gems of the 6th Ray are primarily those ruled by Neptune, but also the ones ruled by Ketu. Neptune stones, which are best set in silver, are the purple and violet stones. They include Amethyst, Sugilite, and Purple Tourmaline. The stone for Ketu is Chrysoberyl Cat's Eye.

6th Ray Mantra: At this point there is not a Sanscrit Astrological mantra for Neptune since Vedic Astrology does not normally include interpretations of the planet. It does, however, have a mantra for Ketu. It is Om Katave Namaha. Repeat mantras audibly or mentally at least 108 times and 1-2x a day.

6th Ray Organs and Body Parts: 6th Ray persons can have sensitivity in their feet and occasional foot problems. Those 6th Ray natives that are particularly ungrounded or do a lot of psychic work can also suffer from weakness in the kidney/adrenals, especially the right kidney, which rules over fire and the male or yang energies in the body. By being ungrounded for a prolonged period a person can become excessively yin. This can have the effect of water damaging the fire, the root of which is the kidney/adrenals. The excessive yin can also damage the functioning of the thyroid.

6th Ray Treatment

6th Ray Counseling: To be fulfilled 6th Ray persons need to be on a path that culminates in wearing away the ego and transcending into a higher consciousness. Service, spiritual disciplines, and shamanism are attractive ways to accomplish this goal. 6th Ray persons can also become deluded by certain beliefs and ideals that are destructive to them, so healing for them sometimes requires a de-programming.

6th Ray Color Therapy: For kidney/adrenal dysfunction broadcast a red light over the lower back. To stimulate Thyroid function shine an orange light over the Thyroid area. Red and black colored foods have been previously mentioned. Purple and violet foods include eggplant, purple grapes, purple onions, purple cabbage, purple plums, purple bell peppers, purple broccoli, globe artichokes, purple grapes, etc.

6th Ray Sound Therapy: Use soothing music set to the note E. "Cosmic Music," wherein the listener can lose him or herself in the music, work best to get a 6th Ray person back into alignment. When broadcasting Red light play note G and for Orange light play note A.

6th Ray Meridian Therapy: Use points on the Kidney and Heart Meridians. The kidney and adrenals can also be tonified and balanced by points on the Ren and Du Meridians. Use Large Intestine Meridian points for Thyroid weakness.

6th Yoga Therapy: The devotional nature of 6th Ray persons make them perfectly suited for Bhakti Yoga. Their mystical natures and the desire to merge with a higher consciousness also makes them good candidates for Raja Yoga, the yoga of deep meditation, as well as Laya Yoga, the yoga of absorption in sound and light.

The 7th Ray of Alchemy and Transformation

7th Ray Colors: 7th Ray colors are colors associated with transmutation, magic, and alchemy. They include black, red and green. Violet, which is the last color of a spectrum and the point of transition to a higher spectrum, is also a color of transmutation associated with the 7th Ray.

7th Ray Lords and Ladies: Since the 7th Ray is an odd numbered and male ray, one of its lords is Sanat Kumara, the primeval embodiment of the male principle. The other 7th Ray Lords and Ladies are specifically associated with alchemy and destruction and transformation, which are two sides of the same coin. Lord Shiva and Goddess Kali are the Lord and Lady of destruction and transformation in the

Hindu pantheon. Saint Germain is the lord of the 7th Ray in the Ascended Masters tradition. Baphomet, the dark goat deity of the Knights Templar that is a symbolic representation of the Kundalini, as well the patrons of the Templars, "Two Johns" - John the Baptist and John the Divine - are all Lords of the 7th Ray. John the Baptist was the embodiment of the Holy Spirit or Kundalini when on Earth, and John the Divine became the Cupbearer of the Baptist's power after it moved through Jesus Christ. The Two Johns are the patrons of Freemasonry and the Secret Societies of Europe that practice alchemy and/or teach the philosophical secrets of the art.

7th Ray People: These are the sorcerers, magicians, shamans, yogis, prophets, alchemists, and Kundalini masters, who work with power. The higher evolved 7th Ray natives awaken the inner Kundalini power and use the energy for transforming themselves and others. **Positively**, 7th Ray persons use power to evolve and heal themselves and others. They practice white magic, yoga, shamanism, and seek to learn the esoteric mysteries. They want to know what is behind the creation, i.e., what are the underlying forces that govern the universe. Their inquiry leads them into the study of metaphysics, astrology (the study of the planetary forces), psychology (what's at the root of the human psyche) and even Quantum Physics (how matter is produced from the Source). **Negatively**, 7th Ray persons can seek to control and dominate persons. They can be dictatorial and direct their power into black magic. These people do not control the energy that naturally builds in the sexual area (7th Ray persons are born with a lot of sexual energy because their alchemical power will eventually feed off their sexual fluids). Rather than move the energy up for spiritual evolution they move it out through their excessive sexual activity. Their inability to move the energy upwards can also cause them to build it up to such an extent that they become volatile and explosive.

7th Ray Urges and Desires: The higher evolved 7th Ray persons desire to transform and heal themselves and others. They also have the urge to learn and teach the mysteries. The lower evolved 7th Ray natives have the urge to control others and use their power for self-centered purposes.

7th Ray Mental Tendencies: 7th Ray natives have deep and penetrating intellects. They have incredible perceptive ability and can understand what is underneath the surface of human behavior, as well as what invisible forces govern the physical universe. Some have clairvoyant power to see a person's past lives, as well as what will occur in the future. These people are both scientific as well as keenly intuitive, and some are even of genius caliber. They have a penchant for ferreting out some forgotten wisdom, solving an abstruse mystery, or discovering a long hidden artifact.

7th Ray Emotional Tendencies: 7th Ray natives can suffer from intense anger if the transformative Kundalini fire in their system is not able to move without obstruction or find an exit out of the body. The lower evolved ones will also get very angry if others are insubordinate to their control, or if their power and control is not adequately deferred to and respected. 7th Ray persons can also succumb to depression, especially manic depression or bi-polar syndrome, as well as certain forms of psychosis, such as megalomaniac schizophrenia.

7th Ray Spirit Animal: The 7th Ray spirit animal is the snake or serpent, the secretive and very wise creature that continually renews or resurrects itself by shedding its skin. 7th Ray persons often have dreams or visions of serpents. Such milestones presage that the person is or soon will be undergoing a transformation and receiving the wisdom of the serpent. Such a vision could also denote that the person has or will soon have an awakened serpent power or Kundalini.

The snake is, therefore, the power animal of the 3rd , 5th, and 7th Rays. The difference is that while 3rd , 5th Ray and 7th Ray persons all inherit the creative and destructive powers of the serpent, the 7th Ray native also inherits its *transformational* powers, as well as its *Gnostic* and *Intuitive* wisdom.

7th Ray Chakras: 7th Ray natives have very active 1st and 2nd chakras, both of which are related to power. The first chakra is the home of the Kundalini power and the second chakra controls the sexual fluids that the Kundalini feeds off of and transmutes once it is awakened. A 7th Ray person's second chakra also supports their penetrating intellects and intense psychic ability Lower evolved 7th Ray natives have a very difficult time controlling their second chakras and indulge in excessive sexual activity. The higher evolved 7th Ray people have chosen to preserve their sexual fluids and transform them into spiritual power. These persons also have active 6th and 7th chakras, which become activated by the Kundalini that rises to the top of the head and activates the two-thirds of the brain which are normally dormant.

7th Ray Planets and Zodiacal Signs: The principal Zodiacal Sign associated with the 7th Ray is Scorpio, the sign of death, magic, alchemy, and the Kundalini. 7th Ray persons have the sign Scorpio as their Ascendant and are governed by both Mars and Pluto and the 3rd and 7th Rays. Pluto, the planet of the re-born Phoenix, is the principal planet aligned with the 7th Ray. Pluto, which is named after the god of the fiery underworld, rules the fiery transformative forces within the human body. In Vedic Astrology the 7th Ray is also associated with Rahu, the North Node of Western Astrology, which reveals the direction of one's evolutionary destiny. Rahu, the Dragon's Head, is a transformative power that alchemically transforms and teaches the lessons an incarnate soul needs in order to move to its next level of evolution. But it is only necessary to understand the nature of Rahu if you are going to delve deeper into a person's Vedic chart than just determining their Ascendants.

7th Ray Gems: These stones are colored the alchemical colors of black, red, green, and violet. The black stones include Smokey Quartz and Onyx, but the best are

Black Tourmaline, which works powerfully on through the electro-magnetic field to activate the Kundalini in the etheric body, and Obsidian, which is volcanic glass and thus contains the fiery, transformative power of volcanoes. The best transformative green stones include Emerald, Green Tourmaline, and Malachite. The best violet or dark purple transformative stones include Amethyst and Purple Tourmaline. Clear Quartz, which has a fiery nature by virtue of being composed of tetrahedron molecules, is also transformative and can benefit 7th Ray people. All 7th Ray stone can be set in gold and worn as a pendant of ring. Green stones should be worn on the little finger, red stones on the ring finger, and black stones on the middle finger.

7th Ray Mantras: There is not currently a Sanscrit mantra for Pluto. The mantra for Rahu is Om Rahave Namaha. Repeat mantras audibly or mentally at least 108 times and 1-2x a day.

7th Ray Organs and Body Parts: The lower torso, especially the sexual organs, are ruled over by the 7th Ray. 7th Ray persons can often suffer from sexual-organ disharmony and illness, such as venereal disease. Their excessive sexual activity and urge to control others can negatively effect their kidney/adrenals, as well as exhaust the essence of their body, known in Chinese Medicine as the Jing. The Jing supports the entire body and when it is weak or depleted the whole body can suffer. Jing, which is stored in the kidneys, is inherited from the parents. When it is completely depleted or used up a person dies. If you are born to parents with good longevity then you will normally receive an abundance of Jing from them and live a long life.

The 7th Ray is also associated with the liver, since this is the organ directly related to the smooth flow of the life force in the body. 7th Ray persons, since they have an abundance of life force power moving through them (the Kundalini is a form of life force they can easily get their life force congested. This congestion causes fire in the liver that then manifests in the body as excess heat, high blood pressure, anger, and headaches.

7th Ray Treatment

7th Ray Counseling: To feel fulfilled 7th Ray persons need to be involved with vehicles through which they can develop and channel their power, such as magic, shamanism, and yoga. They should also be involved in the field of transformation and alchemy, and they should enroll in the study of the esoteric and occult to get a deeper understanding of existence. 7th Ray persons are not content with a normal worldly life. They seek deep and intense experience – even experience that may be considered taboo. They also are not content unless they are gaining a grasp on the hidden mysteries of life, such as those taught within the Mystery Schools. The lower evolved natives will be very attracted to black magic and possibly perverted sexual or ritualistic experiences. Most all 7th Ray persons will have strong sexual impulses which need to be constructively channeled. They should daily enroll in some spiritual practice or physical exercise to keep their excessive energy from becoming blocked up and causing explosive anger and possibly violence.

7th Ray Color Therapy: For sexual organ problems broadcast a red light over the base of the torso (front or back), and an orange colored light over the area of the sexual organs. If there is infection or venereal disease, use a blue light. It is also good to completely bath a 7th Ray person in green light in order to promote the smooth flow of life force in the body and balance the liver. And a violet light is helpful to activate the transformational forces in the body while keeping a 7th Ray native's thoughts elevated to Heaven rather than downwards.

7th Ray Sound Therapy: Bathe the body in the note G while using drums to harmonize the first and second chakras. This will be beneficial unless the 7th Ray person is feeling an overabundance of energy, heat, and/or anger. You would then want to use more soothing music in the note of E while broadcasting blue light. When using Violet light play note F#.

7th Ray Meridian Therapy: For 7th Ray persons use both the Du and Ren Meridians, the two channels that connect with the kidneys and act as channels for the Jing and Kundalini. Also use the Liver Meridian points to balance the flow of the life force.

7th Ray Yoga Therapy: It is good for 7th Ray persons to practice Hatha Yoga daily in order to move the life force and keep it from congesting. Kundalini Yoga, the yoga designed to move and awaken Kundalini, is specially designed for 7th Ray natives. Jnana Yoga is also helpful for 7th Ray natives as it satisfies their desire to understand the nature of the universe and the goal of life.

A Note on the Human Body and the Ray Colors

The human body can be divided into three zones, each of which is ruled by one of the Three Rays of Essence. The First Blue Ray governs the area from the shoulders to the top of the head. This is the region of the brain that governs and makes decisions for the rest of the body. The Second Yellow-Gold Ray governs the middle of the torso, a region where information and experiences are digested and one achieves wisdom. And the Third Red Ray governs the lower part of the torso, from the abdomen downwards, which includes the Source Chi and the Adrenal Glands that energize and move the body. The Rays of Aspect are modifications of the Three Rays of Essence and govern sub-areas within these large three regions.

The Rays: Chakras, Planets, Signs, Gems, Mantras, & Deities

Rays	*Chakras*	*Planets*	*Signs*	*Gems*	*Mantras*	*Lords/Ladies*
1st Ray Will & Power Blue	1st/2nd 5th 6th, 7th	Saturn Sun	Capricorn Aquarius Leo	Blue Sapphire Blue Topaz Lapis Lazuli Ruby, Garnet	Om Sanischarya Namaha Om Suryayai Namaha	Sanat Kumara Master Morya St. Michael Brahma
2nd Ray Wisdom Golden Yellow	3rd 6th 7th	Jupiter	Sagittarius Pisces	Yellow Sapphire Yellow Topaz Citrine Quartz	Om Brihaspataye Namah	Sananda Kumara Vishnu, Avatars John the Baptist Kuthumi
3rd Ray Action & Creativity Red/ Orange	1st/2nd 3rd 4th	Mars Sun	Aries/Scorpio Leo	Red Coral Carnelian Ruby, Garnet	Om Kujaya Namaha Om Suryayai Namaha	Sanat Kumara Rudra, Kali Mahachohan
4th Ray Love, Beauty & Harmony White/Pink	1st, 2nd 3rd 4th 5th	Venus Moon	Taurus/Libra Cancer	Diamond Pearl/Moonstone Clear/Pink Quartz Pink Tourmaline	Om Shukraya Namaha Om Chandraya Namaha	Sananda Kumara Divine Mother Krishna/Avatars Serapis Bey
5th Ray Healing & Technology Green	3rd 4th 5th 6th	Mercury Uranus	Virgo Gemini Aquarius	Emerald Green Tourmaline Green Peridot Malachite	Om Budhaya Namaha	Sanat Kumara Thoth-Hermes Saraswati, Athene Hilarion
6th Ray Devotion & Mysticism Purple	1st, 2nd 6th	Neptune Ketu	Pisces	Amethyst Sugilite Cat's Eye	Om Katave Namaha	Sananda Kumara Kwan Yin Avalokiteshwara Lady Nada
7th Ray Alchemy & Transformation Violet, Black	1st, 2nd 3rd 6th, 7th	Pluto Rahu	Scorpio	Meteorite Bl. Tourmaline Amethyst Hessonite Garnet	Om Rahave Namaha	Sanat Kumara Shiva/ Kali John the Baptist St. Germain

The Rays: Urges & Emotions

Rays	*Urges*	*Positive Traits*	*Negative Traits*	*Mental Tendency*	*Emotions*	*Professions*
1st Ray Will & Power Blue	To Rule To Organize To Control	Align w/God's Will Organized Warrior for Righteousness	Arrogant Egotistical Dictatorial Rigid	Inflexible ideas Scientific Intuitive	Depression Fear Anger	Politicians Mayors, Senators Organizers CEOs, Bosses
2nd Ray Wisdom Golden Yellow	To Understand To Teach To Serve	Serving others Wisdom Oriented Align with God's Will	Controlling Arrogant Dogmatic	Philosophical Intuitive	Anger Depression Over Optimistic Compassion	Minister, Priest Philosopher Spiritual Guide Guru/Teacher
3rd Ray Activity & Creativity Red/Orange	To Create To Lead To Shine	Creativity Leadership Initiative Pioneering	Lack follow-thru Controlling Over Aggressive Egotistical	Scientific Intellectual	Frustration Anger Raucous Joy	Athlete Musician, Painter Outdoor Guide Builder, Inventor
4th Ray Harmony, Love & Beauty White/Pink	To Nurture To Love To Relate, Unite To Beautify	Diplomacy Serve Others Sociable Protective	Materialistic Indulgent Needy Overly Attached	Intuitive Imaginative Practical	Worry Sadness/ Grief Depression Moody	Diplomat Therapist Counselor Healer
5th Ray Technology & Healing Green	To Communicate To Understand To Heal, Balance To Serve	Inovative Serve others Discrimination	Critical Arrogant Skeptical Judgmental	Intellectual Scientific Practical	Nervousness Worry	Doctor, Healer Inventor Electrician Plummer, Builder
6th Ray Devotion & Mysticism	To Merge To Serve, Sacrifice To Worship To Transcend	Divine Love Self Sacrificing Compassionate	Escapism Victim Complex Overly Idealistic Ungrounded	Intuitive Philosophical Imaginative	Confusion Overwhelm Depression Psychosis	Monk, Renunciate Psychic, Channel Healer Teach Meditation
7th Ray Alchemy & Transformation Violet, Black	To Transform To Control To Wield Power To Understand	White Magic Transforms Self Uses power to heal, help others	Black Magic Dictatorial Vindictive Explosive	Intuitive Scientific Philosophical	Anger Psychosis Depression	Renunciate Magician Alchemist Yoga Teacher Kundalini Adept

The Rays: Sensitive Organs, Healing Colors, Notes, Channels & Yogas

Ray	Organs	Tissues	Colors	Notes	Channels	Yogas
1st Ray Will & Power Blue	Kidneys Adrenals Pituitary Heart	Bones Teeth Brain Ears	Dark Blue Red Black	E G	Kidney Du Ren	Karma Yoga Jnana Yoga
2nd Ray Wisdom Gold, Yellow	Liver	Blood Eyes Tendons	Yellow Green White	B C	Liver Gall Bladder	All Yogas
3rd Ray Action & Creativity Red/Orange	Heart Adrenals	Tongue Muscles Shen	Red Orange	G A	Heart Kidney	Hatha Yoga Jnana Yoga
4th Ray Beauty, Love & Harmony White, Pink	Lungs Stomach Heart Kidneys	Throat, Skin Muscles Shen	White, Blue Yellow Green, Pink Indigo, Black	D, E B C	Lung Stomach Heart Kidney	Bhakti Yoga
5th Ray Healing & Technology Green	Intestines	Nervous System	Green Yellow Lemon	C B	Lung Sm Intestine Lg Intestine	Hatha Yoga Jnana Yoga
6th Ray Devotion & Mysticism Purple	Feet Pineal Kidneys Liver	Brain Ears Eyes	Purple, Violet Dark Blue Black Green, Yellow	F# E C, B	Kidney Du Liver, GB	Bhakti Yoga Raja Yoga
7th Ray Alchemy & Transformation Violet, Black	Adrenals Sex Organs Liver	Sex Fluids Jing Chi	Red Black Violet	G F#	Du Ren	Kundalini Yoga Jnana Yoga Hatha Yoga

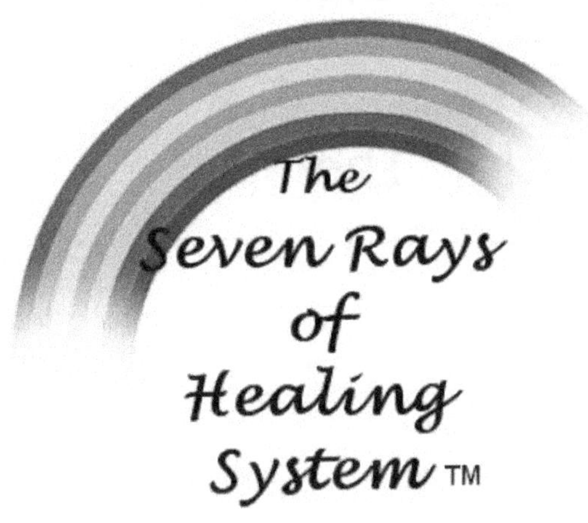

Chapter 3
Seven Rays
Color and Sound Healing

Color and Sound Healing are two of the pillars of the Seven Rays of Healing System. Through these modalities alone a person can fully align themselves and their organs with their their appropriate rays.

Seven Ray Color Therapy

When you have determined a person's ray you can immediately suggest that they consider spending regular periods under lights that will broadcast the color of their ray(s) onto them, that they drink structured water that has been saturated with the color of their ray(s), that they wear clothing the color of their ray(s), and paint the walls of their rooms the color of the ray(s), etc. Becoming immersed in the color of their personal ray(s) will help them remain physically healthy, emotionally peaceful and aligned with their destinies.

Color Healing Theory

Many of the regions where the Seven Rays of Healing migrated to following the demise of the Pacific Continent of Lemuria produced their own system of correspondences between the rays, organs, chakras and seven colors. In the chart below the color/organ systems of two of these countries, India and China, are shown.

Organ	Ray	Hindu	Chinese	Chakra
Liver	2-Yellow	Yellow	White	3/4 Yellow Green
Heart	4-White Pink	Red	Red	4 Green
Stomach	4-White	White	Yellow	3 Yellow
Lung	5-Green	Green	White	4,5 Green Blue
Kidneys	1- Dark Blue	White Red	Black	1,2 Red Orange
Intestines	5- Green	Red	Red White	2,3 Yellow Orange

The General Physiological Effects of the Colors

Besides being the color of a person's ray, the colored light chosen for broadcasting over any person or organ is also determined by the natural physiological effect of that color. These are listed below. As you can see, the effects of the Four Secondary Colors include the effects of the two Primary Colors each is the union of.

The Effects of the Three Primary Colors

Blue: Cooling, Sedating, Calming, Stagnating, Moisturizing, Astringent, Activates Intuition.
Red: Heating, Activating, Stimulating, Moving, Drying, Dispersing.
Yellow: Astringent, Coagulating, Digestant, Moving, Drying, Stimulates Intellect.

The Effects of the Four Secondary Colors

Orange: Red and Yellow united. Both Activating and Astringent.
Green: Yellow and Blue united. Balances Yin and Yang. Calming, Astringent, Coalescing
Indigo: Dark Blue. Deeper effects of Blue. Very Sedating, Very Cooling, Activates Intuition
Violet: Blue and Red united. Both Activating and Calming. Cooling. Stimulates Intuition, Alchemically Transforming.

The Effects of the Other Colors

White: Clarifying,
Pink: Calming, Soothing
Black: Retention
Purple: This color **is** Violet & Yellow united and carries the physiological effects of both. Activating, Calming, Transforming. Activates Gnostic Centers.
Lemon: Yellow and Green unites. Stimulating and Balancing.

The Effects of the Colors on the Organs

Below is the effect of each color on the individual organs.

Liver

Yellow: Moves the energy, or Chi, of the Liver
(Good for stress, migraine headache. Gives smooth flow of Chi in body)
White: Clarifying, helps Liver purify the blood and toxic emotions
Green: Helps Liver to Coalesce (build) and cleanse blood. Releases both bile & blocked emotions.

Heart

White: Clarifies Heart emotions
Pink: Soothes, heals Heart emotions. Opens Heart to give/receive love
(Relieves Psychological and Emotional Issues)
Red: Strengthens, Stimulates Heart muscle
Green: Soothes Heart, Mind & Emotions. Promotes Physical, Emotional & Mental Balance
(Arrhythmia, Psychological and Emotional Problems)

Stomach

Yellow: Stimulates Digestion; Moves Chi of Stomach; Drying of excess fluids
(For Indigestion. Calming to Stomach)
White: Clarifying of enzymes and emotions (grief). Dries excess fluids
Also:
Lemon: Calms Stomach; Heals Ulcers. Assists Digestion

Lung

Green: Facilitates harmonious respiration; Healing to Lung tissue
(Calms Cough, Good for Asthma, Bronchitis, Pneumonia)
White: Clarifies and cleans Lungs.
Blue: Cools Lungs. Calms Lungs. Moisturizes Lungs.
(Use for Dry Cough and as Expectorant for Congested Lungs)
Lemon: For productive cough

Kidneys

Blue: Cools infected Kidneys & Urinary Bladder; Coagulates Jing/Sexual Fluids;
Generates Kidney Yin (increases coolness and fluids in entire body)
Red: Moves Kidney Chi; Stimulates Adrenal Glands; Generates Kidney Yang
(increases heat and energy throughout entire body).
Black: Strengthens Function; Retains body fluids; Retains Sexual Fluids;
Strengthens Urinary Bladder
Also:
Orange: Stimulates, Moves and Coagulates
(Relieves Menstrual Cramps and Controls Heavy Menstrual bleeding)

Intestines

Green: Calms, Heals Intestines; Astringent; anti-diarrheal.
Red: Warms Intestines; Moving to blockages; Drying.
(For Cold Diarrhea, Cold Constipation))
Yellow: Stimulates; Digestant; Astringent; Moving.
White: Clarifies; Purifies Intestines
Orange: Activating and Astringent
And also:
Lemon: Activating and calming.
(Mild Laxative)

Color Light Therapy Tools

There are many tools and machines you can acquire for Color Therapy. Some of the more basic tools are presented in this and future chapters.

Light Sources

Colored Light Bulbs: You can use common colored light bulbs and switch them throughout the tonation. They should be at least 60-75W strength. Light bulbs with very high wattage have not shown to have a substantially greater or more beneficial effect on the body than those with lower wattages. There are also multi-colored bulbs available for purchase online that have as many as 16 different colors and can be changed by a remote device.

Colored Gels: Colored gels can also be purchased through theater supply companies, such as Rosco. They either come in large sheets or squares and need to be cut to size to fit over the light source you are using. They can also be cut into slides and then projected onto the body through projectors. Some companies featured on Amazon.com offer complete sets of colored gels that have already been made into slides.

Projectors: Color gel slides can either be inserted directly into old-time projectors and then beamed onto a person, or individual colors can be transmitted from a laptop computer to a projector and then broadcast onto the body. In the latter case the projector can be set on a table or attached to a tripod and beamed directly onto the person's body. Put all the colors you will use during a tonation into a Power Point presentation and then simply move to the Power Point slide with the color you want to transmit through the projector. To create an assortment of colors in your Power Point you can simply download the various colors you want off of the Internet.

These three light sources are featured on the following page.

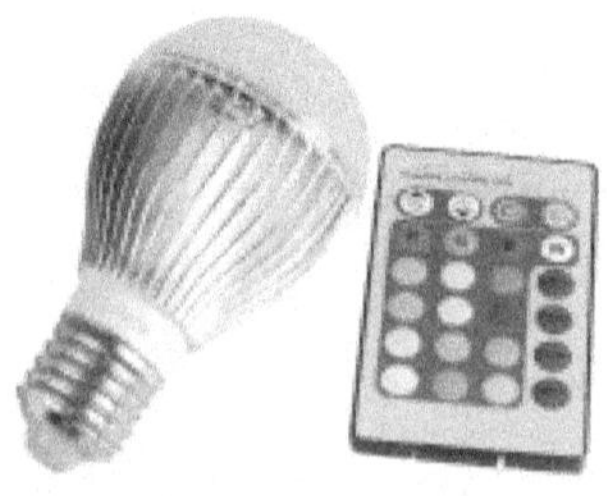

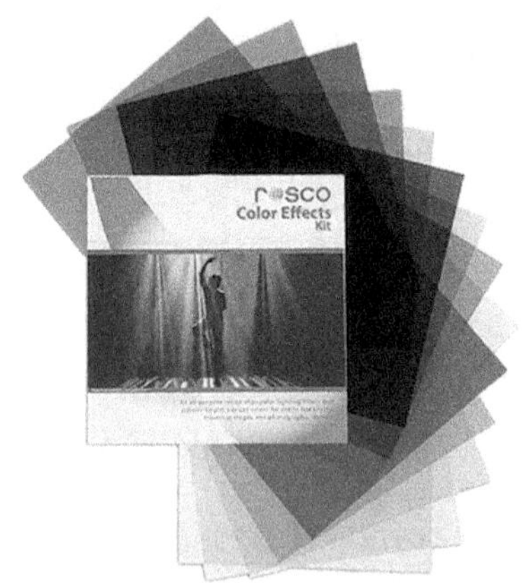
rosco
Color Effects
Kit

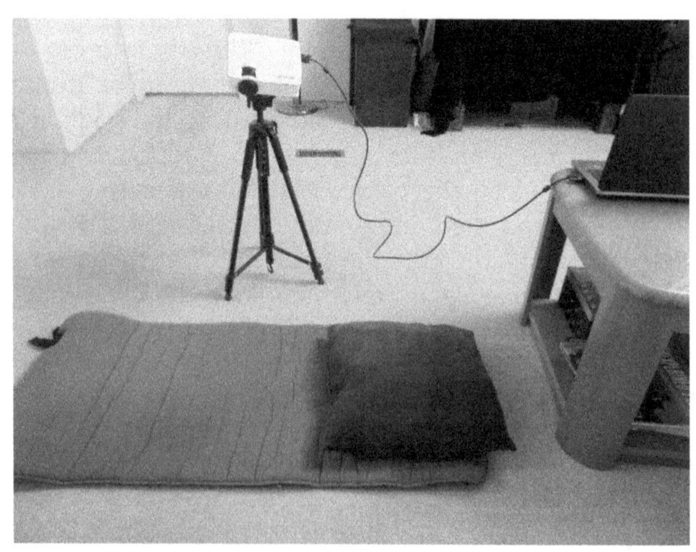

The Rules of Color Light Therapy

A Color Light Therapy session is called a "Tonation" because you are vibrating the body with colors of different tones.

Length and Frequency: A tonation should last a minimum of 30-45 minutes, but can last as long as you would like. If the health problem is acute (recent) then consider a longer tonation and at least 2-3 times a day. If the problem is chronic (long standing), consider giving an average length tonation, but do so on a regular basis. Try to administer at least one tonation a day.

Day or Night: Tonations using the lower frequency colors (below Green) are ideally administered morning and afternoon because they will be stimulating to the body and mind. A stimulating tonation can make it very hard for the person to relax and sleep if given later in the day. But tonations using the higher frequency colors (above Green) can be administered anytime, day or night.

Expose Skin: If possible, a tonation should be broadcast directly onto bare skin. This will give the best results. If much of the body is to be tonated and exposed, then the therapy room should be amply heated

Eyes Open: During a tonation, when possible the patient should have their eyes at least partly open to catch the color rays. Then the color ray can travel along the optic nerve to the brain and stimulate a reaction in that organ. This is only possible if the patient is sitting up and/or lying either on their side or back while receiving the tonation.

Direction of Body: If possible during a tonation the patients head should be north and their feet south. This will keep them in alignment with the Earth's electromagnetic field.

The Tonation Zones of the Human Body

Now you will learn where to broadcast the colored lights on the human body. You can broadcast your lights systemically to cover the entire body and/or over specific zones of the body.

Systemic Tonations over the Entire Body

Anytime you give a person Color Light Therapy first consider bathing their bodies in the color of their birth ray(s), even if you do not feel that they are out of alignment with their ray(s). You can also work systemically at any time for other purposes using the follow colors:

Red: Heats up entire body. Energizes body. Increases Yang, Chi.
Can cause body to perspire to cleanse blood and reduce fever.
Blue: Cools down and slows down body processes. Calms, relaxes.
Eliminates toxins; Antibacterial; Increases Yin, blood, fluids, etc.
Green: Calms, balances and heals body. Also has an Alchemical Effect
on the body and internal organs.
Violet: Alchemically Transforms entire body and all internal organs.

Color Therapy and the Three Body Regions

Just as when the Primal Dragon first divides itself into its polarity as the first two Rays of Blue and Yellow, the human body can also be initially divided into Yellow and Blue Zones. The union of Blue and Yellow is Green, **so the body is actually divided into the three colors of Blue, Yellow, and their intersection or overlap as the secondary color of Green.**

You can also divide the torso into three parts with each part corresponding to the color of one of the first three rays: Blue, Yellow and Red. All the organs contained in the blue region will respond favorably to blue, those in the yellow region will respond favorably to yellow, etc.

Both 3-fold divisions are shown on the following page. As you can see both yellow and green are colors for the middle region, and the organs in middle torso respond favorably to both. Similarly, both red and yellow are prescribed for the lower region where organs respond favorably to both colors.

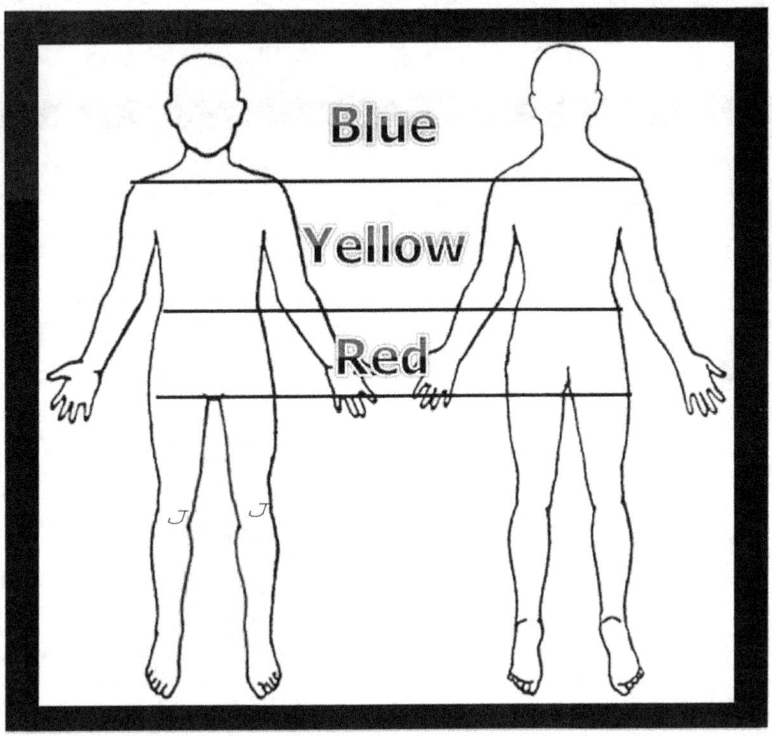
Blue
Yellow
Red

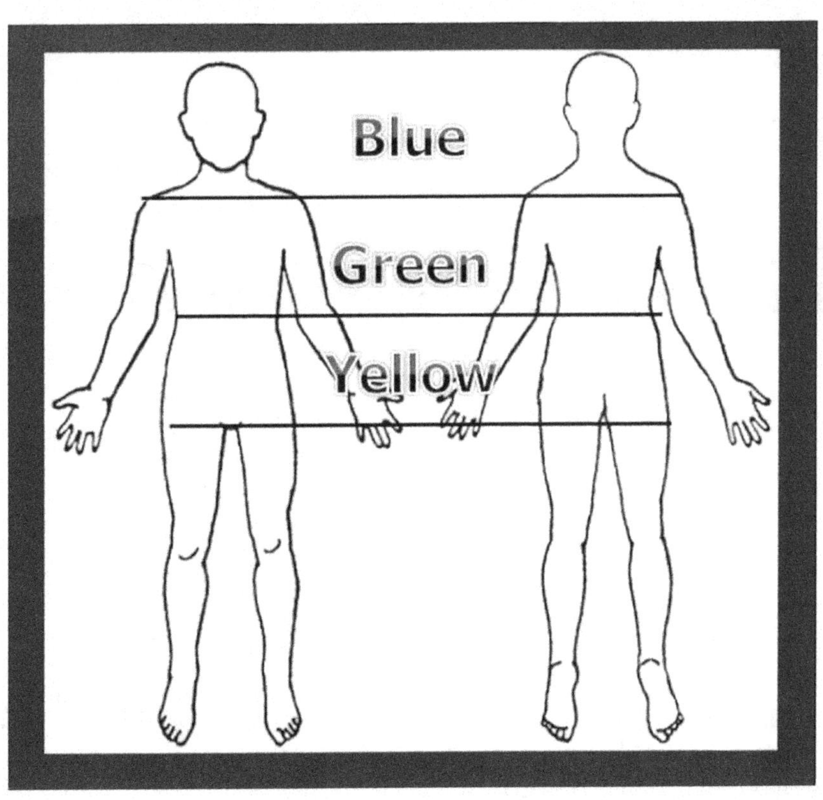
Blue
Green
Yellow

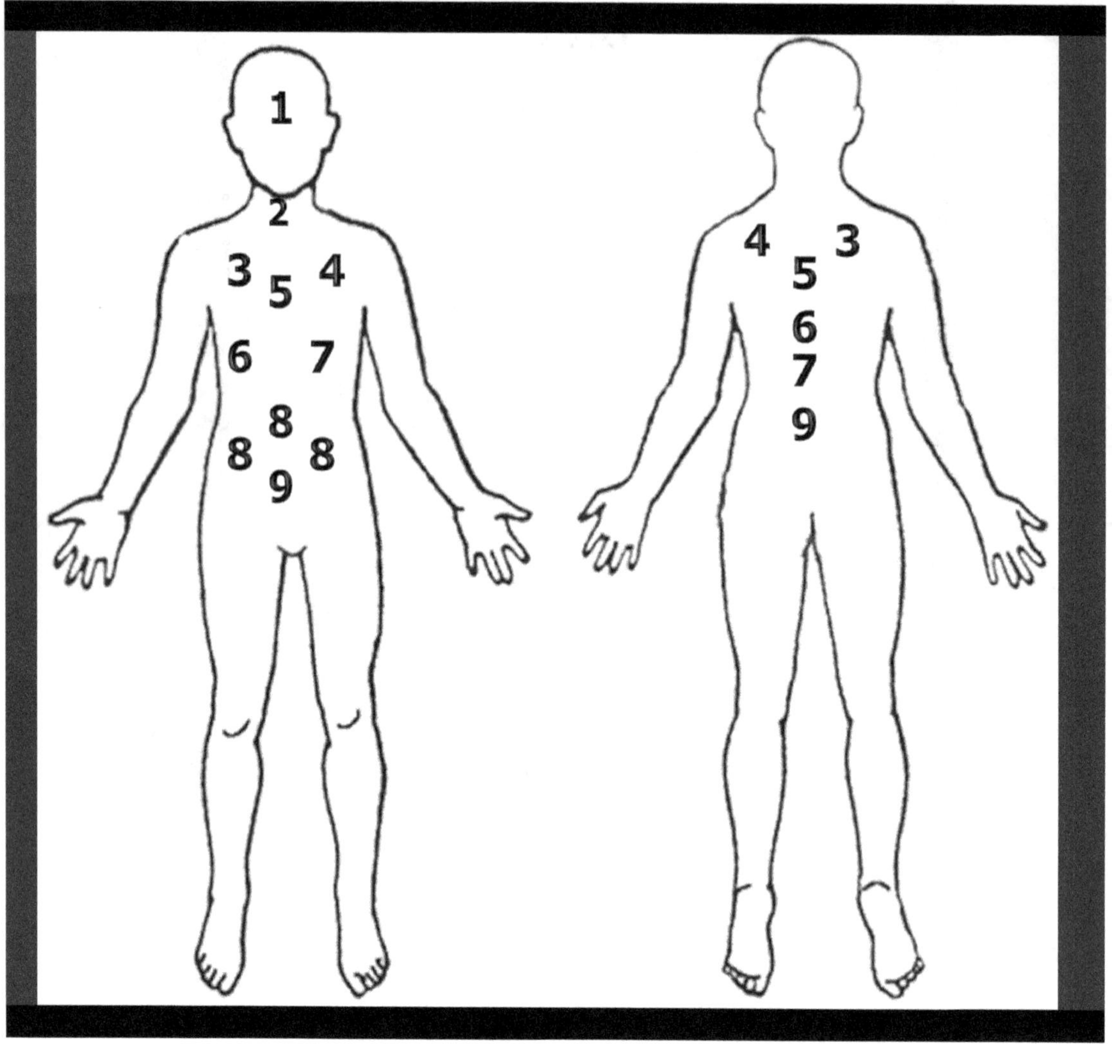

KEY

1- Head, Pituitary, Pineal, Third Eye, Brain
2 - Throat
3, 4 - Lungs
5 - Heart

6 - Liver, Gall Bladder
7- Stomach, Spleen
8 Upper - Small Intestines
8 Lower - Large Intestines
9 - Kidneys, Adrenals Urinary Bladder

Specific Tonation Zones of the Head and Torso

The torso and head regions are further divided up into zones. The above charts reveal the locations of these zones on the front and back of the body. Thus, when tonating the face you would broadcast your light on the Head Zone #1. When treating the stomach you would tonate the Stomach Zone #7 on the front and/or the back.

Color Therapy with Colored Water

Water that is tonated provides an excellent source of color for those working with specific colors. **The colored water can be consumed throughout the day thereby reinvesting the body with the therapeutic colors it needs.**

Making Colored Water

To make colored water you can fill a transparent glass container with filtered water and then broadcast colored lights onto it. The time you spend broadcasting a color should not be less than one hour. You can make colored water this way while at the same time you are giving a tonation to a client. Place the water so it is receiving the broadcasted color at the same time it is being beamed onto the body zone. **You can also place water in a colored transparent container and set it in the Sun.** The rays of the Sun will then transmit the color to the water. Keep in the Sun for at least one full day.

Color Therapy with Crystals and Gems

Crystals and Gems make excellent long-term Color Therapy tools that will continually broadcast their color frequency 24/7. They can be worn on the body as pendants, necklaces, rings, bracelets, etc. and/or they can be held or placed on the body during times of therapy and alchemical spiritual work.

Like Colored Lights that give the best results when broadcast onto bare skin, colored crystals and gems also give their best results when worn directly on the skin. In general, a crystal or gem will become stimulated when set in gold, although any of them can also be set in silver. However, the best metal for milky white Moon stones is silver, because silver is the metal of the Moon.

For the best results a crystal or gem should be of good quality and clarity; and they should be at least 2 carats in size. If this is not possible because of budget restrictions, at least make sure that the stone is clear with few or no inclusions (additional elements or substances trapped inside the stone).

These are the recommended healing stones for each color
Red Stones: Ruby (best, Garnet, Red Tourmaline, Fire Opal
Orange Stones: Red Coral, Carnelian, Fire Agate, Orange Sapphire, Orange Sapphire
Yellow Stones: Yellow Sapphire, Yellow Topaz, Citrine Quartz, Yellow Tourmaline
Green: Emerald, Gr.Tourmaline, Green Serpentine, Green Jade, Malachite, Adventurine
Light Blue: Turquoise, Aquamarine
Dark Blue: Blue Sapphire, Lapis Lazuli, Azurite
Violet: Amethyst
Purple: Sugilite, Purple. Tourmaline, P. Sapphire, Purple Fluorite

Clear Quartz Crystal: "The Seven Ray Stone"

Quartz Crystals have been called"Crystallized White Light" and "Full Spectrum Stones."They vibrate at the white frequency which, as the synthesis of all the colors, can balance and harmonize all the color-coded elements, organs and chakras of the body.

There are many other reasons Quartz Crystals are considered perfect healing stones. In ancient times they were known as "Fire Stones" because their piezoelectric properties can generate light (placing pressure on their surface generates a flow of electrons) and **they also emanate fiery energy that can stimulate a person's internal alchemical fire that is both healing and deeply transformative.** On the molecular level they are composed of tetrahedrons, which is one of the five Platonic Solids associated with the element of fire, and the fiery property of a Quartz Crystal is also ascribed to the angle of its termination, which is usually approximately that of the Great Pyramid, 51o 51'. This makes them a vehicle for the generation of "fire in the middle" (pyr--a-mid) which in the human body is the fiery Kundalini.

A six-sided Quartz Crystal also creates perfect balance in the body because their molecules also unites as a six- pointed star, which is the Sacred Geometrical form of perfect balance. And they also balance the human DNA because, like it, their atoms also create a double-helix formation.

Quartz Crystals also move and amplify energy. So they can be placed on areas of the body where energy is blocked, such as the Liver when that organ processes blocked physical and emotional toxins, or any other place in the body where intense pain exists (all pain is blocked Chi). When using single terminated crystals, turn the points towards a weak organ to send it energy, and away from an organ that is experiencing acute pain. If you are using crystals that are terminated at both ends, either end can point towards the organ for directing energy too or from the organ. Also, since Quartz Crystals amplify energy, any tonation administered with them will generate additional energy to enhance and magnify the result of the tonation.

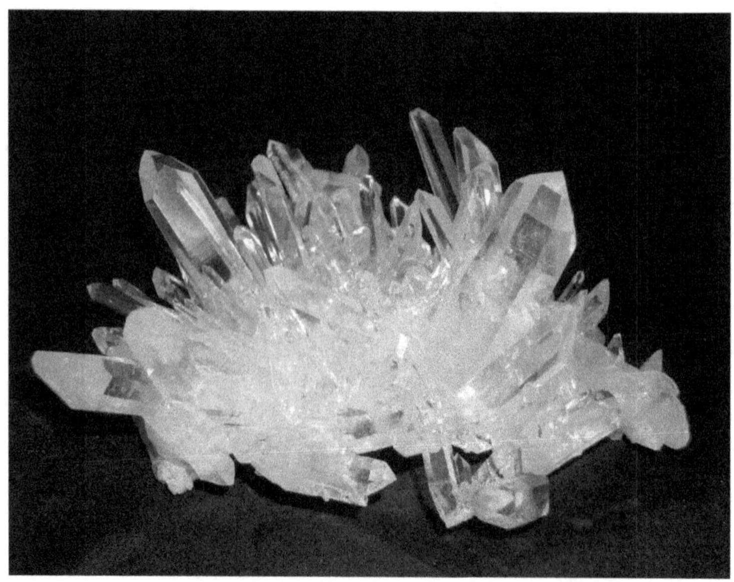

Alchemical Stones

Alchemical Stones are used to get a deeper, more profound and longer lasting healing of a person and/or an organ than other stones. They especially work on the deeper etheric/emotional levels to clear the emotional components of a health condition. This is a list of some efficacious alchemical colored stones.

Alchemical Black and Red Stones

All black and red stones naturally vibrate the Kidneys and Adrenals and the underlying Root Chakra, which is the seat of the alchemical force of Kundalini. When the Kundalini is activated all organs and all parts of the body get alchemically transformed.

BlackMeteorites

The best black stones for alchemy are meteorites. They include Nickel-Iron Meteorites and the lighter black Tektites. **Meteorites were used in the Mediterranean mystery schools during initiation rites designed to unite the polarity and awaken the inner serpent fire.** The fiery Meteorites were believed by the ancients to have been created by the union of water and fire, or the male-female polarity, and could thus engender a similar union within a candidate for initiation. They were also identified as manifestations of the Goddess Venus, whose legends asserted that she had descended from the heavens as a ball of fire that landed in the Mediterranean Sea and then rose up in a cloud of steam as a beautiful woman. Thus, both Venus and her sacred meteorites were the union of the polarity as water and fire, and Heaven and Earth.

The black color of meteorites can itself awaken the Serpent Fire. And when their strong electromagnetic fields interface with an individual's personal electromagnetic field they can indirectly activate Kundalini.

Other Alchemical Black and Red Stones

After meteorites, the best black stone is Black Tourmaline, which contains bands or striations that both emanate a black color frequency and powerfully stimulate the bands of energy in a person's electromagnetic field. Another efficacious black mineral is Obsidian which, as volcanic glass, possesses the natural alchemical fire of a volcano. Other good black stones include Smokey Quartz and Onyx. as for red stones, the darker a stone is in the red spectrum the better it is for activating the Root Chakra. In this category are dark Ruby, and the many versions of dark red Garnet, such as Pyrope Garnet.

Alchemical Green Stones

Green stones have a natural alchemical propensity to balance the inner polarity, and ultimately to unite within the body to produce the alchemical force. Alchemical Green Stones can be placed anywhere on the body, and over any organ, to produce a deep alchemical healing and purification.

Leading the list of Green Alchemical stones are Moldavite and Emerald. Moldavite is a Tektite Meteorite found in Moldavia Czechoslovakia. It has a very similar effect as Iron Meteorite to activate Kundalini, with the added effect of healing and opening the Heart Chakra. The vibration of Emerald is that of Thoth-Hermes, the patron of Alchemy, who engraved the 13 precepts of alchemy on an Emerald Tablet. **Of the semi-precious green stones, Green Tourmaline and its sibling, Watermelon Tourmaline, are excellent because they both possesses a green color and striations to activate the electromagnetic field.** Green Jade is a good alchemical stone that can lead to immortality, which is why the early Chinese alchemists would consume it as a powder and bury their dead with it. Other efficacious green stones include Peridot, Malachite and Aventurine. Malachite, which means "Emotional Release," is one of the best minerals for alchemically healing and releasing blocked emotions. such as green Moldavite.

Alchemical Violet Stones

Violet, the premier stone of the 7th Ray, has the power to alchemically transform a person or organ and raise them to the next higher octave. **Any violet stone possesses this property, and each can be set over any organ or part of the body to facilitate its alchemical transformation.** The best known alchemical violet stones are Amethyst and Violet/Purple Tourmaline.

A good way to alchemically transmute an organ or chakra is to roll an Amethyst Crystal Ball in a clockwise direction on the skin covering them.

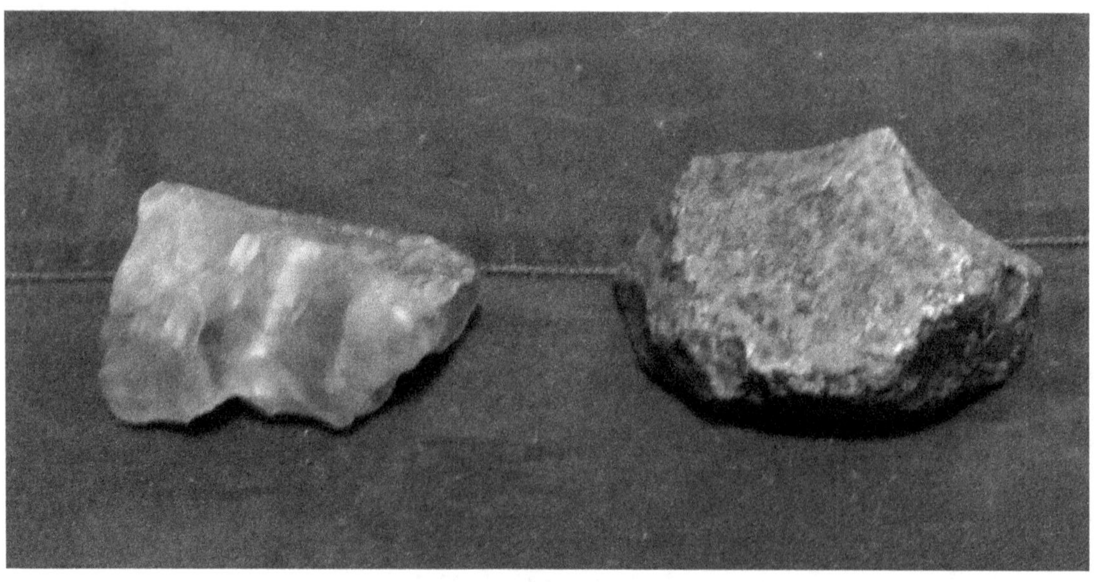

Moldavite Tecktite and Nickel-Iron Meteorite

Color and Gem Therapy Chart

Color	Ray	Chakra	Organs	Gems	Alchemy Stones
Black	7th	1st	Kidneys	Onyx Smokey Quartz Obsidian Bl.Tourmaline	Meteorite Bl.Tourmaline Obsidian
Red	1st, 3rd	1st	Kidneys/ Adrenals Heart	Pyrope Garnet R. Tourmaline Ruby Fire Opal	Pyrope Garnet R. Tourmaline Ruby
Orange	3rd	2nd	Kidneys/ Adrenal Intestines	Red Coral Fire Agate Carnelian Orange Sapphire O.Tourmaline	Red Coral O.Sapphire O.Tourmaline
Yellow	2nd	3rd	Liver Stomach/ Speen Intestines	Y. Sapphire Y. Topaz Citrine Quartz Y. Tourmaline	Y. Sapphire Y. Tourmaline
Green	5th	4th	Heart Liver Lung Nerves Brain	Emerald Gr. Tourmaline Malachite Moldovite Adventurine	Emerald Gr. Tourmaline Malachite Moldovite
Blue	1st	5th, 6th	Pituitary Kidney Thyroid	Bl Sapphire Bl Topaz Turquoise Azurite Lapis Lazuli	Bl. Sapphire Azurite
Violet/ Purple	6th, 7th	6th, 7th	Pineal/ Third Eye Kidneys	Amethyst Sugilite P. Tourmaline Alexandrite Flourite	Amethyst P. Tourmaline

Seven Ray Sound Healing Therapy

Sound Healing therapy is a powerful therapy on its own and makes a perfect adjunct to Color Therapy. As shown below each color corresponds to a note and sound frequency. The color and Sound can be broadcast together for a more comprehensive and powerful tonation.

Color	Note	Frequency
Red	G	392
Orange	A	440
Yellow	B	466
Green	C	523
Blue	D	587
Indigo	E	622
Violet	F#	740

Tools for Seven Ray Sound Healing Therapy

There are many tools that can be used for Seven Ray Sound Healing Therapy. The most common and easiest to work with are speakers, which you can set on either side of a person undergoing therapy and then broadcasting upon them the appropriate note or healing sound. Tuning forks are also excellent tools especially when seeking to get the unbroken vibration of a tone channeled onto the body or directly to an organ being treated. Frequency Counters are also very effective although the pure frequency being broadcast can often be unsettling when listened to for a long period of time. Try broadcasting their piercing frequencies in conjunction with soothing music you play in the background. And, finally, live instruments can be played during the time of therapy. Certain instruments, such as drums, when played with their associated colors of red or orange can be very healing to an organ or chakra. Some instruments, such as Crystal and Tibetan Bowls, are very exacting and specific in effect because they are tuned to specific notes. See the following page for color/organ/ray/note/instrument correspondences. For those serious about adding Seven Ray Sound Healing Therapy to their treatments, full sets of Crystal and Tibetan Bowls calibrated to all the seven notes can be purchased and used by themselves or in conjunction with Seven Ray Color Light Therapy. Some Crystal Bowls, called Practitioner Bowls, are made specifically to be held by the therapist over the person or organ being treated.

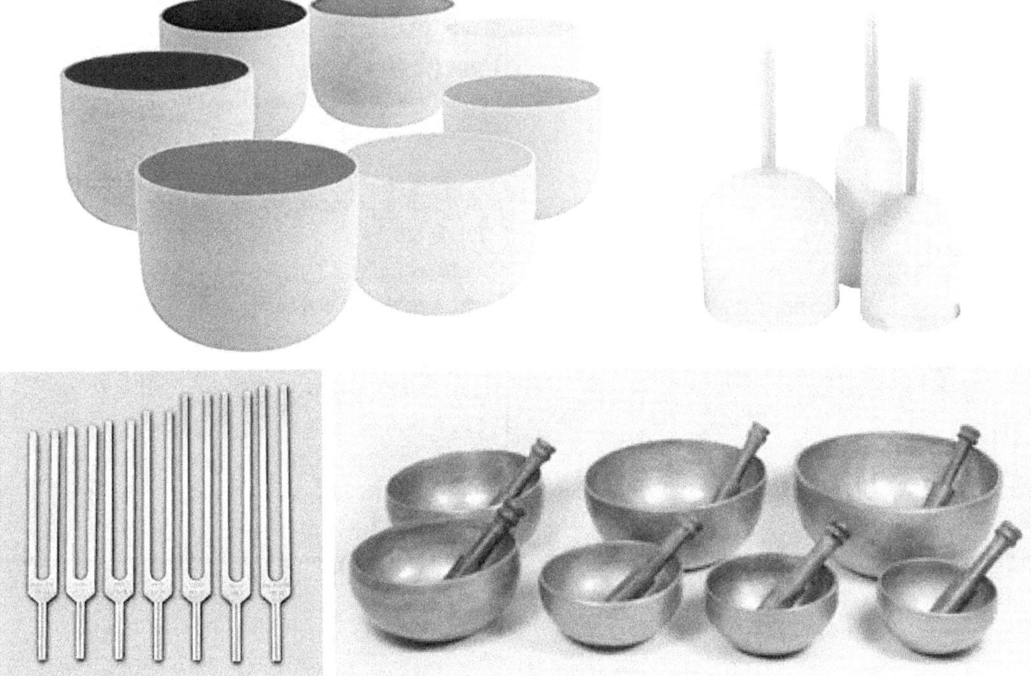

Sound and Color Therapy Chart

Color	Chakra	Note	Instruments/ Genre	Mantra
Red	1st	G	Deep Bass Drums/Hand Drums Crystal/ Tibet Bowl/Fork tuned to G Bass Shamanic Rattles & Drums Bass Djeridoo Tibetan Chanting	BAM
Orange	2nd	A	Bass-Tenor Drums/ Hand drums Crystal/ Tibet Bowl/Fork tuned to A Shamanic Rattles & Drums Tenor Djeridoo, Light Percussion Tibetan Overtone Chanting	VAM
Yellow	3rd	B	Tibet/Crystal Bowls/forks tuned B Shamanic Rattles, Hand Drums Tenor Djeridoo Harp, Piano, Flute, Violin Low-Mid Range Notes	RAM
Green	4th	C	Harp, Piano, Flute, Violin Mid-Range Notes Tibet/Crystal Bowl/Fork tuned to C	HAM
Light Blue	5th	D	Harp, Piano, Flute, Violin Upper Notes Tibet/Crystal Bowl/Fork tuned to D Classical Music	YAM
Indigo	6th	E	Harp, Flute, Piano, Violin High Notes Tibet/Crystal Bowl/Fork tuned to E "New Age" Synthesized Music Classical Music	OM
Violet	7th	F#	Harp, Flute, Piano, Violin High Notes Tibet/Crystal Bowl/Fork tuned to F# "New Age" Synthesized Music Inspiring Classical Music	OM

Mantras and Seven Ray Sound Therapy

Mantras are sound vibrations that are also excellent to use for Seven Ray Sound and Light Therapy. To receive the healing and transformative effect of mantras they can be sung live as bhajans (sacred chants) and/or as recorded selections on CDs that are broadcast into a room via speakers. They can also be simply repeated out loud or silently by a therapist, practitioner or patient in order to heal and raise consciousness during a treatment. A patient or practitioner of Japa (mantra repetition) can either vocalize a mantra so it is heard audibly, which is known as repetition on the Vaicari level, or it can be repeated mentally on the Madhyama level of sound. Madhyama is the level of sound that vibrates in the heart. A mantra repeated in this level has a much stronger effect on the patient or practitioner than repeating it audibly.

Thus, when working with a client you can either play a CD of the mantras that correspond to the body area being worked on, or you can audibly chant or continuously repeat them. You can also instruct your client to repeat the mantra mentally and thereby elicit an even stronger healing.

The following are some full spectrum mantras that can be broadcast into a healing space, and/or be repeated by you and/or your client. They can played or repeated throughout a treatment that addresses one organ, many organs, or the entire body. These can be called "Seven Ray Mantras" because they resonate with all the Seven Rays.

OM: The Seven Ray Mantra

OM is the "Mother Sound" of creation. It is the synthesis of all the sounds of all the Seven Rays, and recognized to be the primal sound from which all the other sounds of creation emerged. OM is the sound vibration of life force, which was the first manifestation of energy or matter, and its vocalization can actually generate life force. This truth is explicit in one of the names of OM, "Pranava," which means "that which produces prana (life force). Because of this property to generate prana OM - and its cousin sound of AMEN - is repeated at the beginning and end of prayers. Its generation of life force helps to bring the desires contained in the prayers into manifestation.

As the synthesis of all the sound frequencies of color and the Seven Rays, OM can be played, chanted or mentally repeated in a healing space during an entire Seven Ray Healing treatment no matter what part of the body is being healed.

OM is the primal name of the Goddess, which is emanated from the Infinite Spirit as pure energy or life force at the beginning of time. OM or AUM denotes the Goddess who is Spirit united with Matter (OM) and wields the three powers of Creation, Preservation and Destruction (AUM).

The Sri Yantra (next page) is the Yantra (geometrical form body) of both the Goddess and the OM. It is beneficial to place images of the Sri Yantra in your healing space as it will generate a vibration of perfect balance while also generating life force. This will greatly enhance your practice of healing.

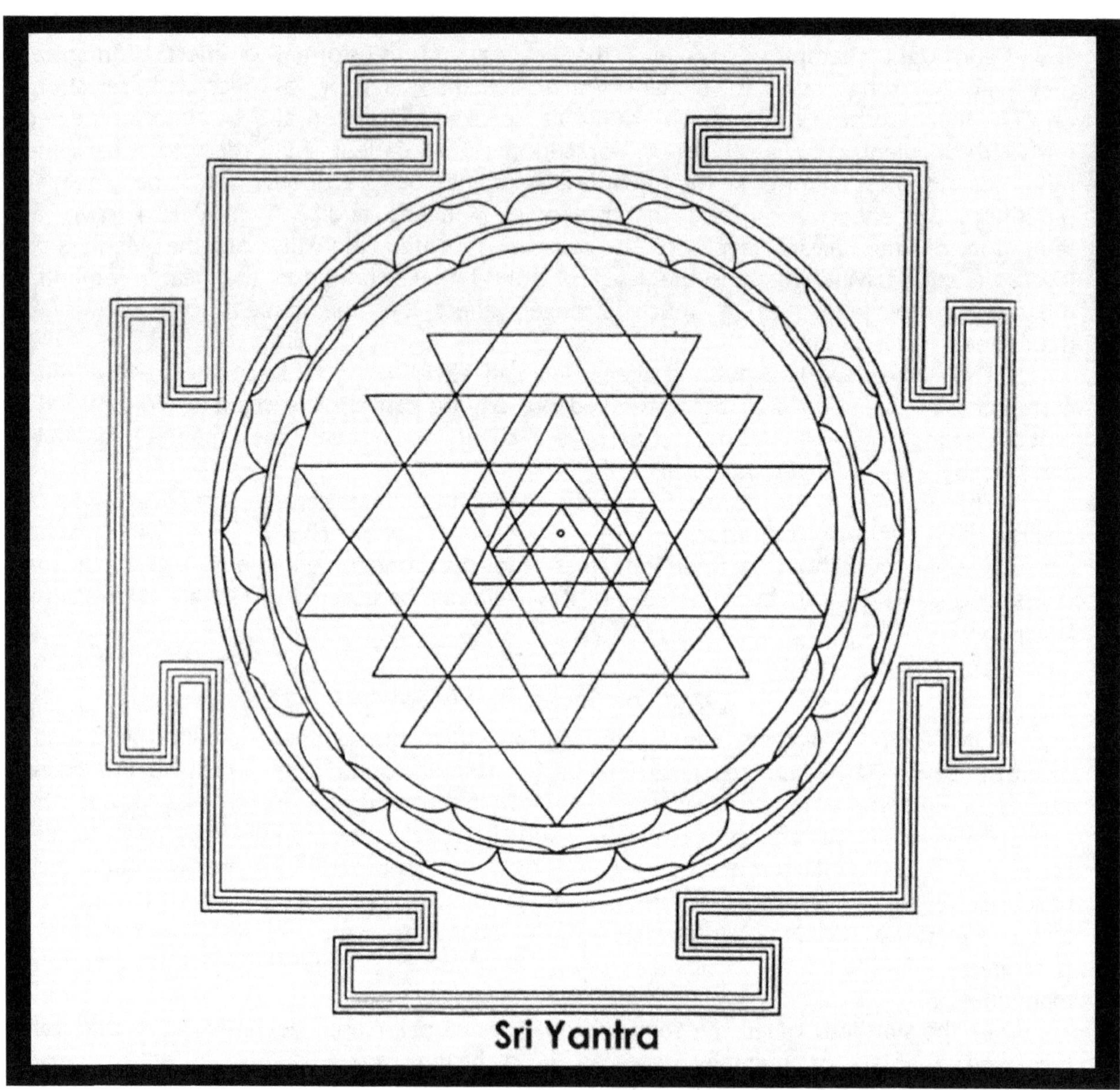

Sri Yantra

OM NAMAH SHIVAYA

"Salutations of Shiva" (the Infinite Spirit and One's Inner Self)

The mantra OM NAMAHA SHIVAYA is another mantra that is inclusive of all Seven Rays and all Colors and can be that can be played, chanted or mentally repeated in a healing space during an entire Seven Ray Healing treatment. OM NAMAHA SHIVAYA is the sound frequency of the Goddess as pure energy when She becomes divided into the 7 Rays and the five elements of matter. The syllables of the mantra corresponds to each of the Seven Chakras and their corresponding colors and rays.

OM

The sound of OM resonates within both the 6th and 7th Chakras.
It is associated with the Divine Mind

NA

NA resonates within the Root Chakra and is associated with the Earth Element

MA

MA resonates within the 2nd Chakra and is associated with the Water Element

SHI

SHI resonates within the 3rd Chakra and is associated with the Fire Element

VA

VA resonates within the 4th Chakra and is associated with the Air Element

YA

YA resonates within the 5th Chakra Root and is associated with the Aether Element

By playing or repeating OM NAMAHA SHIVAYA during a Seven Ray Healing treatment all the chakras and all the five elements that comprise the physical body are purified and alchemically transformed.

THE GAYATRI MANTRA

Om
Bhur Bhuva Svaha
Tat Savitur Varenyam
Bhargo Devasya Dheemahi
Dhiyo yonah Prachodayat

(OM) OM (Dheemahi) We meditate (Bhargo) upon the Spiritual Effulgence (Varenyam Devasya) of THAT Supreme Divine Reality (Savitur), the Source (Bhur, Bhuva, Svaha) of the Physical, the Astral and the Heavenly Spheres of Existence. (TAT). May THAT Supreme Divine Being (Prachodayat) enlighten (Yo) our (Dhi Yo) intellect (so that we may realize the Supreme Truth).

The Gayatri Mantra is another Seven Ray Mantra that is inclusive of all frequencies associated with all the Seven Rays and 7 Colors. Since it resonates in many different worlds and dimensions, it will address all levels of a person, including their physical, emotional, and mental bodies. It can also be played, chanted or silently repeated during the entire length of a Seven Ray Healing session.

Lalita Sahasranam: The Thousand Names of the Goddess

A third chant that can be played in your healing space that will keep the energy charged and facilitate healing is the *Lalita Sahasranam*. **This chant contains 1000 names of the Universal Goddess, and includes names associated with all Her Seven Rays.** Each name is an attribute and a power of the Goddess. When played in proximity of a person they are bathed in the healing presence and power of the Goddess Herself. The chant be can purchased online as a CD.

Any long Sanscrit chant like *Lalita Sahasranam* is efficacious because it contains all the 50 letters of the Sanscrit alphabet. Each letter vibrates one of the 50 petals that collectively surround all the chakras from the Ajna Chakra downwards (the Root Chakra has 4 petals, the 2nd Chakra has 6 petals, etc.). Each petal is associated with both an ability and special wisdom. When they are all vibrated a person is fully charged and activated on all levels. This is the value of a sacred language like Sanscrit, and why it is used for spiritual work and healing. A sacred language will vibrate parts of you to unleash wisdom and power while at the same time ascending and expanding your consciousness.

The *Lalita Sahasranam* is traditionally recited or broadcast in the presence of the Sri Yantra, which is the Sacred Geometrical form of the Goddess. Together, they fill a room with the pure essence of the Universal Goddess and Her immense healing power.

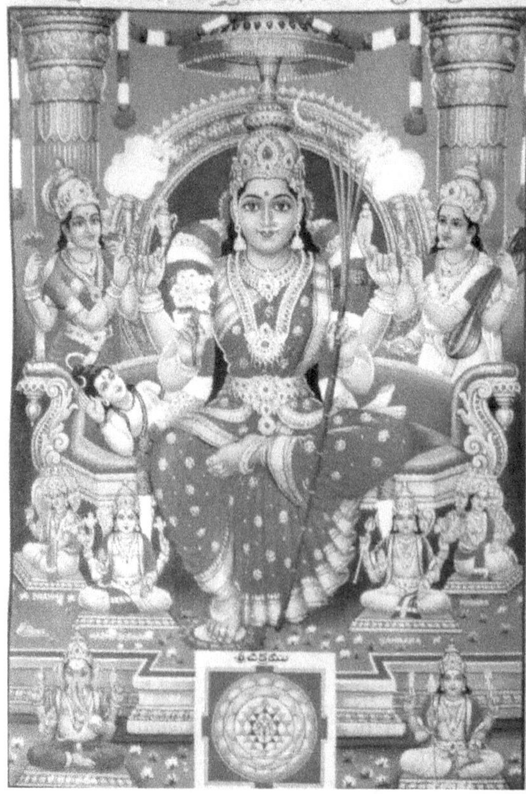

Goddess Lalita

Mantras for the Chakras

These individual mantras for each chakra can be broadcast over speakers or repeated audibly or mentally by you and/or your client.

LAM - 1st Chakra
VAM - 2nd Chakra
RAM - 3rd Chakra
HAM- 4th Chakra
YAM - 5th Chakra
OM - 6th, 7th Chakra

Mantras for the Seven Rays and their Planets

Each of the Seven Rays is associated with one or two of the planets of the Solar System. Thus, when healing and balancing an individual's personal ray, or the ray of an organ, the corresponding spirit of the planet associated with that ray can be invoked and placated with its mantra.

Each of the following mantras can be repeated during a Seven Ray Healing treatment and/or throughout the day by the person who is in need of balancing the associated planetary spirit. They can also be repeated often by a person to align with their ray and its planetary spirit.

A person repeating these mantras should repeat them in cycles of 108. This is a sacred number associated with the Goddess and healing. To keep track of their repetitions a practitioner of Japa can use a mala (rosary). Begin with the bead next to the "Guru" bead (the largest, most prominent bead). When the Guru bead is finally reached then 08 repetitions of the mantra have been completed. Most malas are composed of Rudraksha Seeds that work to purify the blood when they are held for Japa and/or worn on the body.

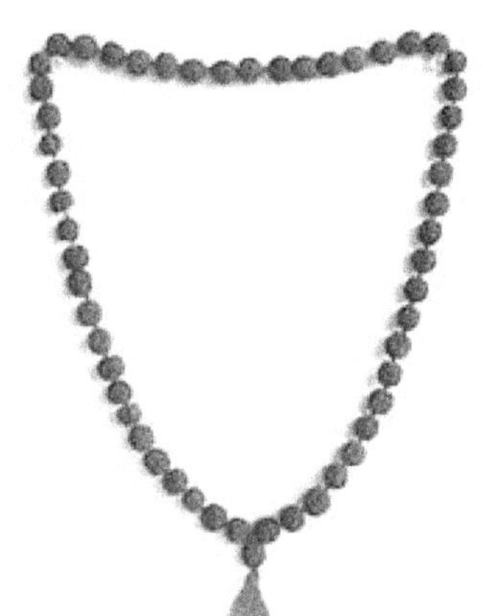

Rudraksha Mala with prominent "Guru Bead"

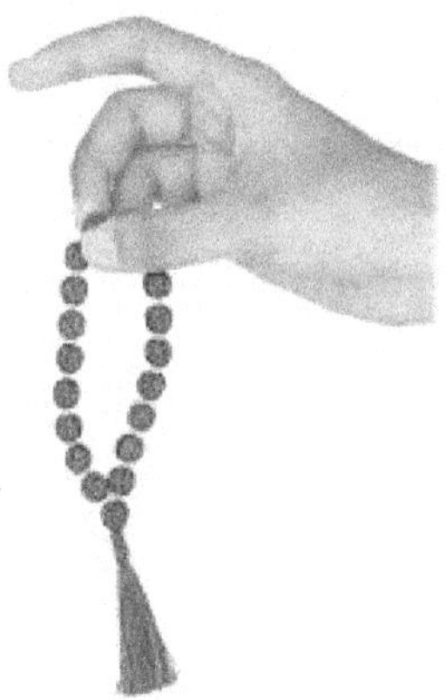

With each repetition of a mantra a Rudraksha bead is moved ahead using thumb and middle finger

Ray	Color	Planet	Mantra
1st Ray	Blue	Saturn "Sani"	Om Sanischarya Namaha
2nd Ray	Yellow	Jupiter "Guru"	Om Brihaspataye Namaha
3rd Ray	Red/ Orange	Mars "Kuja" Sun "Surya"	Om Kujaya Namaha Om Suryaya Namaha
4th Ray	White/ Pink	Venus "Shukra" Moon "Chandra"	Om Shukraya Namaha Om Chandraya Namaha
5th Ray	Green	Mercury "Buddha"	Om Buddhaya Namaha
6th Ray	Purple/ Violet	Ketu	Om Ketave Namaha
7th Ray	Violet	Rahu	Om Rahave Namaha

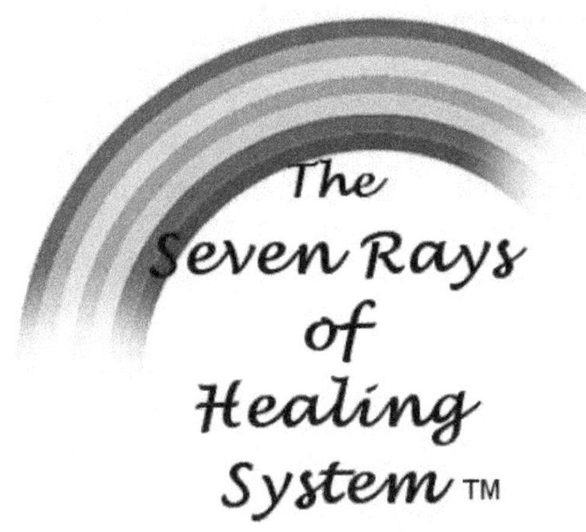

Chapter 4
The Inner Organs
DDiagnosis and Treatment

In this chapter we will explore the Rays, Emotions, Exoteric and Esoteric Functions and Treatment of the Inner Organs. But before we focus on each organ individually we will cover the Three Treasures, which are the three vital substances or essences that keep all the organs strong and functioning properly. A weakness or lack of any of the Three Treasures can weaken all the organs, so an initial evaluation of them is a good first step in any diagnosis. This wisdom comes directly from Chinese Medicine.

The Three Treasures: Chi, Jing, and Shen

Chi, Blood, and Jing, are known as the Three Treasures because they are so valuable to the body. When they are abundant you are blessed with health and strength, and when they are depleted you become weak and possibly dis-eased. The Three Treasures are inter-related; when one of them becomes depleted so do the other two.

Chi is simply life force. It is the energy in your body that drives all the organs and bodily processes. When your Chi is low, your energy and bodily processes become sluggish. When your Chi is depleted, your organs cannot perform the functions they are intended to and dis-ease eventually sets in.

Chi comes into the body through the air we breath and the food we eat. It is manufactured by the digestive organs and taken in by the Lungs. It is also produced by the Jing (the essence of your body), and it can be depleted by a weakened Shen (a weak mind; see below).

Jing is the liquid essence of your body. It manifests as sexual or seminal fluid, as well as bone marrow. Jing, which principally dwells in the Kidneys, is the essence inherited from the parents; when it is completely depleted, a person dies. Jing can, however be somewhat replenished throughout life through the food we consume, but a person's Chi must be sufficient to support the digestive organs to create Jing. Jing is the most refined form taken by fully digested food.

Jing can be transmuted into Chi through the stimulation of the Adrenal Glands, which have a heating influence on the body. Jing can also become Chi or spiritual energy (a higher frequency of Chi) when it is heated up through sexual relations and certain spiritual exercises. When the Kundalini is awakened through spiritual practices, for example, it feeds off the Jing and transmutes it into itself. Then, as spiritual energy, it rises up within the body and performs the work of alchemically transforming a person into a divine being.

Jing can become depleted through too much stress and a weakened Shen. It is also depleted through the consumption of alcohol, tobacco, and other toxic substances. Since Jing supports the functioning of the brain, when it becomes depleted a person loses his or her ability to think clearly and the Shen (mind) suffers. A weakened Jing can ultimately result in a lack of ability to see or hear.

Shen dwells within the heart. It is roughly translated as Spirit and Mind, which are inter-related. In the East it is understood that when the Spirit is calm, the Mind is inactive and peaceful, and vice versa. When a person's Shen is strong, they are calm and focused, but when the Shen is weak, they become easily distracted with worries and develop an overactive mind. In order for the Shen to be strong, the Chi and Jing must also be strong. It is impossible to have a calm and peaceful mind when one's energy is depleted, or one's brain is not functioning properly.

When working with patients with mental problems the Shen must always be taken into consideration. A depleted and unstable Shen is a contributing factor behind most all mental problems, including schizophrenia.

If you discover weakness in any the Three Treasures you will know immediately that there is a weakness in one or more inner organs. A weakness of Chi can be caused by an imbalance of the stomach/spleen or lungs, but as you will discover as you read on it could also be the result of an imbalance in the intestines, heart and/or kidneys. A weakness of Jing often points to a kidney imbalance, but it could also be the result of stomach/spleen issues. And issues with an unstable Shen are usually related to the heart, but they could also be influenced by the stomach/spleen dysfunction.

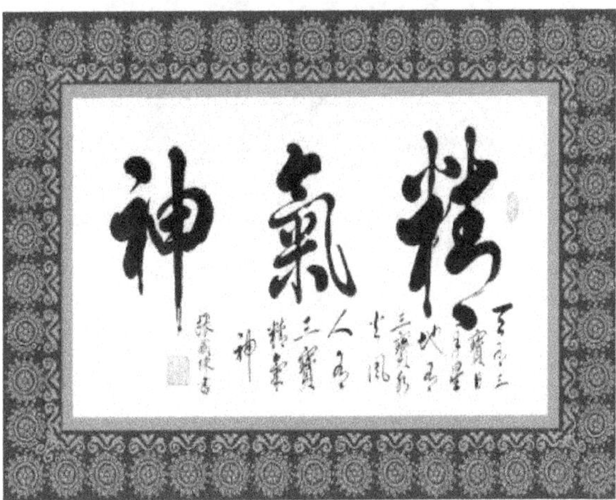

Jing, Chi, Shen

The Inner Organs

Rays, Emotions, Exoteric and Esoteric Functions and Treatment

Having covered the Three Treasures we can now present the functions of the inner organs. The exoteric functions of the organs include their physical, emotional, and mental functions, while the esoteric functions refer to the organs' spiritual functions. Each organ is also associated with an emotion; when a person over indulges in an emotion it will adversely affect the corresponding organ, and when a person chronically experiences the same emotion, it is a sign that the corresponding organ is probably imbalanced.

In the next two pages are anatomy maps to help you locate the organs in the body.

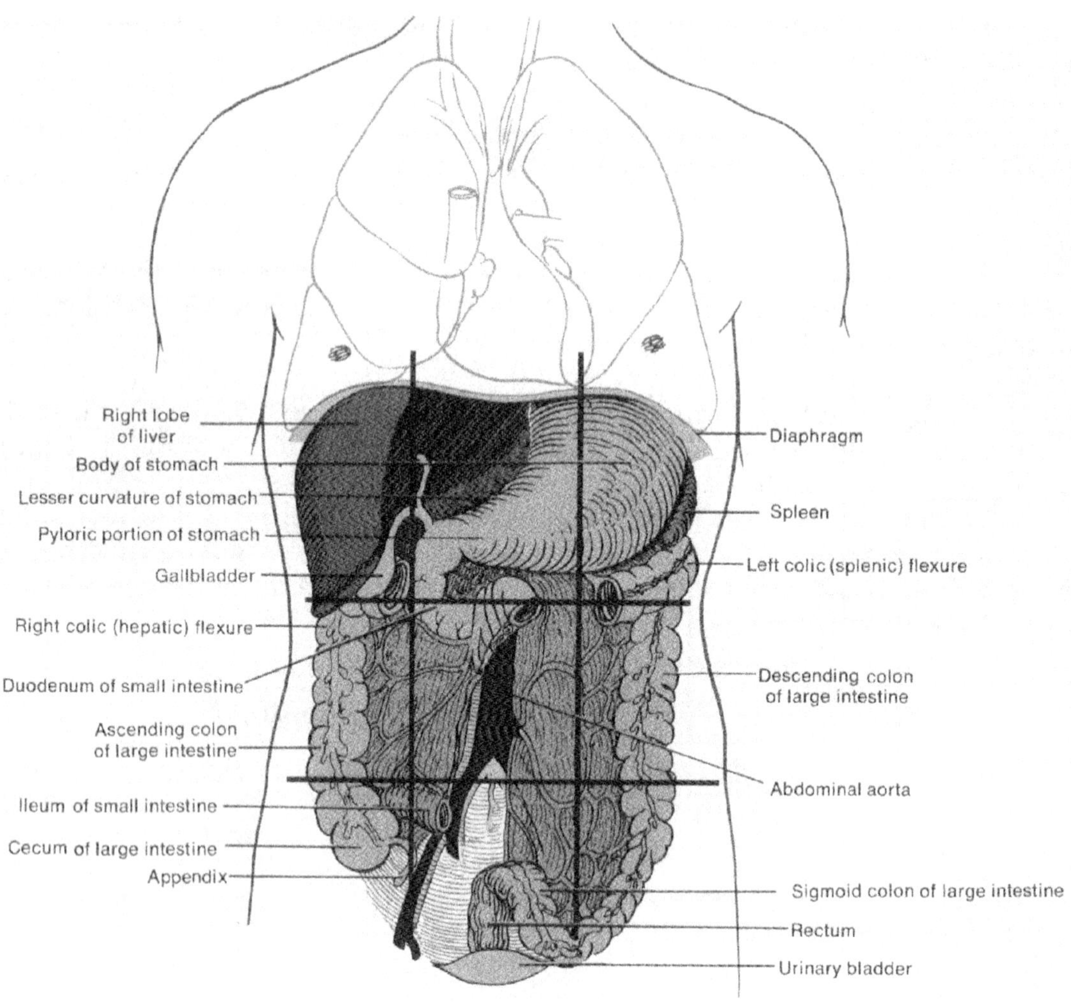

The Organs in the front part of the Abdominal Cavity

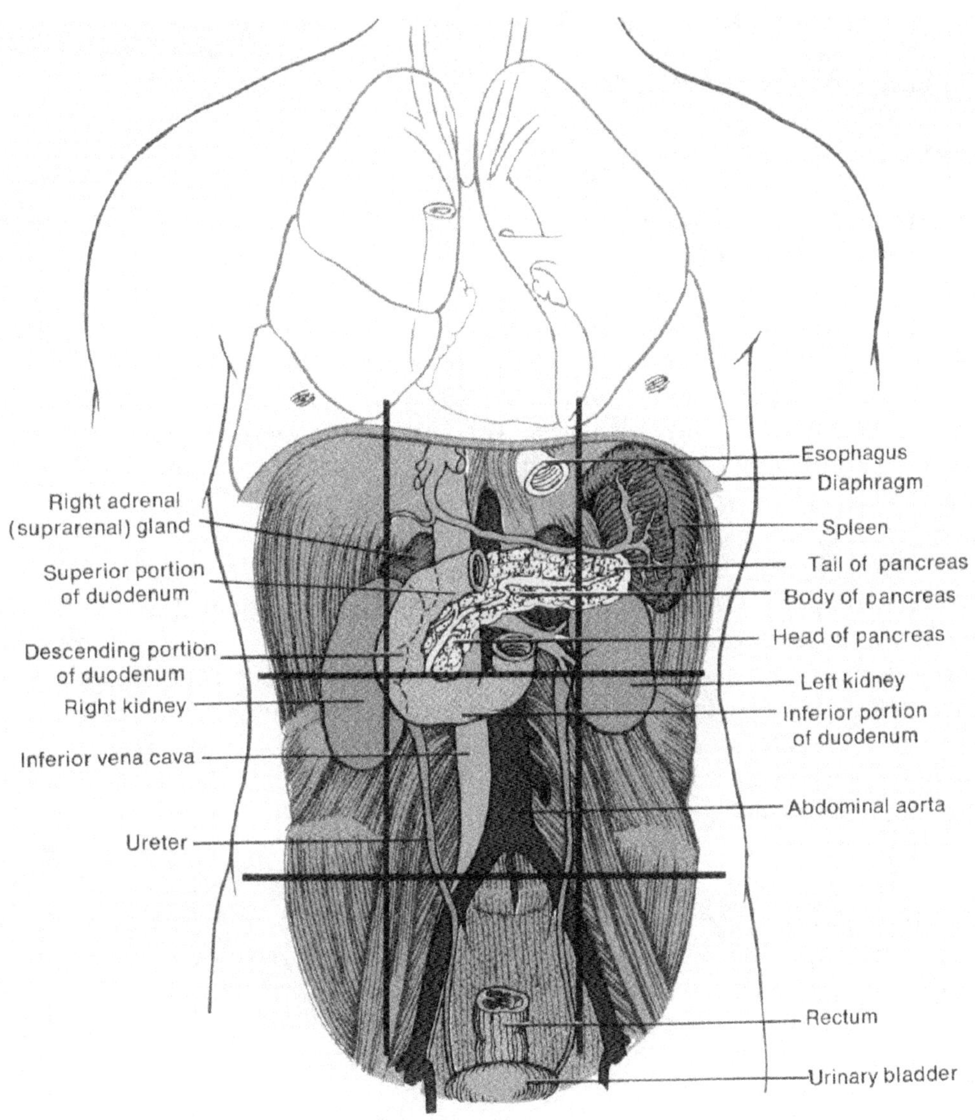

The Organs in the back part of the Abdominal Cavity

The Liver and Gall Bladder

(They are united as one organ in Chinese Medicine)

The Ray: The Liver and Gall Bladder are governed by the 2nd Ray.

Colors: Yellow, Green, Lemon.

The Emotion: The principal emotion that can injure the Liver, as well as indicate Liver disharmony, is anger.

Exoteric Function: The functions of the liver include: 1. Producing, cleansing and moving the blood 2. Overseeing the smooth flow of Chi in the body.

1.The Liver manufactures the various proteins in the blood, so weak blood or anemia can signal Liver weakness. The Liver filters the blood and breaks down toxins. When too many toxins enter the blood stream, the Liver becomes overworked and disharmony of the organ often results. The Liver also moves blood, so stagnant blood can signal Liver disharmony.

2. The liver oversees the smooth flow of Chi in the body. When it functions properly there is a peaceful movement of energy in the body similar to what one experiences after stretching exercises. But when a person experiences prolonged stress, the liver does not properly perform its function of moving Chi and tightness in the muscles occurs (especially the shoulders and neck). If stress continues, the Chi becomes bottled up within the liver and causes heat (blocked energy always eventually turns to heat), which rises to the head and produces a stress headache. Blocked Chi will also promote expressions of anger, which is the principle emotion associated with liver disharmony.

Esoteric Function: The liver is the seat of the emotional body, so virtually all emotions – especially those that are not processed and released - are captured and stored by it. The liver is the storehouse of emotions from this life and other lives, so when working with someone on an emotional and/or spiritual level always address the liver. As the body's filter, the Liver also processes toxic emotions. When a person experiences an abundance of unresolved and intense emotions over a period of time, the Liver will become congested and the organ will begin to show signs of imbalance.

Since the emotional body is inter-related to the astral body, a weak liver can make it difficult to stay grounded in the physical body. There may be an involuntary tendency to astral project or to take astral journeys.

In relation to its intimate connection to the 2nd Ray, when the liver is functioning properly a person can make clear decisions and plan for the future. But when it is malfunctioning a person can find it difficult to steer a steady course through life.

Symptoms of Liver Disharmony: The liver rules over the eyes, tendons, and nails, so any noticeable difficulty reflected in these parts of the body can indicate a liver imbalance. Liver related eye problems include sensitive eyes and both near and far sightedness. Hard or inflexible tendons can denote liver problems, as can brittle, ridged, or disfigured fingernails.

The color yellow is associated with the liver, and a yellow jaundiced complexion can indicate liver disharmony. Jaundice is usually associated with a malfunction of the bile. Jaundice is often accompanied by a bitter taste in the mouth. A bitter taste is a sure sign of liver disharmony whether it is accompanied by jaundice or not. Often, a liver afflicted person is literally bitter towards the world.

Since the liver rules over the smooth flow of Chi in the body (the Chi is moving smoothly when you are relaxed and peaceful), symptoms of liver imbalance include tight muscles, anger, stress headaches and migraines (headaches that occur on the sides of the head).

The liver is related to almost all negative emotional expression, because such emotions cause the Chi to become blocked up in the body. If the Chi remains blocked up for a period of time, a liver afflicted person will eventually succumb to depression, which is a symptom of chronically "depressed" Chi.. Blocked Chi in the Liver will eventually turn into fire; the afflicted person will then become angry and the fire will eventually rise to the head to cause a headache. Depression and anger are both related to the Liver. In this regard, it is said that "depression is anger turned inwards"

Treatment for a malfunctioning Liver

Color Therapy: Since the Liver vibrates to the 2nd Ray and is aligned with the Third or Manipura Chakra, the color yellow can be broadcast over the Liver to rebalance the organ (Zone #6). The Liver, which also influences ones emotional state, is also allied with the Fourth or Heart Chakra, and thus responds to the color green. Green is always the color to use with someone if they are experiencing an inordinate amount of intense emotion.

Taste: Each organ has a taste associated with it. If a small amount of food with the taste corresponding to an organ is taken internally, the organ will become stronger, but if too much of the same taste is taken in the organ will be weakened.

The beneficial taste for the Liver is the sour taste. Therefore, sour foods, such as sour fruits, are beneficial for the Liver as long as they are not taken in very large quantities. Probably the best sour fruit for the Liver is the lemon because it combines the yellow color with the sour taste, both of which benefit the Liver.

Foods: Sour foods, as mentioned, benefit the Liver. Carrots, which benefit the eyes, the organ ruled over by the Liver, assist the Liver. Beets, which enhance the Liver blood, also support Liver function.

Herbs: There are a growing number of herbs on the market to heal and promote Liver function. A couple common western herbs are Milk Thistle and Dandelion Root. These can be taken as pills or in a tea. The best Chinese herb for the Liver is Bupluerum. You can usually find Bupluerum in a combination with other Chinese herbs. A popular and easy to find Chinese combination for the Liver is Xiao Yao Wan. This combination is particularly good for those who have a congested Liver due to processing too many food and/or emotional toxins.

Gems: Both yellow and green stones are good for the Liver. The yellow stones include Yellow Sapphire, Yellow Topaz, and Citrine Quartz. The green stones include Emerald and Green Tourmaline. In order to correct Liver disharmony, these stones can be placed directly over the Liver during a healing session, and/or they can be worn by the afflicted person as a ring or pendant.

Alchemical Gems: Alchemical Gems are stones that have a special property in purifying and transforming a person. The best alchemical stones for the Liver include Malachite and Green Tourmaline. Malachite, which means "emotional release," is the best stone to use to release blocked emotions in the Liver. Green Tourmaline will both balance and alchemically transform the Liver. It will also unite the Liver to the Heart and dissolve all blocked emotional resentments in divine love.

Acupressure Points: Points on the Liver Channel, especially Liv 3, are good for balancing the Liver. Since it is favorable to work with the Heart when balancing the Liver, also use H 7 (Heart 7). And LI 4 (Large Intestine 4) is good because it helps release blocked Chi in the upper part of the body. These points, and their locations will be covered in Chapter 5.

The Heart

The Ray: The Heart is associated with the 3rd Ray and plays a role in the creative/destructive physical activities of the 3rd Ray.

Colors: Red, Green, Pink.

The Emotion: The emotion of joy dwells within the Heart. When the Heart is open, one's expression of joy comes naturally, but when the Heart is closed a person cannot experience the natural and spontaneous joy of life.

Exoteric Function: The Heart pumps blood throughout the body.

Esoteric Function: The Heart is the seat of the Shen. The Shen is the Spirit and the Mind. When the Spirit is quiet, so is the Mind. All psychological illness is related to the heart, and indicates an imbalance related to the organ.

The Heart and Liver are interconnected; treat them together. When the Liver driven emotions run high, then the Spirit or Shen in the Heart is unsettled and one's mind becomes overactive. And when the mind is overactive the emotions tend to flare up. Therefore, when treating the Liver for any disorder, always treat the Heart simultaneously, and vice versa.

Symptoms of Heart disharmony: The Heart rules over the tongue and lips through pumping the blood; any irregularities to these, such as purple lips and tongue, is a good indication of a heart disorder. The heart also rules over the blood vessels and anomalies to these vessels, such as an irregular pulse, can also denote a heart problem. Other common symptoms of a heart disorder include: Chest and arm pain; irregular heartbeat; difficulty breathing; an overactive mind; and psychological disorders.

The emotion associated with the Heart is joy. When the heart is open, one experiences a natural joy, but when joy becomes raucous or destructive, damage can occur to the heart.

Treatment for a malfunctioning Heart

Color Therapy: The principal color for the Heart is the color of the 3rd Ray, red. The color red should be used principally to treat a weakened physical Heart. To calm the Shen and emotions related to the Heart use the colors green and/or pink, which are associated with the Heart Chakra. Broadcast colors over Zone #5

Taste: The Heart is benefited by the bitter taste. So recommend a small quantity of bitter foods for persons with Heart ailments.

Foods: When treating a person with a weak Heart recommend warming soups, especially those containing garlic, which is an excellent herb for the Heart and Circulatory System.

Herbs: Garlic is an excellent Heart herb, especially for those with high blood pressure. Hawthorne Berry is also good for most Heart and Circulatory System problems. Ginseng can be prescribed for those with a weak heart.

Gems: Use red stones, such as Ruby and Garnet, to strengthen the physical Heart. Use green and pink stones, such as Rose Quartz and Rhodachrocite, to calm the Shen and sooth the emotions. These stones can be placed directly over the Heart during therapy and/or worn as a pendant or ring.

Alchemical Gems: Green and Pink Tourmaline will sooth the heart while also opening the Heart to divine love. Green and Pink Tourmaline can also be used together as Watermelon Tourmaline.

Acupressure Points: Points along the Heart Meridian are helpful, especially H7 (Heart 7). Liv 3 (Liver 3) should be used when there are emotional problems related to the Heart (relationships, lack of joy, etc.) Stomach and Spleen points, such as St. 36 and Spl 6, will help generate blood to nourish the Heart and calm the Shen. (See Chapter 5)

The Kidneys and Adrenal Glands

(They are united as one organ in Chinese Medicine)

The Ray: The Kidney/Adrenals are governed by the 1st, 3rd and 7th Rays.

Colors: Dark Blue, Black and Red.

The Emotion: The emotion associated with the Kidneys is fear.

Exoteric Function: The Kidneys clean the blood. They also keep a balance of certain minerals in the blood stream.

Esoteric Function: The Kidneys produce and store the Jing, the seminal essence that supports all the bodily processes. And the Kidneys are also the seat of the Source Chi, which is roughly synonymous with the energy released by the Adrenal Glands. The Kidneys are the "pilot light;" they store and continually release the power that fuels all the other organs. They are, therefore, the foundational and most important organ. Their food is the Jing, the material essence of the body. When the Jing is completely used up, a person dies.

The Kidneys create a trinity with the Heart and Liver. Together, they represent the first three and most important Rays. To affect the best cure, all three organs should be addressed in every treatment. The Kidneys are a person's root energy; the Heart governs their Spirit and Mind; and the Liver oversees their emotional body. If all these three parts of a person are not healed and healthy, complete and permanent healing cannot take place.

Kundalini Activation: The Kidneys are the location of what is called in China the "Moving Chi between the Kidneys," and in India it is known as the Mundane Kundalini. The Mundane Kundalini is the primal life force located in the lower torso that fuels all the bodily processes. In doing so, it divides into its male and female components and then becomes anchored in the body by the left and right Kidneys, which alternately control the female (cooling, slowing down) and male (heating, speeding up) metabolic processes in the body. The Kidneys accomplish this through the two subtle energy Meridians or Nadis that connect to the left and right Kidneys, known in China as the Ren and Du Meridians and in India as the Ida and Pingala Nadis. When the Mundane Kundalini moves through the Ren Meridian or Ida Nadi the bodily processes are slowed and the organs are given rest while becoming "cool." But when the Mundane Kundalini moves through the Pingala Nadi or Du Meridian, all bodily processes are speeded up and the inner organs become active and "hot." The Mundane Kundalini moves alternately through these primary energy vessels in 90 minute cycles, so at any given time of the day your organs are either fiery and active, or cool and inactive. Meanwhile, you are breathing alternately through the left and right nostrils, which connect to the Ida and Pingala Nadis respectively. The only time that the Chi from the air or the Mundane Kundalini below moves evenly through both energy vessels is between 4 and 6 AM. This is the time when the body is most balanced, and the time that is most efficacious for meditation.

The Kidneys are the physical organs most closely associated with the awakening of the Spiritual Kundalini. The Spiritual Kundalini is the same as the Mundane Kundalini; but it is a life force of higher frequency. It normally resides in a latent state at the base of the spine while waiting for the moment when a person is ready to know his or her true nature as a living god or goddess. The Spiritual Kundalini can become awakened when complete equilibrium of the male and female energies exists in the body, such as between the hours of 4-6 AM and/or when a person has evolved into a fully androgynous human being with a perfect balance of masculine and feminine tendencies. Or, it can be awakened by bringing inhaled Chi down to the lower abdomen and holding it there until it turns into fire. This retention creates a spark that travels to the base of the spine to awaken the Spiritual Kundalini.

Once it is awakened, the Spiritual Kundalini feeds off the Jing just as the Mundane Kundalini did, however it converts the seminal fluid into pure spiritual energy. The Spiritual Kundalini then rises up the center channel in the body, the Sushumna Nadi, and the person is able to breathe equally through both nostrils. The body is now continuously in a state of balance. When the Spiritual Kundalini rises up the central energy vessel in the center of the spine it pierces the seven charkas and purifies (unblocks) all the 72,000 energy vessels in the body. All diseases then leave the person, because, as it is said in China, "all disease is caused by blocked energy." Physical immortality can then be attained. When the Spiritual Kundalini finally merges into the crown of the head, the Sahasrara Nadi, the person looses his or her individual identity and merges their consciousness into the Infinite. He or she is now in Nirvana and has the option of returning to a more individualized consciousness to help uplift the world, or remaining forever merged in their quintessential infinite nature.

Symptoms of Kidney disharmony: Through its rulership of the Jing, the Kidneys govern the brain, or as the Chinese say, it "forms up the brain." When the Kidney Jing is weak, the brain does not get its requisite nourishment and hearing loss results. Dizziness or "spacey ness" can also manifest. Kidney Jing deficiency is most commonly seen in older persons who after many years of life have depleted their inherited Jing and thus lost a good percentage of their brain functioning. Such persons often display hearing disabilities, as well as dizziness and loss of short-term memory. Kidney Jing deficiency is also seen in persons who have been under stress for a long period of time, or persons who have been battling a chronic illness. The Jing, which governs and creates the immune system out of itself, will eventually become depleted after a prolonged illness. But the easiest and most common road to a depleted Jing is through excess sexual activity. This is more a problem for men, who loose a little of their Jing every time they ejaculate, than it is for women. Men need to be conscious of this truth and seek to conserve their seminal fluid in order to remain to in good health.

The Jing also manifests as the head hair and the bones. If the head hair is scant or the bones are brittle, Kidney Jing deficiency must be considered. Men who become bald at an early age usually have a lot of male hormones and masculine fire in their bodies. Their excessive male fire burns up the watery Jing, causing these men to go pre-maturely bald and even lead to an early death.

The lower back, known as the "Palace of the Kidneys," is the region of the torso wherein the kidneys reside. When the kidneys are weak, the lower back is chronically sore and weak. This can be seen commonly in older persons whose Jing is depleted. They often contract chronic lumbago. A general rule is: **the stronger and more abundant the Jing , the stronger are the Kidneys and the parts of the body they support - the back, bones, brain and immune system.**

The Kidneys rule the Urinary Bladder. When weak the Kidneys can cause water retention in the Urinary Bladder and systemic edema (excess water in the tissues).

Chronic low energy is a definite sign of Kidney weakness, since the Kidneys supply the root energy to the entire body. Along with low energy, weak Kidneys can engender a weak immune system response; and they can promote weak knees. Boxers are often warned against having sexual activity before a fight in order to prevent weak knees.

The emotion associated with the Kidneys is fear. The owner of weak Kidneys is likely to have numerous fears and phobias regarding life. They are also likely to be lacking in willpower, because as mentioned in the previous lesson, the Kidneys are the home of the 1st Ray of Will and Power.

Treatment for Malfunctioning Kidneys

Color Therapy: The darker and lower frequency colors, such as black and red, nourish the Kidneys and their corresponding Chakras, the First and Second Chakras. Red is more stimulating and activating to the Kidneys than is black, but black is better for nourishing the Jing. A very dark blue, which is nearly black, can also be used to balance the Kidneys because of their relationship to the 1st Ray and the deep blue sea. Broadcast colors over Zone #9.

Taste: The taste that supports the Kidneys is the salty taste. A little salt is good but a lot will sedate the Kidneys.

Food: Salty food, such as seafood, will nourish the Kidneys. Foods of a black color, such as black beans, also nourish these organs. Black bean soup is a good Kidney food. Some black foods, such as black coffee, will stimulate the Kidneys but eventually weaken them.

Herbs: Black herbs support the Kidneys. The best Chinese herb is cooked Rehmannia, which is dark black in color. The best Chinese patent medicine for weak Kidneys is Eight Flavor Tea Pills. Red herbs are also good for deficient Kidneys, especially Red Ginseng; either Chinese or Korean Red Ginseng is good. Ginseng will tonify not only the Kidneys, but all the organs. For water retention and edema caused by weak Kidney function, use Uva Ursi, Horsetail, or Nettles.

Gems: Place black or red stones over the Kidney area, or wear them as rings or pendants. Obsidian, Smoky Quartz and Garnet are all good Kidney balancing stones. Red stones, such as Bloodstone, are more activating for both Kidney and sexual functioning, but black stones are more nourishing to the Kidneys.

Alchemical Stones: To stimulate the transmutation of the Kidneys and activate the higher frequencies of the Spiritual Kundalini, use Black Tourmaline and Meteorite. The high concentration of Iron Ore gives Meteorite powerful stimulating and electromagnet properties. Meteorites were considered extremely sacred around the Mediterranean Sea and used for initiation purposes in the mystery schools. Obsidian that is high quality can also be used for Kundalini activation. Since it carries the energy of fiery transformation, it can awaken the power of fiery transformation within the body. Use red stones to stimulate Kidney related fears and release them, and use black stones to transform fear into power.

Acupressure Points: Points on the Kidney Channel, especially K3 (Kidney 3), help balance Kidney function and nourish Jing. Ren 4, 6 nourish Jing and Source Chi (Mundane Kundalini) respectively. Du 4 is also good for supporting Jing and Chi. Generally speaking, the points on the Ren Channel, through which the female energies flow, will support and build up the feminine or water essences in the body, such as Jing, while the points on the Du Channel, through which the male energies move, will stimulate Chi or Mundane Kundalini and support the active functioning of the body's organs. (See Chapter 5)

The Stomach and Spleen

(They are united as one organ in Chinese Medicine)

The Ray: These organs are governed by the 4th Ray.

Colors: Yellow, Lemon.

The Emotion: The Stomach/Spleen are associated with the emotion of worry.

Exoteric Function: Although western physiology recognizes the Spleen as a blood filter, in the east both the Stomach and Spleen are said to work together to digest and assimilate food. Because of their function in the digestion process, the Stomach and Spleen are said to assist in the production of blood and Chi.

Symptoms of Stomach and Spleen disharmony: If the Stomach/Spleen are not working right a person will experience chronic digestive ailments. This could manifest as abdominal bloating, indigestion, stomachache, gas and flatulence. A weak Stomach and Spleen could also reveal itself as a chronic loss of appetite and, eventually, a lack of energy because not enough food is being transformed into blood and Chi.

The emotion associated with the Stomach/Spleen is worry, and when these organs are weak the afflicted person could tend to chronically worry. Conversely, if a person is a chronic worrier his or her Stomach/ Spleen will be injured.

Because of their association with the blood, pale lips (indicating weak blood) can be a sign of Stomach and Spleen weakness. Weak muscles resulting from lack of blood and Chi can also result.

Treatment for Malfunctioning Stomach and Spleen

Color Therapy: The best color for Stomach and Spleen disharmony is yellow. Broadcast over Zone #7.

Taste: The sweet taste corresponds to the Stomach/Spleen. A little sweet taste is beneficial to the appetite and digestion, but a lot will weaken it. Unfortunately, in the west we have a tendency to have large, sweet deserts, which weaken the Stomach/Spleen when we need them the most.

Food: For weak Stomach/Spleen and debilitated digestion, feed the body warming semi-sweet soups with well-cooked grains. Spicy soups with ginger or other stimulating spices will build up the power of the Stomach/Spleen and assist them in digestion. In general, warming foods with or without spices are best for assisting the Stomach/Spleen in their digestive functioning. Spices should especially be eaten with foods in a hot and humid climate, as the Stomach/Spleen will be weakened by such an environment.

Herbs: Yellow and spicy herbs, such as Ginger and Ginseng, are excellent to build up the digestive power of the Stomach/Spleen. Licorice Root is also good, and makes an excellent combination with Ginger as Licorice and Ginger Tea (equal parts of each). For indigestion, use Peppermint Tea.

Gems: Place yellow stones, such as Citrine Quartz, over the Stomach area for Stomach/Spleen disharmony, and/or wear these stones in a ring or pendant. Blue stones can be placed over the area for Stomachache in order to sedate the energy of the organ. As a general rule, red color or red stones stimulate and heat up an area or organ, while blue color and blue stones will cool and sedate an area or organ.

Alchemical Stones: Milky stones, such as Moonstone and Pearl, will transform the emotional worry associated with the Stomach/Spleen.

Acupressure Points: Points on the Stomach and Spleen Channels should be used. Use St36 (Stomach 36) by itself or in conjunction with Spl6 (Spleen 6). Spl4 and P6 (Pericardium 6) are also a good combination for most digestive problems. LI 4 (Large Intestine 4) can also be used indigestion and bloating. Ren 13 is the best point for stomachache. (See Chapter 5)

The Lungs

The Ray: The Lungs are governed by the 5th Ray.

Colors: White, Yellow and Lemon

The Emotion: The Lungs are associated with extreme sadness or grief.

Exoteric Function: The Lungs receive Chi from the air. Part of the Chi is circulated through the body via the blood, while another portion of it is sent down to the Kidneys and stored. If the Kidneys are weak, then they cannot grasp the descending Chi and the afflicted person is not able to breathe deeply. Asthmatic conditions often result.

Symptoms of Lung disharmony: When the Lungs are weak one suffers from shortness of breath, and can easily contract colds and coughs. As mentioned above, chronic difficulty in breathing deep can, however, be a symptom of Kidney weakness. Look for other Kidney deficient signs.

The Lungs rule over the skin pores. If a person perspires easily, he or she may be suffering from weak lungs. The Lungs give the pores the strength to hold in the fluids.

The Lungs also rule over the body hair, as opposed to the head hair, which is ruled over by the Kidneys. If a person is lacking hair over their arms and legs, it could be the sign of Lung weakness.

It is said that the "Lungs open to the Nose," therefore, running nose or abnormal nose problems could be a sign of a Lung imbalance.

The emotion associated with the Lungs is grief. If a person cries easily and copiously, they could be suffering from weak lungs. Conversely, if a person has been experience a lot of grief for a prolonged period of time, they could end up weakening their Lungs.

Treatment for Malfunctioning Lungs

Color Therapy: Since it is aligned with the 4th Ray, white light benefits the Lungs. For cold Lungs or Lung symptoms associated with Colds, broadcast a red light over the Lungs. For heat in the Lungs, such as infectious conditions with yellow sputum, such as Bronchitis, use a blue light. Broadcast colors over Zones #3,4.

Taste: The spicy taste is associated with the Lungs. A little spice in the diet nourishes the Lungs, but a lot will dry them out and harm them.

Foods: Spicy food is good for the Lungs. Give spicy soups to convalescents. The Lungs and Stomach/Spleen are often afflicted at the same time by such illnesses as colds and flues. Spicy soups are the best foods at such times as they benefit both the Stomach/Spleen and Lungs.

Herbs: Many of the same herbs benefit both the Lungs and Stomach/Spleen, such as Ginseng, Ginger and Peppermint. Ginger Root is especially good for coldness in the Lungs, and Peppermint is good for heat in the Lungs and infectious conditions. Use Ginseng as an overall tonifier for the Lungs.

Gems: 4th Ray white gems, such as Pearl and Moonstone, are supportive to the Lungs. For cold Lungs, wear red stones, for hot Lungs, place blue stones over the Lung region and wear them as rings or pendants.

Alchemical Gems: The white stones will balance and transform the emotional grief associated with the Lungs.

Acupressure Points: Use points on the Lung Meridian, such as L9 (Lung 9), for Lung ailments. For cough, use L7 and LI 4 (Large Intestine 4). Also use UB13 (Urinary 13) on the back for any Lung disorders. When a person experiences Lung ailments associated with colds and flues, their entire shoulder and neck region will often become blocked up. Message this area and get the Chi properly flowing again.

The Small and Large Intestines

The Ray: The Intestines are associated with the 2nd and 5th Rays and the color yellow. The 5th Ray is the most intellectual and the most intimately related to assimilation, especially the assimilation of information.

Colors: Yellow, Lemon

The Emotion: Worry, excessive mental activity and analyzing will weaken the Intestines.

Exoteric Function: The Small Intestine completes the digestion and assimilation of food begun by the Stomach. The Large Intestine separates the useful substances from the waste material and then passes the resulting waste to the rectum.

Symptoms of Intestine disharmony: When the Small Intestine is not functioning properly food is not properly digested and assimilated. The result is gas and abdominal distention. When the Large Intestine does not perform its function properly the afflicted person may contract diarrhea or constipation.

Treatment for Malfunctioning Intestines

Color Therapy: Yellow is a good color to balance the Intestines. It is particularly useful for enzyme weakness and assimilation problems. Broadcast a red light for coldness causing constipation or diarrhea and a blue light for infectious diarrhea and dysentery. Broadcast colors over Zone #8.

Taste: Spicy taste will assist in the release of Intestinal enzymes, but too much spicy taste will harm the Intestinal lining. Astringent taste is good for loose stools and diarrhea.

Food: Warming and spicy foods are good for diarrhea caused by coldness in the body. Astringent black tea and dry toast is good for abundant loose stools and both hot (infectious) and cold diarrhea. For dry and cold constipation (older persons get this a lot), eat warming grains or vegetables and drink warming soups and teas, including black tea, to warm-up and move the energy in the Intestines. Roughage from fruits is good for constipation and to clean out the Intestines when the person is constipated but not cold.

Herbs: For cold diarrhea, warming and spicy herbs, such as Ginger Root and Peppermint, are helpful. For abdominal bloating and gas, consider Fennel Seed and Anise, and for constipation give the patient Fennel Seed and/or Cascara Sagrada.

Gems: Place yellow stones over the lower abdomen for assimilation problems, and/or wear yellow stones set in a ring or pendant. For cold diarrhea, place red stones over the area, and for hot diarrhea or dysentery, place blue stones over the region.

Alchemical Stones: Use yellow stones to transform and improve a person's assimilation abilities.

Acupressure Points: You can use LI4 (Large Intestine 4) for all Intestinal problems, including diarrhea, constipation and dysentery. St 25 (Stomach 25) connects directly to the Intestines and is also excellent to use for intestinal disharmony. Two other stomach points that can be used for any intestinal ailments are St 36 and St. 37. Of these, St. 36 will generally be the stronger. (See Chapter 5)

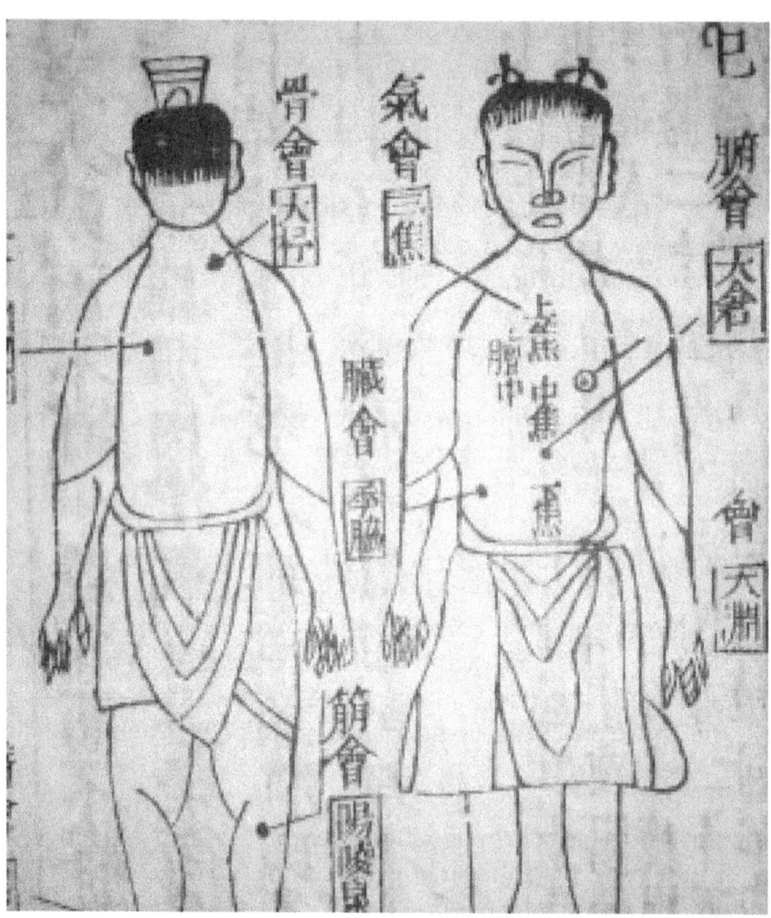

The Exoteric Functions of the Organs

Organs	Functions	Emotions	Ray	Tissue	Color	Taste
Liver/ Gall Bladder	Makes/Moves Blood Causes even flow of Chi in body	Anger	2nd	Eyes Tendons Nails	Yellow Green	Sour
Heart	Moves Blood Seat of the Shen, Mind	Joy	3rd	Tongue	Red Green	Bitter
Kidneys/ Adrenals	Cleans Blood Balances Salt Levels Stores Jing, Essence Source Chi Seat	Fear	1st	Ear Bones Brain Head Hair Immune System	Dark Blue Red Black	Salty
Stomach/ Spleen	Digests Food Produces Chi Helps to make blood	Worry	4th	Lips Tongue Muscles	Yellow	Sweet
Lungs	Receives Chi Disperses Chi	Grief	4th	Nose Body Hair	White Yellow	Pungent Spicy

The Esoteric Functions and Alchemy of the Organs

Organ	*Esoteric Functions*	*Chakras*	Alchemy on Organ *Stones*	*Influence*
Liver/ GB	Balancing Organ Balances flow of Chi & Blood Seat of Astral/Emotional Body Seat of Jnana Shakti, Decision Making	3rd	Malachite Green Tourmaline	Release and Transformation of Emotions Good Decision Making Ability
Heart	Commanding Organ Seat of Shen-Spirit Seat of Ego	4th	Pink, Green Watermelon Tourmaline	Release Emotion Open Heart Activate Intuition Calm Spirit
Kidneys/ Adrenals	Seat of Kundalini Shakti Seat of Iccha Shakti, Will Seat of Body Yin and Yang	1st, 2nd	Black Tourmaline Meteorite	Activate Kundalini Transmute Fluids (Jing) into Alchemical Force

Diagnosis and Treatment of the Organs

Organs	*Symptoms*	*Gems*	*Points*	*Herbs*	*Foods*
Liver/ Gall Bladder	**Side pain, Anger, Bitter Taste Side Headache, Eye, Nail problems Uncontrolled Emotion, Depression**	**Green Stones Yellow Stones**	**Liv 3 L.I. 4 H. 7**	**Milk Thistle Dandelion Root Bupluerum**	**Lemon Carrots Beets**
Heart	**Chest, Arm pain, Irregular pulse Blue Lips, Shortness of breath Psychosis, Depression, Dizzyness**	**Red Stones Green Stones Pink Stones**	**H 7, Liv 3 Spl 6, St 36 UB 15**	**Hawthorne Berry Ginseng Garlic**	**Warming Soup w/Ginger, Garlic**
Kidneys/ Adrenals	**Low Back pain, Edema, Fear Chronic Low Energy, Weak Knees Weak Immunity, Dizzyness**	**Dark Blue Stones Red Stones Black Stones**	**K 3 Ren 4,6 Du 4 K 1**	**Rehmannia Ginseng Uva Ursi, Nettles**	**Seafood Black Beans**
Stomach/ Spleen	**Indigestion, Stomach ache No Appetite, Weak Digestion Bloating, Worry, Low Energy**	**Yellow Stones Golden Stones**	**St 36 Spl 6 Ren 13**	**Ginger Root Peppermint St. Bitters Ginseng**	**Warm, Semi-Sweet, Soup w/Ginger**
Lungs	**Difficulty Breathing, Cough, Cold Flu, Weak Immunity, Grief Perspire Easily, Sparse body hair**	**White Stones Clear Stones Yellow Stones**	**LU 1, 5, 9 UB 13**	**Ginger Root Ginseng Peppermint**	**Spicy soups**
Intestines	**Cold/hot Diarrhea, Constipation Abdominal Distension, Pain Bloating, Abundant Gas**	**Red Stones Yellow Stones**	**St. 25, 36, 37 LI 4**	**Ginger Root Cascara Sagrada Peppermint Fennel**	**Ripe Bananas Toast/Dry bread Whole Grains Black Tea**

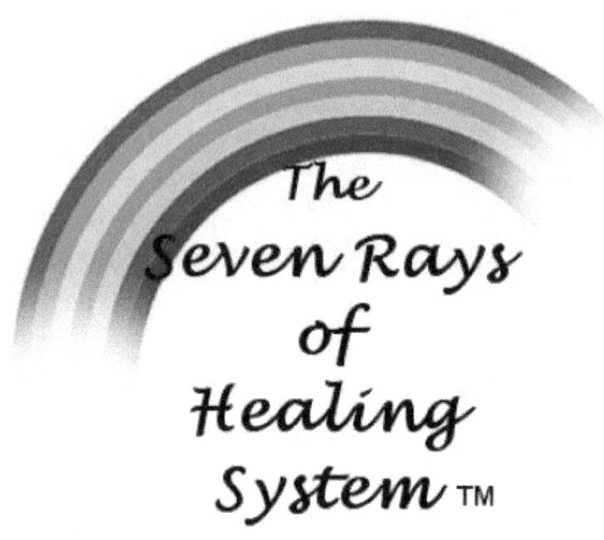

Chapter 5
Seven Ray Healing of the Dragon Body

This chapter will cover the **Dragon Body,** which is the subtle body comprised of energy channels, aka **Meridians/Nadis** and Chakras that the life force, aka **Dragon Force/Chi/Prana,** flows through. The esoteric anatomy of the Dragon Body and how it is associated with the Seven Rays will be presented in detail, followed by its **Chakras** and **Acu-Points,** which are vortexual crossing points of the channels. You will learn how to manipulate these subtle **Dragon Lairs** through acupressure and energy healing to re-establish physical, emotional and mental health. The chapter will end with a presentation of **Windows to the Sky Acupressure**, which is a system of Acu-Points used by the ancient **Taoist Monks** to assist consciousness expansion and psychic awareness. According to legend, both Acupuncture and Acupressure originated with the Taoist Monks, who originally used the therapy on each other to assist in their spiritual purification and evolution.

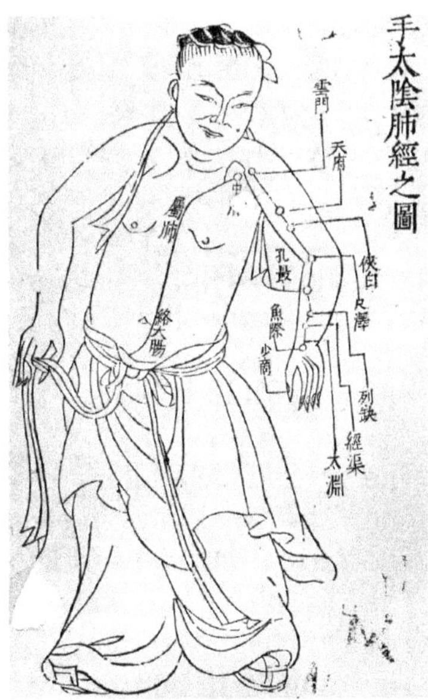

The Dragon Body

The esoteric anatomy of your Dragon Body consists of the subtle energy channels that the life force flows through after it enters the body through the air, water, and food we ingest and then moves to all parts of the body. It also includes the Chakras, the seven energy centers located along the spine that assist in the control and functions of all the glands and organs.

The Meridians or Nadis

The Chinese refer to the subtle energy meridians of the Esoteric Anatomy as Meridians, while the Hindus refer to them as Nadis. The Hindus maintain that there are 72,000 Nadis, and the Chinese recognize 14 Major Meridians and innumerable minor ones.

The Yin and Yang Channels

The two most important subtle energy channels in both the Hindu and Chinese systems are the ones that control the Yin-female and Yang-male balance within the body. These two channels, which are represented by the two snakes that spiral up the Caduceus of Mercury, are **known among the Hindus as the Ida and Pingala Nadis, and among the Chinese as the Ren and Du Meridians.**

When Chi or Prana moves through the Ida Nadi or Ren Meridian the Yin or female energies of the body are activated. This causes the functions of the organs to slow down, and the body becomes cooler and more sedate. The Yin substances or Three Treasures (Chi, Shen, Jing) are manufactured and stored, which is why one name of the Ren Channel is the "Conception Vessel." When Chi or Prana moves through the Pingala Nadi or the Du Meridian the Yang or male energies of the body are stimulated. The functions of the organs speed up and the body becomes hotter and more active. This why the Du Meridna is also known as the "Governing Vessel." Functionally, the Ida Nadi and Ren Meridian correspond to the Parasympathetic Nervous System of Western Anatomy, and the Pingala Nadi and Du Meridian corresponds to the Sympathetic Nervous System. The important Acu-Points on the Ren and Du Meridians, which run up the the front and back of the body respectively, will be will covered later in this chapter.

The 12 Major Meridians

In order to reach the inner organs, the Chi normally moves through 12 meridians, each of which connects to an important internal organ and is classified as Yin or Yang. These 12 Meridians are:

The Yin Lung Meridian
The Yang Large Intestine Meridian
The Yang Stomach Meridian
The Yin Spleen Meridian
The Yin Heart Meridian
The Yang Small Intestine Meridian
The Yin Kidney Meridian
The Yang Urinary Bladder
Meridian The Yin Liver Meridian
The Yang Gall Bladder Meridian
The Yin Pericardium Meridian
The Yang San Jiao Meridian

*The Pericardium Meridian connects to the Pericardium, the protective sack that surrounds the Heart, and its points are normally used to influence Heart related imbalances. The San Jiao Meridian does not connect to a specific organ but empowers all the important organs of the torso that influence water metabolism, including the Kidneys, Stomach/Spleen, and Lung.

The Dragon or "Kumara Body" and the Seven Rays

Your Dragon Body of Meridians and Chakras is your inheritance from the Lord of the Seven Rays, Sanat Kumara. Legend has it that the Kumaras worked together in the creation of the human body and its etheric double, the Dragon Body. It was in the Dragon Body that Sanat Kumara placed a spark of himself at the base of the spine as the Mundane and Spiritual Kundalini. The Mundane Kundalini is another name for Chi or Prana; through it Sanat Kumara keeps the body alive and functioning. The Spiritual Kundalini is the name of the alchemical force at the base of the spine that once awakened leads one to enlightenment. Through placing it in the Dragon Body Sanat Kumara ensured that every person could achieve the same level of wisdom and power as himself and ultimately achieve immortality. This is why an alternate name of the Dragon Body is the Kumara Body. When it is fully developed via the Spiritual Kundalini you become the forever-young, powerful and wise Kumara.

Like Sanat Kumara, the Lord of the Seven Rays, the Dragon or Kumara Body is the synthesis of the Seven Rays. The Seven Rays manifest in it as the Seven Chakras and the 14 (2x7) Major Meridians. Correspondences between the Rays, Meridians and Chakras are shown in the chart on the following page. Each Ray governs one primary chakra and one meridian, as well as numerous secondary ones.

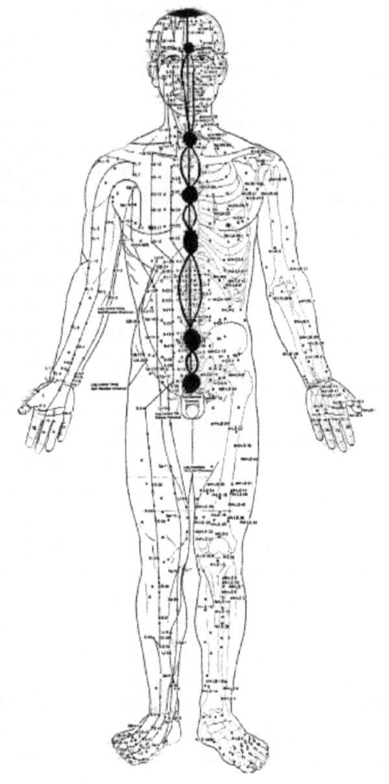

RAYS	CHAKRAS	MERIDIANS
1st Ray	1st Chakra Secondary (2,5,6)	Du Channel Secondary (Kid/UB
2nd Ray	3rd Chakra Secondary (4,6)	Ren Channel Secondary (Liv/GB)
3rd Ray	2nd Chakra Secondary (1,3,4)	Stomach/Spleen Secondary (Kid/UB)
4th Ray	4th Chakra Secondary (2,6)	Heart/ Sm.Intestine Secondary(Per/SJ)
5th Ray	5th Chakra Secondary (3,4,6)	Lung/ Lg.Intestine Secondary (Spl.St)
6th Ray	6th Chakra Secondary (4,2,7)	Pericardium/S.J. Secondary(Heart/SI
7th Ray	7th Chakra Secondary (1,2,6)	Kidney/ U.Bladder Secondary(Du)

Life Force Energy Flow

Life force is continually flowing from the sky to the Earth and from the Earth to the sky. The Yang energies come from the Sun above and the Yin energies come from the cool Earth below. Your body acts as a conduit for this Yin/Yang energy flow.

In order to understand the energy flow in your body stand up and raise your arms straight above your head. The Yang energies from above always move down the back of your body to the floor, so the Yang Meridians begin at the back of your hands. The Yin energies of Earth always rises up at your feet and move up the front of your body, so the Yin Meridians begin at the front part of your feet.

Yin and Yang Meridians

The 12 Major Meridians and their associated organs are paired. Every Yin Meridian and organ is paired with a Yang Meridian. The paired organs are:

Yin Lung Meridian -- Yang Large Intestine Meridian
Yang Stomach Meridian -- Yin Spleen Meridian
Yin Heart Meridian - Yang Small Intestine Meridian
Yin Kidney Meridian -- Yang Urinary Bladder Meridian
Yin Liver Meridian -- Yang Gall Bladder Meridian
Yin Pericardium Meridian -- The Yang San Jiao Meridian

The six Yin Meridians connect with the "Yin" organs. The Yin organs produce and store one of the Three Treasures. The six Yang Meridians connect with inner "Yang" organs. The Yang organs that are involved with functional activity of the body but do not store and produce one of the Three Treasures.

The 6 Yin Meridians and their organs:

Lung Meridian connects to the Lungs, which capture and hold essential Chi.
Spleen Meridian connects to the Spleen, which produces Chi and blood
Heart Meridian connects to the Heart, which stores essential Shen
Kidney Meridian connects to the Kidney, which stores and produces Jing
Liver Meridian connects to the Liver that stores and produces blood
Pericardium Meridian – connects to the Pericardium, helps the Heart store Shen

The 6 Yang Meridians and their organs:

Large Intestine Meridian links to the Large Intestine, which moves waste
Small Intestine Meridian links to the Small Intestine, which assists assimilation
Stomach Meridian connects to the Stomach Meridian, which assists digestion
Urinary Bladder Meridian links to the Urinary Bladder, which assists water removal
Gall Bladder Meridian connects to the Gall Bladder, which assists fat metabolism
The San Jiao Meridian connects to the San Jiao, which assists in water metabolism

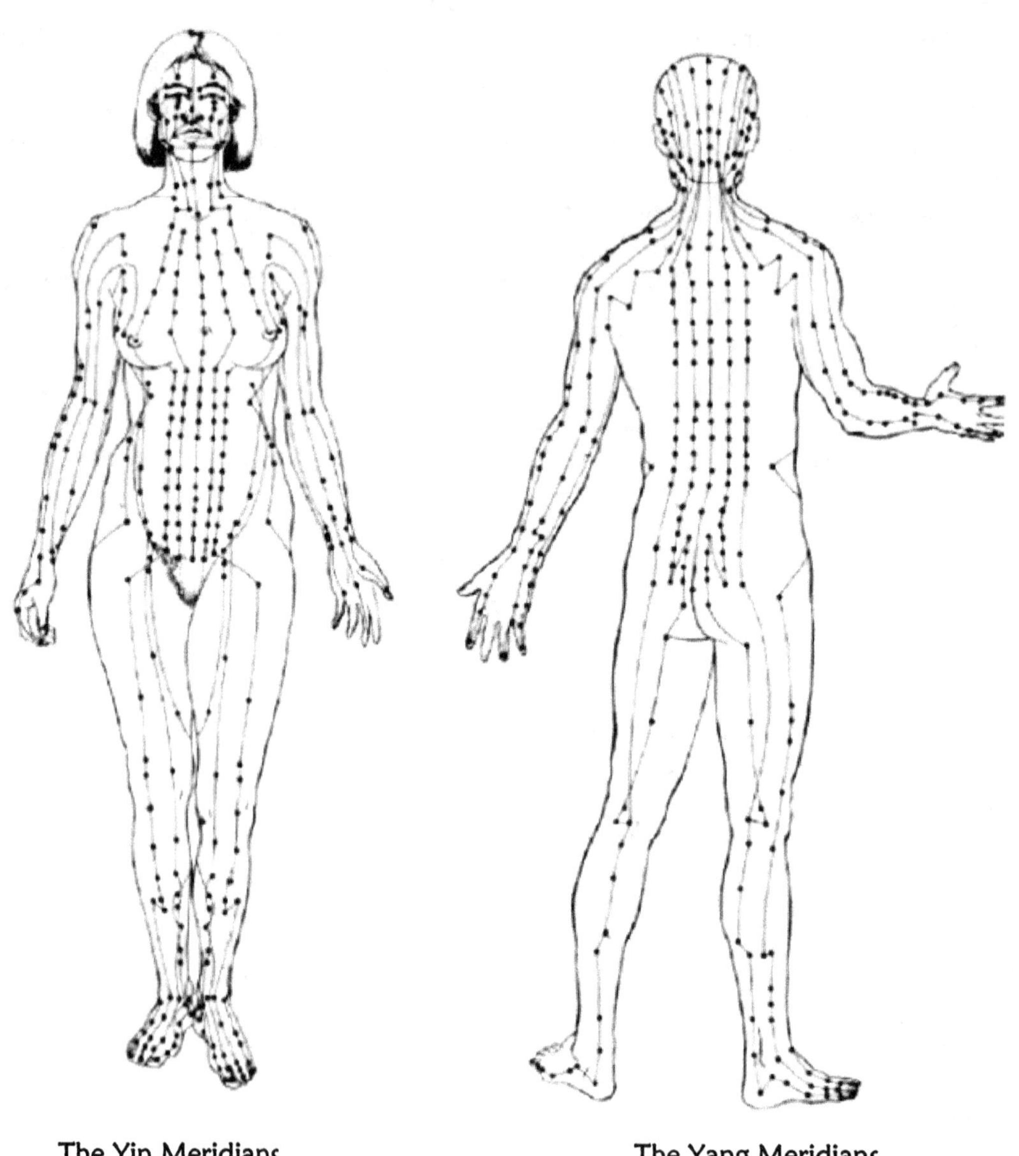

The Yin Meridians

The Yang Meridians

The Chakras and Acu-Points of the Dragon Body

As mentioned, the crossing points of the Nadis and Meridians are the Acu-Points and Chakras. In order to correct the flow of the Chi in the Meridians, and thereby correct imbalances in their corresponding organs, these subtle vortexes are manipulated. In the following pages the locations, functions and healing approaches related to the Chakras and important Acu--points that lie along the 14 Major Meridians will be described in detail.

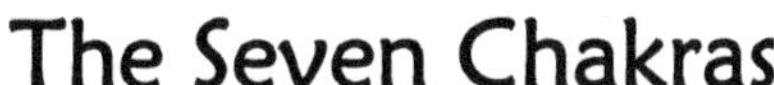

The Seven Chakras

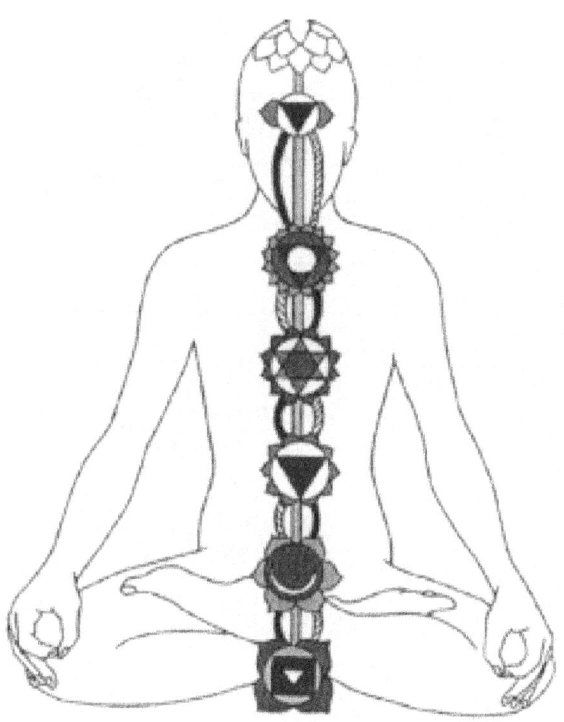

There are 7 major Chakras and numerous minor ones. These 7 Chakras are divided into 3 Yin and 3 Yang Chakras, while the center one, the Heart Chakra, is the union of Yin and Yang. The Yang Chakras, which are the first three charkas, govern physical energy and the lower self or egoic personality. The Yin Chakras, which are the last three, govern the higher self or spiritual nature. The middle Chakra, the Heart Chakra, unites Yin and Yang, lower and higher self together in harmony. When working with the Chakras it is always good to end with the Heart Chakra, as this energy center blends all the bodily energies into a harmonious balance.

There are two effective ways to test whether a chakra is out of balance and functioning either strongly or weakly.

1. Wave a pendulum over it. If after waving it back and forth over a chakra the pendulum swings strongly and in a clockwise direction, then the chakra is healthy, balanced and aligned. But if it swings weakly and/or in a counter-clockwise direction there is an imbalance within it and it needs therapy. If your client is receiving too much energy from the chakra, then consider partially shutting it down by moving your pendulum counter-clockwise over it.

2. Gauge how open and active the chakra is with L-Rods. When using L-Rods hold them by the handles, one in each hand and parallel to each other. As you walk straight ahead towards a standing person aim your L-Rods at one of the person's chakras and watch as they rotate outwards or inwards. If the L-Rods swivel completely outwards, i.e., the left L-Rod moves left and the right L-Rod moves right, then the chakra is functioning strongly. If they move very slowly and only slightly, and/or if they swivel inwards, then the chakra is closed down and/or functioning weakly. Consider therapy to open the chakra.

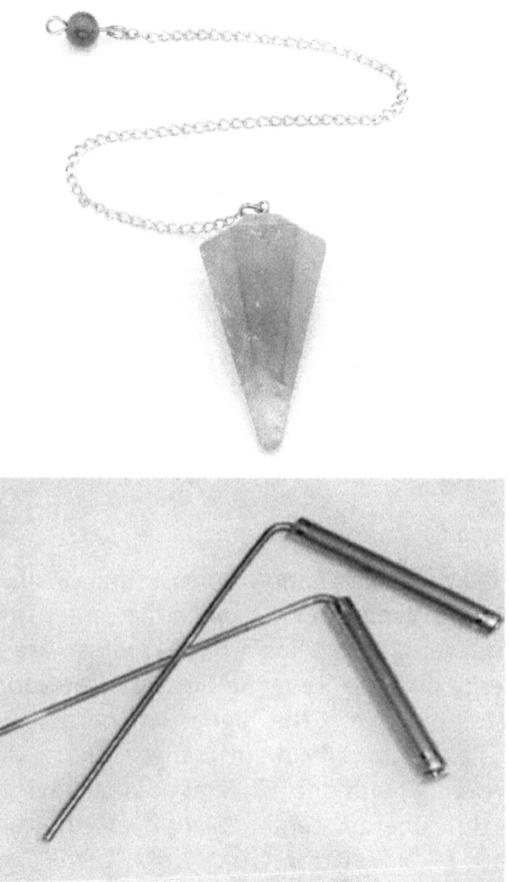

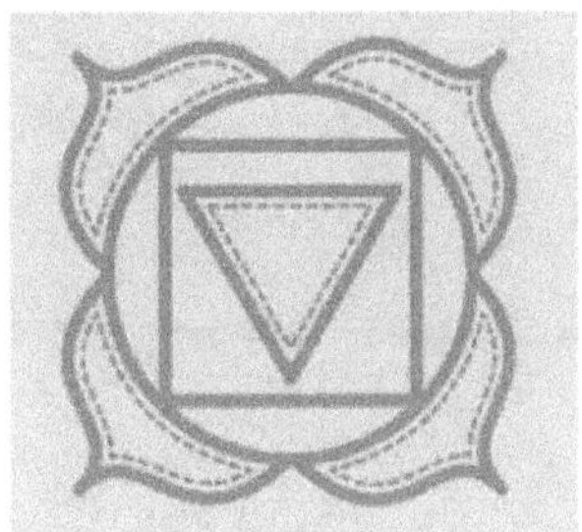

The 1st Chakra

Location: The 1st Chakra is located at the base of the spine.

Function: This Chakra, known as the Muladhara or Root Chakra, governs your root, physical energy. It rules over the Kidneys/Adrenals, which produce the Jing or essence that converts into Prana and thereby fuels all your body processes. In India, it is claimed that the Root Chakra feeds all the 72,000 Nadis with Prana or energy. If a person is chronically low in energy and/or they are having Kidney/Adrenal imbalances, you can work through the 1st Chakra to correct the imbalance.

Element: The Muladhara governs the Earth element in the body, and therefore oversees the creation of hard tissues, such as bones and teeth. Because of its association with Earth, it is this Chakra that keeps people grounded. If a person is having trouble with bones and/or teeth, and/ or they are chronically ungrounded, consider working through the Root Chakra to bring them back into balance.

Emotional and Mental Issues: The Muladhara Chakra governs survival issues. It also governs willpower and fear. If a person is having a difficult time either meeting their survival needs and/or easily give into fear and/ or are lacking in willpower, consider balancing the Root Chakra.

Therapy: To balance the Root Chakra and assist in resolving issues related to it you can use Color Therapy and shine a red light directly over the base of the spine for 20 or more minutes. Do this in conjunction with sound therapy. Vibrate the note G with Crystal/Tibetan Bowls or Tuning forks and/or intone the syllable Lam over the chakra. Or you can play live or recorded drumming music over or near the chakra. Also consider placing red or clear stones on the chakra to balance and empower it, and/or feed your own energy into the Root Chakra by performing Seven Ray Reiki on it (See Chapter 6). You can also twirl a crystal, a wand, or a pendulum over the chakra in a clockwise direction to fully activate it, or in a counter-clockwise direction to close it down. You can, of course, use all the above therapies together, one after the other, in order to affect the most optimum cure.

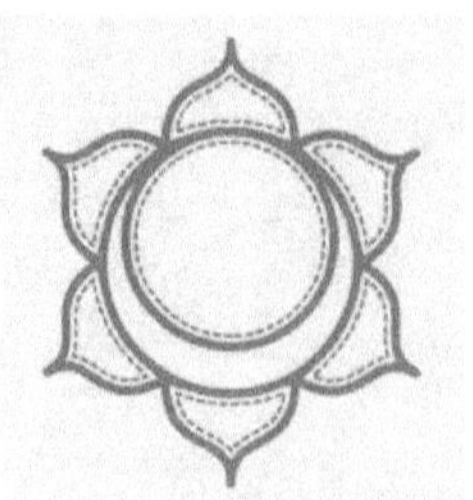

The 2nd Chakra

Location: The 2nd Chakra, called the Svadisthana Chakra, is located along the spine in the area directly behind the sexual organs.

Function: The 2nd Chakra governs the sexual organs, as well as the Urinary Bladder and Large Intestine. They also have some influence over the Kidney Jing. When there are physical problems related to the sexual organs, water elimination, and/or Large Intestines, consider balancing this chakra. And, if the problem is a chronic lack of energy caused by a deficiency of Jing, balance both the 2nd and 1st Chakras. These two Chakras work as a pair, so in general it is good to balance both at the same time.

Element: The 2nd Chakra rules over the Water Element in your body. This is why it has some influence over the Jing, which is the watery essence of the body. When the Water Element is out of balance and there is too little or too much fluid in the body, consider re-aligning the 2nd Chakra.

Emotional and Mental Issues: Since emotional issues are fueled by the Water Element, whenever a person's emotions are consistently extreme, or when they want to be more emotionally sensitive, consider balancing the 2nd Chakra. Since the Water Element also governs intuition, psychic ability and to some extent memory, too much or too little psychic energy and/or memory retention can also be caused by an imbalanced 2nd Chakra. The emotional issues related to the 2nd Chakra are usually related to one's sexual life, so it should be realigned whenever one experiences sexual problems that are emotionally generated, such as sexual abuse.

Therapy: You can broadcast the color orange, and/or place orange gems, over the second chakra region to balance this energy center. Use color and gem therapy along with sound therapy that is broadcast from a speaker, and/or vibrate the note A over the chakra with Crystal/Tibetan Bowls or Tuning forks. Also intone the syllable Bam over it. Play live or recorded light drumming or djeridoo music over or near the chakra. You can also twirl a crystal, a wand, or a pendulum over the chakra in a clockwise direction to fully activate it, or in a counter-clockwise direction to close it down. Also consider Seven Ray Reiki therapy. (Chap. 6) Your hands should remain on the chakra for at least 3 minutes.

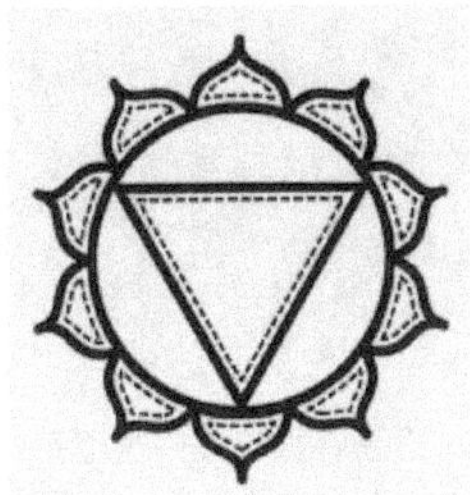

The 3rd Chakra

Location: The 3rd Chakra, called the Manipura Chakra, is located in the region of the Solar Plexus.

Function: The 3rd Chakra governs the Stomach, Spleen, the Small Intestine, and to some extent the Liver. It rules over digestion, detoxification, and assimilation of food. Any Stomach, Spleen, or Liver problem will improve by working through this chakra. You may often find that Stomach and Liver problems occur together because each is linked to the 3rd Chakra. Stress can sometimes adversely affect the Liver, causing anger and headaches, which can then cause a condition known in Chinese Medicine as "Liver invading the Stomach." The manifestations of this condition are indigestion, stomachache, and belching.

Element: The 3rd Chakra rules over the Fire Element in the body, which is why it governs digestion. It is the Fire Element that digests our food. Fire is also associated with stress and anger, the conditions associated with Liver imbalance, and it also rules over the intellect. Too much or too little fire in the body, especially in regards to digestion, anger, and a weak intellect can be corrected through balancing the 3rd Chakra.

Emotional and Mental Issues: Anger is associated with this Chakra, as is the intellect in general, especially in regards to assimilation and retention of information. Working through the 3rd Chakra is an excellent way of strengthening the intellect and improving retention. The 3rd Chakra also rules over the ego. If the ego is too strong or not strong enough, i.e., the person can not make himself or herself sufficiently noticed in the world to succeed, then balance the 3rd Chakra. A weak intellect often accompanies a weak ego, as both are intimately related to the male principle. Strengthen them together through this chakra.

Therapy: The 3rd Chakra can be realigned with Color Therapy using the color yellow, or by placing yellow/gold gems over it. Do this in conjunction with Chakra Music therapy. Vibrate the note B over the energy center with Crystal/Tibetan Bowls or Tuning forks and/or intone the syllable Ram over the chakra. Ram is the name/sound for fire in the Sanscrit language. You can also play Djeridoo and tenor drum music near or over the chakra. Twirl a crystal, a wand, or a pendulum over the chakra in a clockwise fashion to fully activate it or in a counter-clockwise direction to close it down. Also consider using Seven Ray Reiki on the chakra. (See Chap. 6)

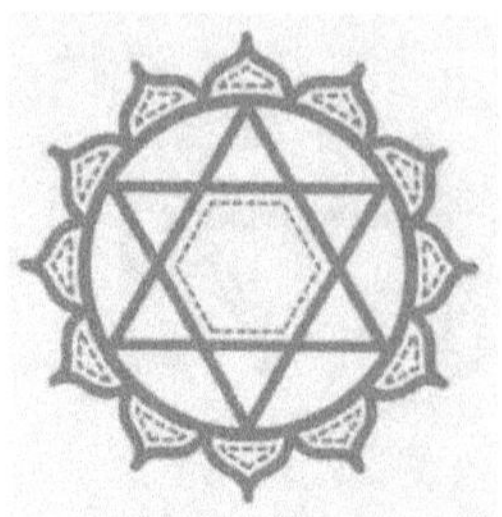

The 4th Chakra

Location: The 4th Chakra, known as Anahata Chakra, is located in the middle of the chest.

Function: The 4th Chakra governs the physical and emotional Heart. It also has some influence over the Thymus Gland and the Liver. For problems related to the Heart, Liver, and Thymus Gland, such as a lack of T--Cell production that weakens the immune system, consider balancing the 4th Chakra.

Element: The Heart rules over the Air Element. It thus influences the mind and intellect, as well as a person's ability to relate to and socialize with others. When a person has difficulty relating to others, balance the 4th Chakra.

Emotional and Mental Issues: The 4th Chakra governs the Heart Shen, a person's spirit/mind, so it influences all mental problems. The emotional issues of the 4th Chakra are principally those related to feeling loved, receiving love, and giving love to others. However any stuck emotions can prevent a person from giving or receiving love, which is why the Liver, the Seat of the Emotional Body, plays a role in the proper functioning of this chakra and why the Heart and Liver should be treated simultaneously. Thus, when a person does not feel love, has difficulty giving love or receiving love, or experiences any overwhelming thoughts or emotions, balance the 4th Chakra. Since giving and receiving love is such a fundamental part of human existence, many diseases are related to blockages in the 4th Chakra. Thus, it is good to always include a balancing of the 4th Chakra in any chakra therapy. Since the Heart is the Seat of Joy, when the 4th Chakra is functioning optimally a person feels love, as well as both joy and spontaneity.

Therapy: Use Color Therapy with green light broadcast over the 4th Chakra, or cover the area with green colored gems and stones. Vibrate the note C over the chakra with Crystal/Tibetan Bowls or Tuning forks and/or intone the syllable Yam. Evocative violin, piano and harp music are very effective to heal and open the Heart Chakra. You can also twirl a crystal, a wand, or a pendulum over the chakra in a clockwise fashion to fully activate it, or in a counter-clockwise direction to close it down. Heart Chakra responds very well to Seven Ray Reiki therapy. (See Chapter 6)

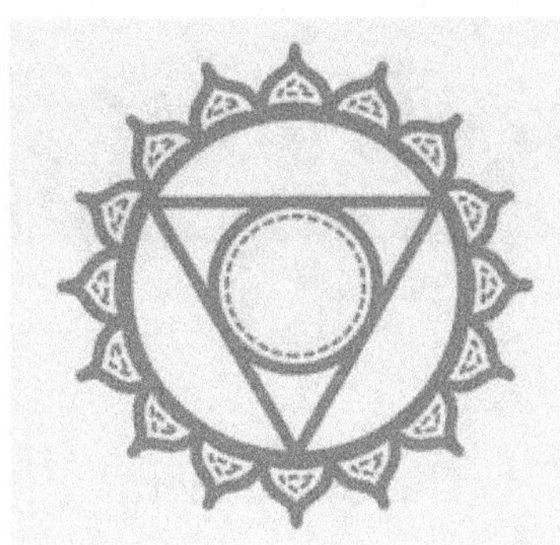

The 5th Chakra

Location: The 5th Chakra, known as Vishuddha Chakra, dwells in the region of the throat.

Function: The 5th Chakra rules over the throat and Thyroid Gland. Throat problems and/or a weak metabolism respond well to 5th Chakra therapy.

Element: The 5th Chakra rules over the Aether Element. This is the element of empty space from which sound or words originate. Any problem with this chakra can manifest as speech difficulties.

Emotional and Mental Issues: This chakra is associated with power, the power that accompanies the spoken word. If a person is feeling dis-empowered it may be because he or she has ineffective communication skills, or they are scared to speak their truth. Consider balancing the 5th Chakra.

Therapy: The 5th Chakra responds to a light blue colored light, as well as light blue or turquoise stones. Use these along with 5th Chakra Music and/or vibrate the note D around or over it with Crystal/Tibetan Bowls or Tuning forks, and/or intone the syllable Ham over the chakra. Consider also playing flute or piano music over or near the chakra. You can also twirl a crystal, a wand, or a pendulum over the chakra in a clockwise fashion to fully activate it, or in a counter-clockwise direction to close it down. Seven Ray Reiki is also effective. (See Chapter 6)

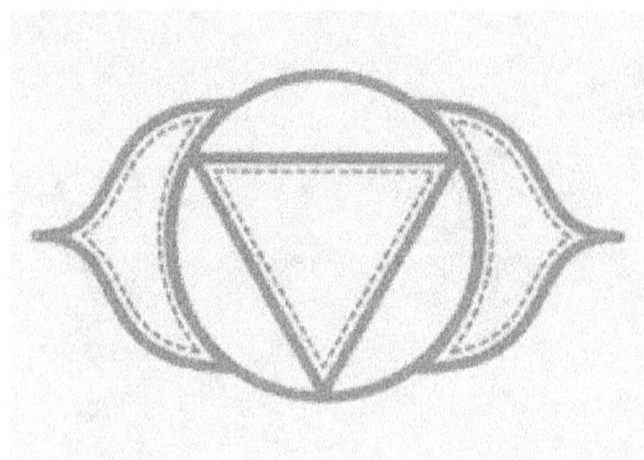

The 6th Chakra

Location: The 6th Chakra, known as both the Ajna Chakra and the Third Eye, is located between the eyebrows.

Function: This Chakra governs the master gland in the body, the Pituitary, so virtually all glandular problems can be improved by balancing it. The 6th Chakra also governs the Pineal Gland, which rules over our sleep cycles. Thus, for sleep related problems, work through the 6th Chakra.

Element: The 6th Chakra is the home of the Divine Mind, which is master over all the physical elements. This is why the 6th Chakra rules over the master gland of the body.

Emotional and Mental Issues: Since the Third Eye is the source of divine wisdom in the body, consider balancing it when your client feels disconnected from any philosophical understanding of life or from divine guidance. The 6th Chakra, when activated, can also give all psychic and clairvoyant powers.

Therapy: Use dark blue or indigo colored lights and/or gems to balance and activate the 6th Chakra. Consider intoning the syllable AUM to balance this Chakra and/or vibrating the note E with Crystal/Tibetan Bowls or Tuning forks. High pitched flute and violin music balances this chakra, and "Cosmic" or synthesized "New Age" music both heals and activates it. Seven Ray Reiki is also a good tool for balancing and activating the 6th Chakra, and formal meditation is excellent for realigning this energy center. You can also twirl a crystal, a wand, or a pendulum over the chakra in a clockwise fashion to full activate it or in a counter-clockwise direction to close it down. See Chapter 6 for information on Seven Ray Reiki Therapy and Chapter 8 for instruction on a Third Eye Activation Treatment.

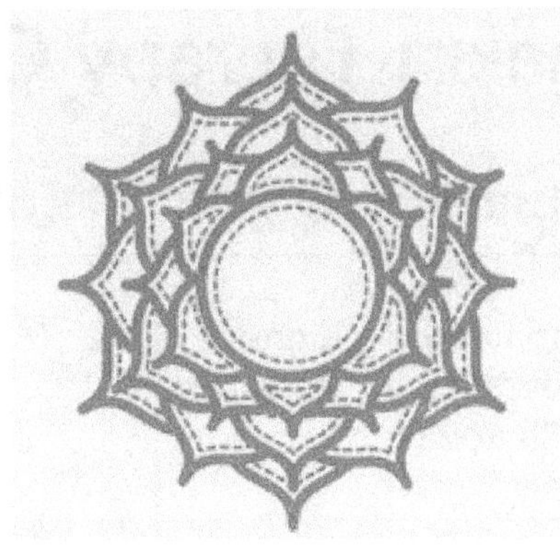

The 7th Chakra

Location: The 7th Chakra, known as the Sahasrara Chakra, or Thousand Petal Lotus, sits at the top or crown of the head.

Function and Element: The 7th Chakra is the seat of Spirit, the pure inanimate consciousness that is the backdrop and invisible foundation for all animate life. Emotional and Mental Issues: The main issue related to the 7th Chakra is the desire to merge and lose oneself in God, the Absolute.

Therapy: Use pure white light, the "color" of quartz crystal or diamond, and/ or gold, the color of wisdom, to balance the Crown Chakra. Violet is also helpful, along with its sound/ note of F# that you can resonate with Crystal/ Tibetan Bowls or Tuning forks. "Cosmic" or "New Age" Music will also assist in balancing this chakra. You can also twirl a crystal, a wand, or a pendulum over the chakra in a clockwise fashion to full activate it or in a counter-clockwise direction to close it down. And always consider Seven Ray Reiki Therapy as a means to heal and balance the chakra. (See Chapter 6)

Chakra Therapy Chart

Chakra	Element	Issues	Organs	Color	Notes	Mantras
1st	Earth	Survival Courage Will Power Fear	Kidneys/ Adrenals	Red	G	LAM
2nd	Water	Sex Creativity Psychic Distress	Sexual Organs Kidneys U. Bladder Intestines	Orange	A	VAM
3rd	Fire	Shyness Power Self Expression Intellect Pancreas	Stomach Spleen Liver Intestines	Yellow	B	RAM
4th	Air	Loneliness Love Peace Mental Illness	Heart Liver Lungs Thymus	Green	C	HAM
5th	Aether	Communication Speech Power Metabolism	Throat Thyroid	Turquoise	D	YAM
6th	Divine Mind	Confusion Faith Psychic Distress Mental Illness	Pineal/ Pituitary Third Eye	Indigo	E	OM
7th	Spirit	Transcendence Dissolution Oneness	Pineal/ Pituitary	Violet	F#	OM

The Important Acu-Points

There are literally thousands of Acu-Points covering the body that are created from the intersections of the 72,000 Nadis. According to Chinese theory, wherever there is a point of tenderness on the body it is an Acu-Point point. However, most acupressure or acupuncture practitioners principally use the points on the 14 major Meridians, and out of all those points there are probably 50 or so that they use consistently. These 50 points are preferred because they have a very strong and immediate affect on the body and the inner organs that their associated meridians connect to.

When locating an Acu-Point look for points of tenderness, as well as anatomical depressions. Many important points lie within depressions along a muscle or bone, as well as where cartilage or adipose (fat) tissue meets a bone.

The location of Acu-Points is expressed in terms of a unit of measurement known as a Cun (pronounced soon). You might, for example, find a point's location described as 2 Cun from the lateral (outer side) of the kneecap, or 3 Cun from the medial (inside) edge of the Tibia. If you are going to go deep into the science of acupressure you will want to do some studying of anatomy in order to accurately find the points. But for those of who do not have a background in anatomy, I will describe the location of points as simply as possible.

You can simply use your hand to measure Cun. One Cun is the distance between the first and second joints of your middle finger. One Cun is also the width of your thumb. 1.5 Cun is the width of your index and middle fingers together. And three Cun is the distance across the middle of all four fingers on each hand. Most points are described as being 1, 2, or 3 Cun away from a bone, an eye, etc, but some are listed as ½ Cun or 1.5 Cun away.

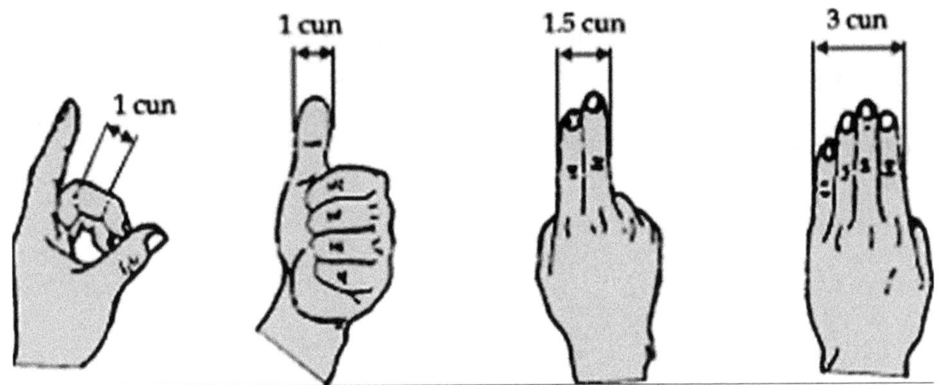

The following are some important points you will want to use. Their location and indications are explained. Each point lies on both sides of the body, so that a point on the right hand has the same location on the left hand, etc. To help locate the points use the charts spaced throughout this chapter, and especially those at the end of it.

Important points along the Lung Meridian

Lu 1 Location: Follow the clavicle (collar bone) to the point it meets the shoulder. Right below that place is a depression. This is Lu 2. Go 1 Cun directly below this depression to find Lu 1.

Indications: Good for most Lung ailments, including cough, shortness of breath, etc. This point can be used effectively **for both acute and chronic Lung ailments.**

Lu 5 Location: Go to the crease of the arm, the crease in the middle of the arm where the upper arm meets the forearm. This is where tendons from the biceps attach to the bone. Flex the arm, feel the tendons of the biceps, and then find a depression at the lateral (outside side of the tendons. This is Lu 5.

Indications: Also good for most Lung ailments, including cough, sore throat, shortness of breath, etc. This point is **particularly good for acute Lung disorders.**

Lu 7 Location: This point is on the Radius bone. It is located on the wrist, in the depression just above the end of the Radius, or where the Radius bone meets the hand. You will find this point approximately 1 Cun above the crease in the wrist as you move up the arm in the direction of the elbow.

Indications: **This is an excellent point for most acute Lung problems.** It is excellent for colds, sore throat, and congested nose.

Lu 9 Location: This point lies at the crease of the wrist, where the arm connects to the hand. Find the crease at the wrist, move towards the thumb until you hit the radial bone. The depression just inside of the bone is Lu 9.

Indications: This point is good for all Lung disorders, but is **best for weak lungs with chronic difficulties.**

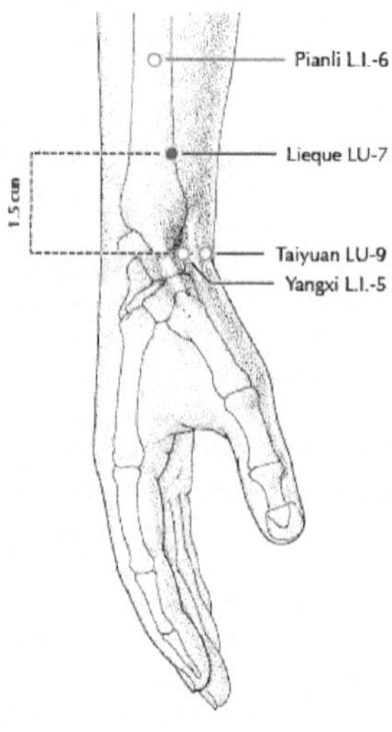

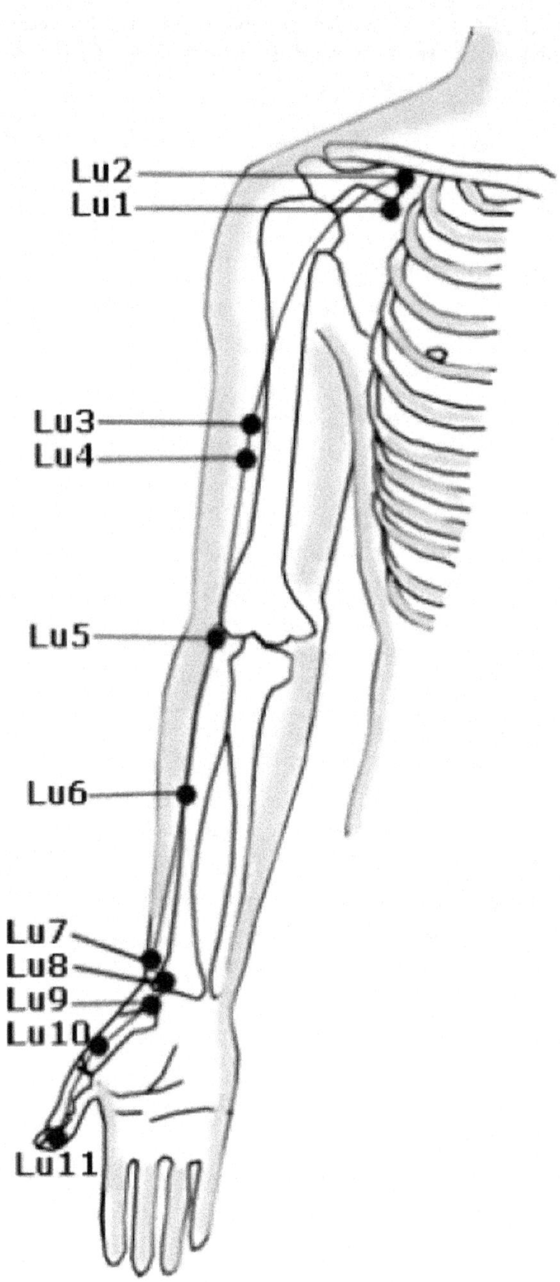
Lu2
Lu1
Lu3
Lu4
Lu5
Lu6
Lu7
Lu8
Lu9
Lu10
Lu11

Important points along the Large Intestine Meridian

L.I. 4 Location: This point is found in the web between the thumb and index finger on both hands. Bring your thumb against your hand and create a bump or bubble in the web of tissue between your thumb and index finger. Press straight down in this bubble and you should get a sensitive sensation. This is L.I. 4.

Indications: This is one of the most important of all points, and one that is commonly known about by both lay persons and professionals because of its influence it relieving headaches. **This point helps relieve headaches because it moves any blocked Chi in the upper part of the body.** All pain, including headache pain, is caused by stuck or blocked Chi. Since emotional stress is the number one offender in blocking pain in the body, **L.I. 4 can also help to relieve emotional stress. And since the Liver is usually involved with emotional stress, L.I. 4 can help move blocked Liver Chi.**

L.I.4 is good for **any kind of Large Intestine problem, including constipation, diarrhea, gas, and dysentery. It is also good for indigestion, nausea, etc.**

Since the Large Intestine Meridian sends a branch to the Lung, it can work with the Lung Meridian to relieve cold and flu symptoms. It can also help relieve sore throat and congested nose because its Meridian passes through the throat and terminates at the nose. Any point, when stimulated, will assist in clearing blockages along the Meridian it is situated on. **For cold symptoms, use this point with Lu 7.**

L.I. 11 This point is located at the end crease of the arm, the crease where the forearm connects to the upper arm. It is located next to Lu 5. Find the place in the middle of the crease of the arm where the tendon of the biceps connect to the bone. Then move laterally (to the outside of the arm) from the tendon until you go as far as you can go before hitting the bone (the place where the Radius meets the Humerus). Just before getting to the bone you will find a depression. You should feel sensitivity when you touch it. This is L.I. 11.

Indications: **This point is excellent for arm and elbow pain. When used with L.I.4 it is also good for moving any blocked Chi in the upper part of the body.**

L.I. 18 Location: On the side of the neck. Start at the Adam's Apple and move laterally (outward) approximately 3 Cun. Move laterally until you feel muscle tissue (the Sternocleidomastoideus muscle), then move the center of the muscle where there is a depression. This is L.I. 18.

Indications: **This is an effective point for neck stiffness, sore throat, goiter (or other disease of the neck, as well as cough.**

L.I. 20 Location: Lateral (to the outside of the nostril. Touch the widest part of the nose, slide down the nostril and then move just ½ inch from the nose. This is L.I. 20.

Indications: **This is an effective point for nasal obstruction and congestion.**

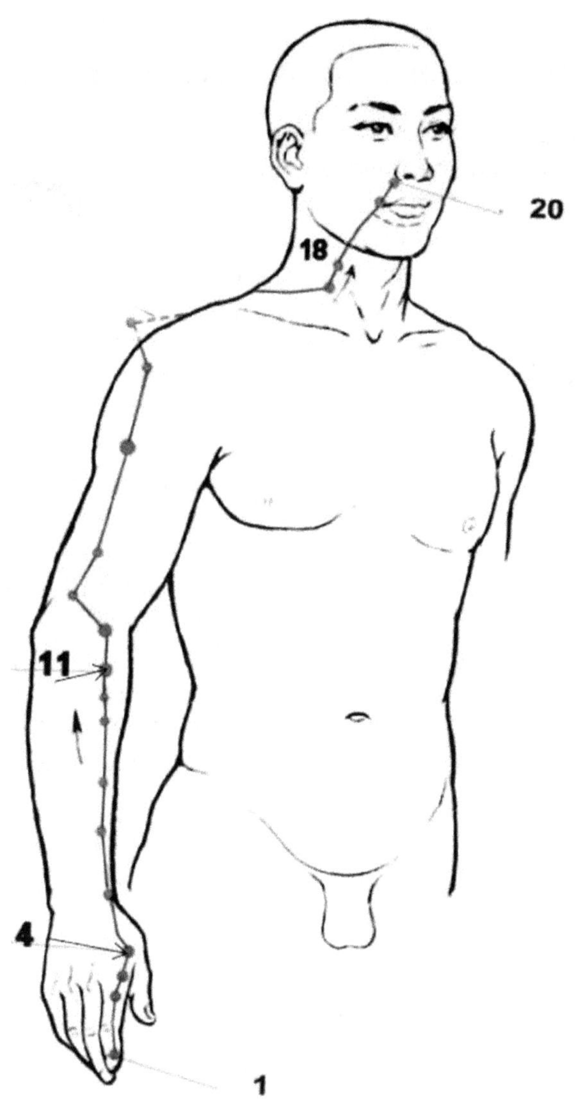
20
18
11
4
1

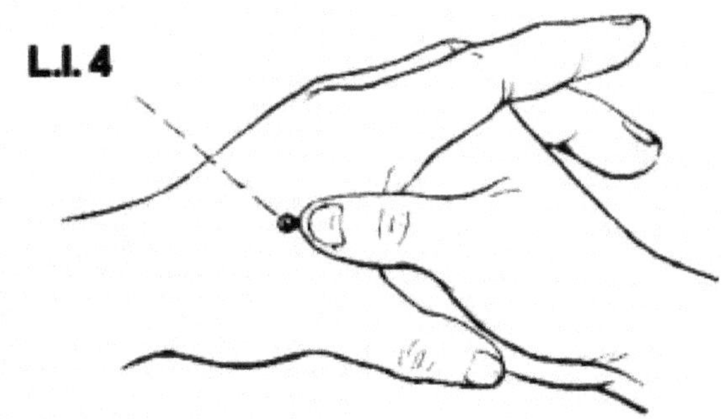
L.I. 4

Important points on the Spleen Meridian

Sp 3 Location: This point is located on the inside of each foot, just below the big toe. With your hand follow the big toe to its base. Where the toe attaches to the foot is a big mass of bone. Move over this mass of bone until you reach the bone that runs along the inside of your foot. This is the 1st Metatarsal bone. Find the fleshy area just below where Metatarsal bone connects to the bone mass. It should be sensitive. This is Sp 3.

Indications: An excellent point **for all Spleen related problems, including poor digestion, abdominal distension, stomachache, no appetite, etc.**

Sp 6 Location: Located on the inside of the lower leg. The point is 3 Cun above the ankle bone and along the edge of the Tibia bone, the main bone of the lower leg. This point is located just off the Tibia, where the bone meets the soft tissue.

Indications: This is one of the most important points in the entire body because it lies at the meeting point of the Spleen, Liver and Kidney Meridians, so technically problems of all three organs can be treated by it.

Sp 6 can be **used effectively for menstrual cramps** because the three Meridians that intersect at Sp 6 also meet again in the menstrual region.

Sp 6 assists in both moving blood and creating blood. **It is an excellent point to use for chronic low energy, anemia, and lack of blood.**

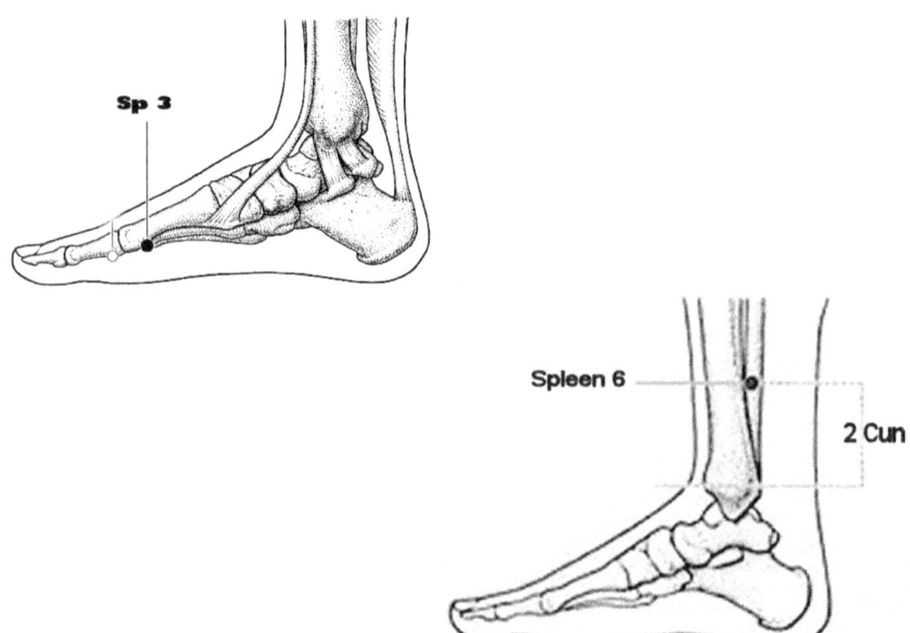

Important Points on the Stomach Meridian

St. 7 Location: This point is located on the side of the face. It is in front of the ear and directly below the "sideburn." Start at the temple and move downwards until you find a depression under an arched bone (Zygomatic Arch). This is St. 7.

Indications: This point is **excellent to use for toothache, stiff or clenched jaw, facial paralysis, and deafness.** It is also good for helping to relax the muscles of the face.

St 25 Location: This point is next to the umbilicus. Find the umbilicus and then move 2 Cun laterally in both directions. This is St. 25.

Indications: An excellent point for **Large Intestine disorders**, including **bloating, constipation, diarrhea, and dysentery.**

St. 36 Location: This point is located on the outer portion of the lower leg. Find the depressions at the base of the kneecap. These are known as Eyes of the Knee. Move 3 Cun below the outer Eye and 1 Cun away from the crest of the Tibia. This is St. 36. There should be some sensitivity if you point location is accurate.

Indications: **This is one of the most important points on the body** and used for many purposes. St. 36 is helpful for **any kind of digestive or elimination problems**, including exotic problems as **Ulcers.** It **treats symptoms associated with both the Stomach and Intestines.** It is also a point to **use for lack of energy, either chronic or acute**, because it helps to produce both blood and Chi.

St. 37 Location: 3 Cun directly below St. 36.

Indications: Very effective for all Large Intestine problems: dysentery, gas, constipation, etc..

St 40 Location: In the middle of the lower leg. Eyeball the middle of the Tibia, which is the area directly between the anklebone and base of the kneecap. Move laterally (to the outside) 2 Cun from the crest of the bone. This is St. 40.

Indications: This is **one of the best points to resolve chronic phlegm problems.** It is also indicated for lower leg pain.

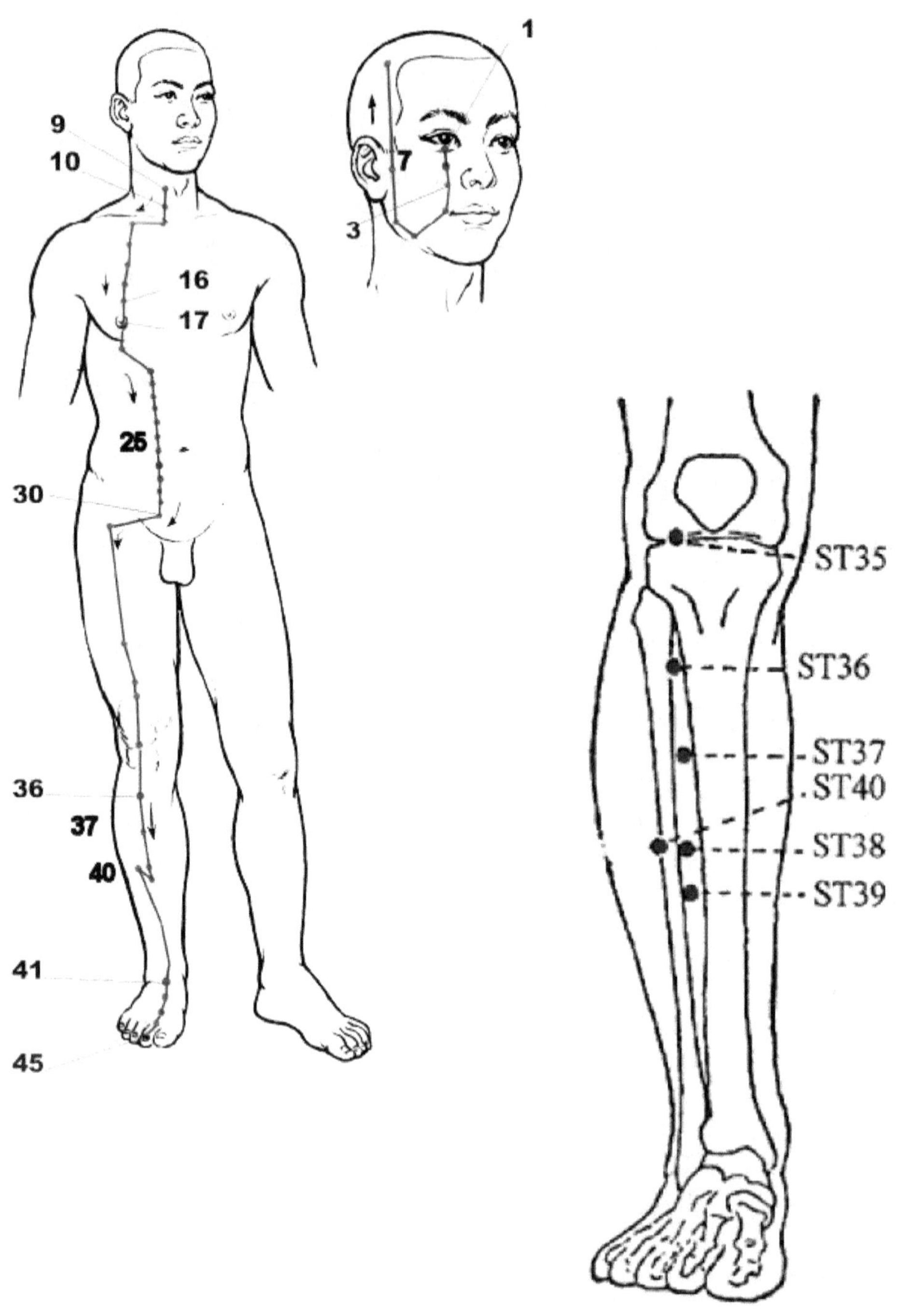
1
9
10
7
3
16
17
25
30
36
37
40
41
45
ST35
ST36
ST37
ST40
ST38
ST39

Important Points on the Heart Meridian

H4 Location: Below the wrist. Find the crease of the wrist. Move to the edge of the Ulna and move up the arm 1 ½ Cun. This is H4.

Indications: An **excellent point for correcting an irregular heartbeat.** It is also good for acute cardiac pain.

H7 Location: At the crease of the wrist. H7 is at the crease of the wrist opposite Lu 9. Find the crease of the wrist, then move your thumb medially (towards the body in the direction of the Ulna bone. When reaching the edge of the Ulna press down in the depression. You should feel some sensitivity. This is H7.

Indications: This point is used to treat **every kind of Heart problem,** including irregular **Heart beat, palpitations, etc., as well as overactive mind and mental illness.** It also treats all kinds of **emotional Heart problems** related to relationships and giving and receiving love. This is **a good point to use in any and all acupressure sessions to sooth the emotions and calm the mind.**

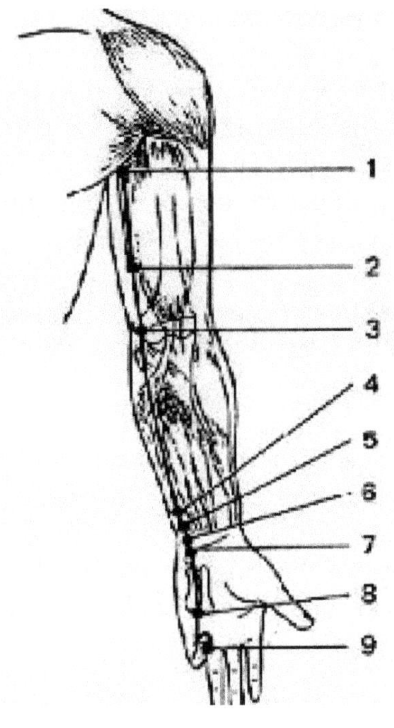

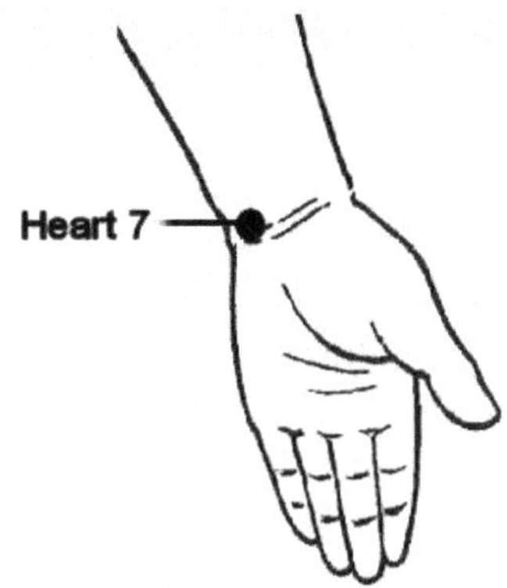

Important Points on the Small Intestine Meridian

S.I. 3 Location: Below the little finger. Follow the little finger to its base. Then move about ½ inch down the hand until you feel a depression. This is S.I. 3.

Indications: **Small Intestine problems, such as poor assimilation and bloating.** Also **neck rigidity, deafness or ear problems,** and headache. This point is also **good for all back problems** as it will unblock any Chi congestion along the back.

S.I. 11 Location: On the shoulder blade (the Scapula. Find the top of the shoulder blade, move to the center of it and then go 1/3 of the way down it. Find a depression. This is S.I.11.

Indications: A good point **for stiff back and neck and pain in the shoulder blade.**

S.I. 12 Location: On the shoulder. This point is directly above S.I. 11. Find the midpoint of the top of the shoulder and then move directly down the back a distance of 2 Cun. This is S.I. 12.

Indication: **This point is good for shoulder pain.**

S.I. 17 Location: On the neck. This point is on the border of the largest muscle of the neck, Sternocleidomastoideus. Find the outer corner of the jaw. Then move to the border of the first muscle you find in the neck. This is S.I. 17.

Indications: **A good point for deafness or ear problems, as well as sore throat**

S.I. 18 Location: Under the middle of the cheek bone in the depression.

Indications: **Facial paralysis, Bell's Palsy, toothache, tightness of facial muscles.**

S.I. 19 Location: In front of the ear. Move your thumb to the middle of the ear and to where it attaches to the face. Have the client slightly open their mouth; you will feel a depression. This is S.I. 20.

Indications: **Good for any kind of hearing or ear problem,** including deafness, ringing in the ears. It is also good for tightness or clenching of the jaw.

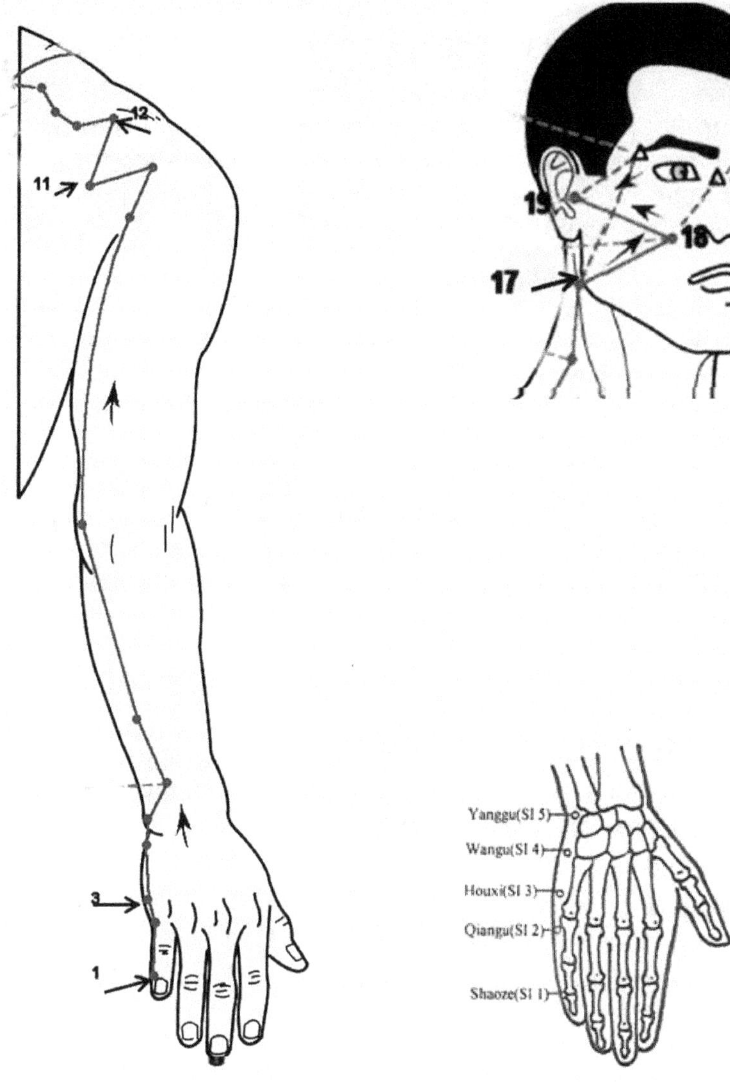
12
11
3
1
19
18
17
Yanggu(SI 5)
Wangu(SI 4)
Houxi(SI 3)
Qiangu(SI 2)
Shaoze(SI 1)

Important Points on the Kidney Meridian

K. 1 Location: On the bottom of the foot. The point is in the center of the foot and one-third of the way down, starting from the toes, where the foot begins to narrow and arch. Go to where the upper red pad meets the white skin, then move your thumb to the center of the foot and feel the depression. This is K.1.

Indications: This is **one of the best points to massage in order to ground a person**. This point activates the Kidney and 1st Chakra function of grounding.

K. 3 Location: Between the medial malleolus (the inner ankle bone) and the Achilles Tendon. Feel for the depression.

Indications: One of the 50 most important points on the body. **Use this point for any Kidney/Adrenal problems**, including low back pain, edema, dizziness, chronic low energy, weak knees, fear, hearing problems, etc. This point is **also good for insomnia, impotence, irregular menstruation, and chronic sore throat.**

K. 7 Location: 2 Cun directly above K.3, located between the bone and the tendon..

Indications: An excellent point for strengthening the Kidneys and Adrenals. **Great for edema, low back pain, chronic low energy**. This is also **an excellent point to cause sweating in case of fever.**

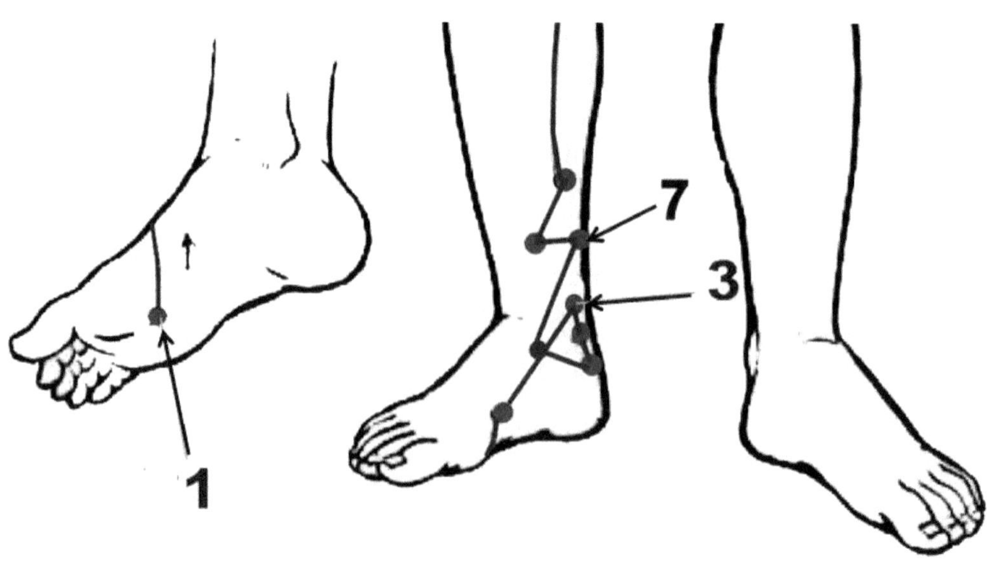

Important Points on the Urinary Bladder Meridian

Note: **This Meridian, which exists next to the spine, is special because it contains important points for almost all the major organs. Just by massaging up and down it or by using laying-on-of hands along it, you can send healing energy to most all the inner organs.**

U.B. 2 Location: At the medial end (towards the center of the body) of both eyebrows.

Indications: **Headache, blurring or failing vision, tired eyes, tightness of the forehead,** etc. This is **a good point to use in a facial massage.**

U.B. 10 Location: At the base of the back of the skull. Find the point at the base of the skull and between the two tendons (Du 16). Move down .5 Cun (Du 15) then move 1.3 Cun on either side of the neck's midline. Feel for a depression. This is U.B.10.

Indications: **Stiffness of the neck.**

U.B. 13 Location: On the upper back. 1.5 Cun on either side of the 3rd Thoracic Vertebrae. To find this point, feel the vertebrae at the very top of the spine. The first one you will feel will be at the base of the neck. This is the 7th Cervical Vertebrae, and below it is the 1st Thoracic. The 3rd Thoracic is two vertebrae below Thoracic 1 (T1).

Indications: **This point is excellent for any Lung disorders.** Briskly massage this point for excess Lung disorders stemming from a cold or flu, and mildly massage it for Lung deficient conditions, like chronic cough.

U.B. 15 Location: 1.5 Cun on both sides of the 5th Thoracic Vertebrae.

Indications: **Excellent for any Heart disorders.** To calm the mind, lightly massage this point or perform laying-on-of hands over it.

U.B. 18 Location: On both sides of the spine, 1.5 Cun from the 9th Thoracic Vertebrae.

Indications: **Excellent for any Liver disorder.** Great for **headaches, emotional stress, anger, etc.**

***Note:** The base of the Scapula or shoulder blade is at the same level as the base of the 7th Thoracic Vertebrae. So instead of beginning at the top of the spine and counting down to find vertebrae low in the back, locate the base of the Scapula, then move across the back to the base of the 7th vertebrae, and proceed.

U.B 19 Location: On both sides of the spine, 1.5 Cun from the 10th Thoracic Vertebrae.

Indications: This point **treats all Gall Bladder ailments, including Gall Stones and jaundice.**

U.B. 21 Location: On both sides of the spine, 1.5 Cun from the 12th Thoracic Vertebrae.

Indications: **Excellent for all Spleen/Stomach related problems, including indigestion, stomachache, etc.**

U.B. 23 Location: On both sides of the spine, 1.5 Cun from the 2nd Lumbar Vertebrae. The Lumbar Vertebrae are the very large vertebrae of the lower back. They are much large than the Thoracic Vertebrae. One way to find this point is to begin at the umbilicus. Trace a line horizontally from the umbilicus to the spine. This is the area of U.B. 23.

Indications: **Excellent for all Kidney/Adrenal problems. It is especially good for tonifying the Kidney/Adrenals and treating chronic low energy and sore back.** This is a good area to rest your hands over to **infuse the body with energy**. The life force you transmit here will go directly to the Kidneys and then to all the other organs.

U.B. 25 Location: On both sides of the spine, 1.5 Cun from the 4th Lumbar Vertebrae.

Indications: **An excellent point for all Large Intestine problems.**

U.B. 36 Location: Where the buttocks meet the upper leg. In the center of the upper leg.

Indications: **Good for Sciatica pain and Hemorrhoids.**

U.B. 40 Location: In the crease behind the knee. This point is located in the depression in center of the crease.

Indications: **Use this point to help relieve all acute backaches.**

U.B. 56 Location: In the very center of the calf muscles. Find the depression.

Indications: **Use this point to relax tight calf muscles.**

U.B. 57 Location: At the center of the base of the calf muscles. Find the depression.

Indications: **Use for tight calf muscles.** Also good for **low back pain.**

U.B. 60 Location: Between the outer anklebone and the Achilles Tendon. Find the depression.

Indications: **Neck rigidity, back pain.** This is **an "aspirin point" good for lowering fevers.**

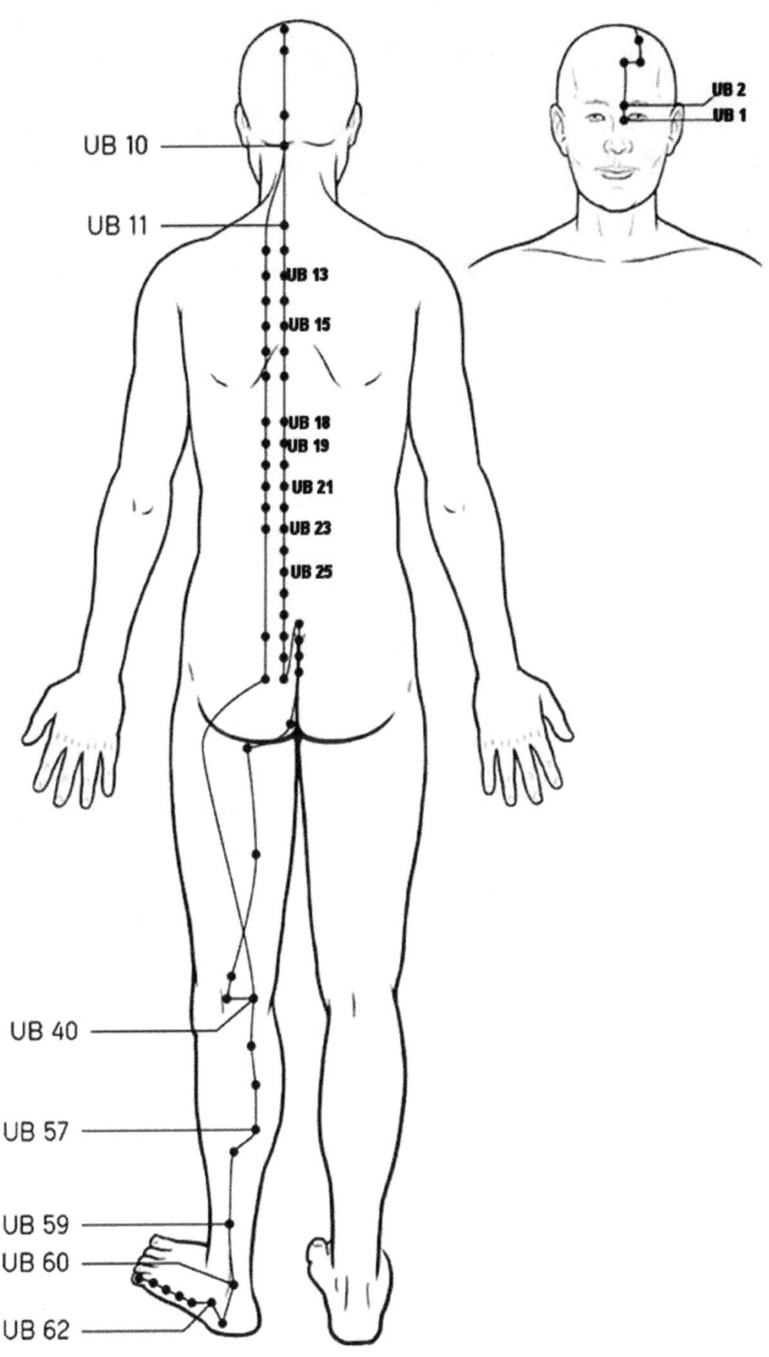
UB 2
UB 1
UB 10
UB 11
UB 13
UB 15
UB 18
UB 19
UB 21
UB 23
UB 25
UB 40
UB 57
UB 59
UB 60
UB 62

Important Point on the Pericardium Meridian

P.6 Location: 2 Cun above the crease of the wrist, towards the elbow. Place your thumb in the center of the crease of the wrist. You will feel two tendons running parallel there. Move your thumb 2 Cun up the forearm. P.6 is 2 Cun above the crease and between the tendons.

Indications: **One of the best points for nausea and vomiting.** Use a strong stimulating massage at the point to decrease nausea and vomiting. You can also **use P.6 to treat any digestive problem.**

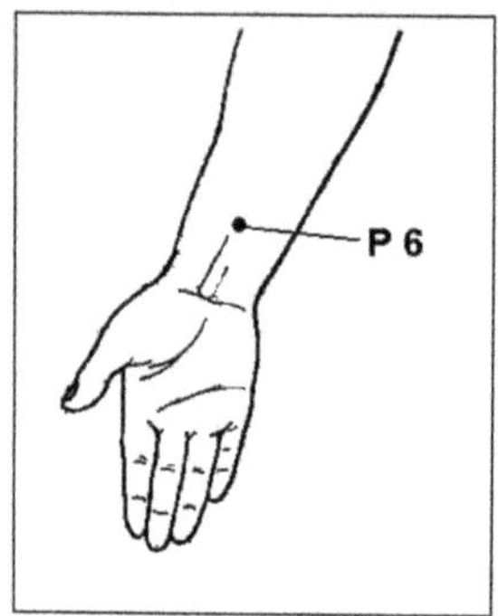

Important Points on the San Jiao Meridian

S.J. 5 Location: Turn hand so it faces down. From the place where the hand joins the lower arm, move up the forearm 2 Cun. Find the depression. This is S.J. 5.

Indications: **Excellent point for constipation. Also good for headache and hearing and/or ear problems.**

S.J. 15 Location: From the top and middle of the shoulder, move down 1 Cun. This point is just above S.I. 13.

Indications: **Tight shoulders and neck.**

S.J. 16 Location: Find the corner of the jaw, then move to the outer border of the Sternocleidomastoideus muscle, the major muscle of the neck. Find the depression. Point is on the opposite border of the Sternocleidomastoideus muscle from S.I. 17.

Indications: **Good point for neck tightness.**

S.J. 17 Location: Right behind the ear lobe, in the depression.

Indications: **Excellent for tightness of the jaw, clenching of teeth, ringing in the ears, and deafness.**

S.J. 23 Location: At the lateral (outside) of the eyebrow, in the depression.

Indication: **Good point for headache.**

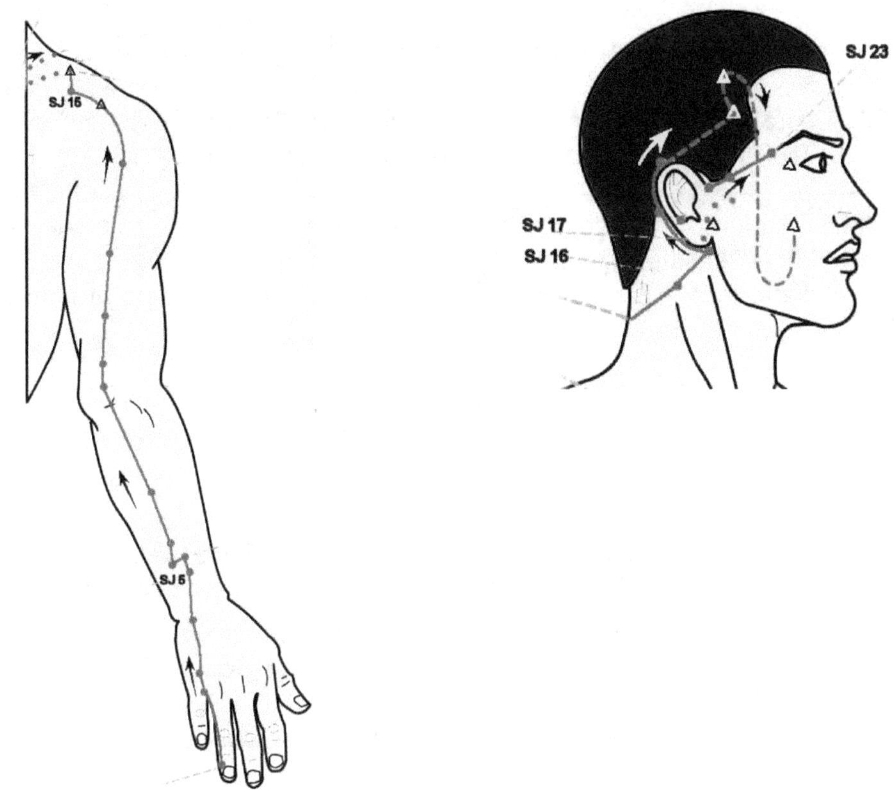

Important Point on the Liver Meridian

Liv 3 Location: On the upper foot. Move your thumb down from the space between the big and second toe. Just below this space you will eel two bones running parallel to each other. Find the deepest depression between these bones. This is Liv. 3.

Indications: **This is one of the most important of all points. It releases all blocked Chi in the lower part of the body, just as L.I. 4 releases all locked Chi in the upper part of the body. Liv 3 and L.I. 4 should be used together to release any blockages of Chi in the body.**

Liv. 3 is **excellent for all Liver problems, including headaches, anger, stress, emotional tension, etc.**

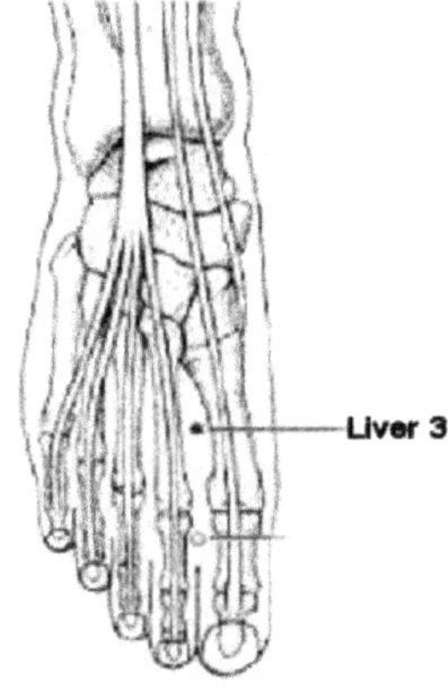

Important Points on the Gall Bladder Meridian:

G.B. 1 Location: Just beyond the outer corner of the eyes. Feel the depression.
Indications: **Good for headache and all eye problems.**

G.B. 5 Location: On the temple. Halfway down the temple and one inch in from the hairline. Feel the depression.
Indications: **Excellent for headaches, especially migraines and temporal headaches.**

G.B. 20 Location: Back of the head. At the base of the Occipital Ridge (the base of the skull). Start at the center of the back of the skull, then slide your hand laterally on either side. You will cross muscle and then there will be large depressions. This is G.B. 20.

Indications: **This is one of the best points for headaches. It is a good one to use for most all kinds of headaches, including stress headaches and migraines.**

G.B. 21 Location: On the shoulder. At the midpoint of the spine and the lateral end of the shoulders, and at the highest point of both shoulders. You should feel some sensitivity here. This is G.B. 21.
Indications: **An excellent point for tight neck and shoulders.**

G.B. 30 Location: The side of the buttocks. In the center of the dimples of the buttocks. Feel a large depression. There should be sensitivity. This is G.B. 30.
Indications: **This is the best point to use for Sciatic pain.**

G.B. 34 Location: In the depression anterior and inferior to the head of the fibula.
Indications: **Excellent point for most Liver issues.** Moves Liver blockage. Relieves side pain, side headache. Good for vomiting, knee issues.

G.B. 36 Location: On the lower leg. Find the lateral "eye of the knee. Move 2 Cun laterally from it and then 2 Cun down the leg. Feel for a depression. This is G.B. 36.
Indications: **An excellent point for any Liver or Gall Bladder problems. Especially good for Gall Bladder symptoms and migraine headaches, or headaches on the sides of the head.**

G.B. 41 Location: On the foot. Flex the foot. You will see a series of tendons. Move your thumb up the foot along the outside of the last tendon (the one that connects with the little toe) until you feel a depression (it is a space between the tendon and a bone). This is G.B. 41.
Indications: **Excellent for headaches, especially migraines.** Also good for neck pain and to stimulate secretion of bile from the Gall Bladder. Also use it for menstrual cramps.

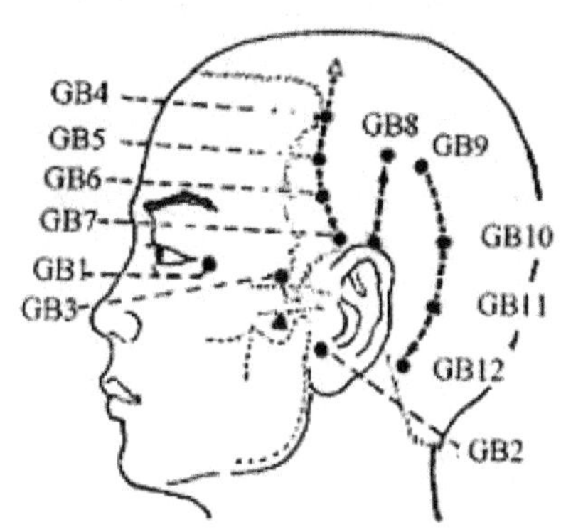
GB4
GB5
GB6
GB7
GB1
GB3
GB8
GB9
GB10
GB11
GB12
GB2

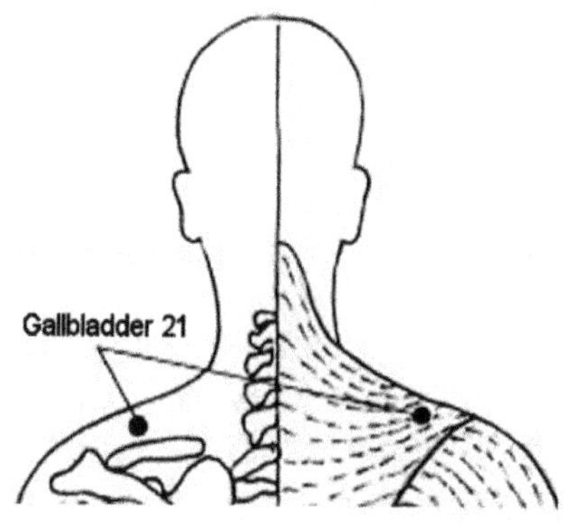
Gallbladder 21

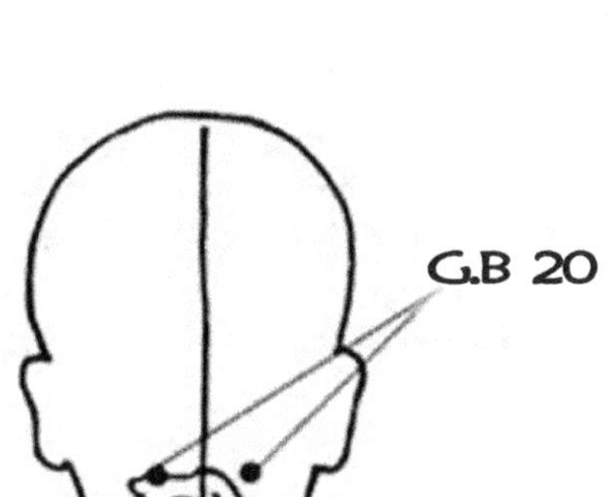
G.B 20

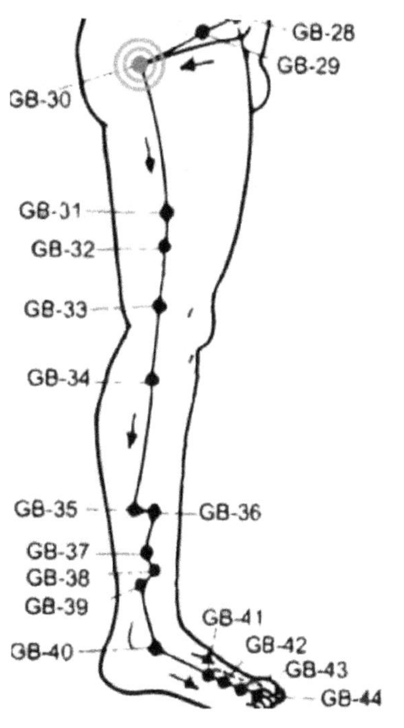
GB-28
GB-29
GB-30
GB-31
GB-32
GB-33
GB-34
GB-35
GB-36
GB-37
GB-38
GB-39
GB-40
GB-41
GB-42
GB-43
GB-44

Important Points on the Ren Meridian

Ren 3 Location: This point is located directly below the umbilicus. Find the umbilicus, then move downwards 4 Cun. This is Ren 3.

Indications: This is **an excellent point to use for all Urinary Bladder problems.** It is **especially good to use for painful urination or involuntary retention of urine.**

Ren 4 Location: 3 Cun directly below the umbilicus.

Indications: **Good point for any menstruation problem, including cramps or irregular cycle. This point reflexes to the Kidney/Adrenals and is a good tonification point of the body. Use for chronic low energy, as well as any Kidney/Adrenal problem.**

Ren 6 Location: 1.5 Cun below the umbilicus.

Indications: This point is called **Qihai (**pronounced Chi-high) and means the "Sea of Chi." This point is your power point, which is called the **Dantien and Hara** in various eastern traditions. It is where martial arts masters get their power from.

This is one of the best tonification points in the body because, like Ren 4, it connects to the Kidney/Adrenals and will build up their store Chi – which then goes to fuel all the other organs of the body. Use this point along with Ren 4 for a good tonification. You can gently massage these points, or you can channel Chi into them through laying-on-of hands therapy. Broadcasting a red light over these points for at least five minutes is another way of sending energy to the Kidney/Adrenals.

Ren 6 can also be used for **any menstruation problem, as well as Large Intestine difficulties.**

Ren 12 Location: This point is located in the exact center of a line running between the umbilicus and the end of the Sternum (the breastbone).

Indications: **Good for any Stomach/Spleen problem, especially stomachache.**

Ren 14 Location: This point is 1 Cun below the end of the Sternum.

Indications: **Good point for all Heart related problems.**

Ren 17 Location: In the middle of the Sternum, level with the nipples. Find the depression on the Sternum. This is Ren 17.

Indications: **Good for cough, especially chronic cough. An excellent point for heartburn.** Also good for resolving excessive phlegm.

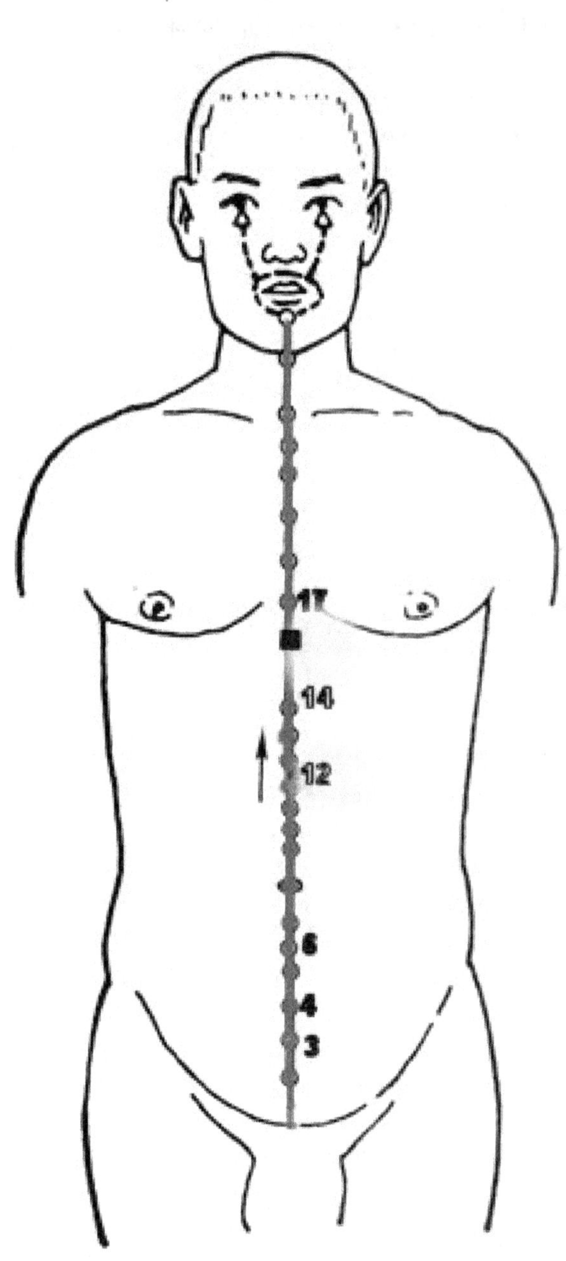
17
14
12
6
4
3

Important Points on the Du Meridian

Du 1 Location: Between the sexual organs and the anus.
Indications: **Excellent point for Prostate Gland enlargement and pain.**

Du 4 Location: Just below the 2nd Lumbar Vertebrae, on the same level as U.B. 23.
Indications: This point, known as Mingmen, the **"Gate of Life,"** moves Chi directly to the Kidney/Adrenals and is therefore **an excellent tonification point**. It is **the Qihai of the back.**

Treat all Kidney/Adrenal problems with Du 4. Since the point is hard to manipulate by hand, you can simply apply laying-on-of-hands therapy over it.

Du 15 Location: .5 Cun below Du 16.
Indications: **Hoarseness of voice.**

Du 16 Location: This point is located just below the base of the back of the skull in the exact center point. Feel for a depression.
Indications: **Headache and neck rigidity.**

Du 20 Location: At the apex of the head. Start with your fingers touching the tops of the ears. Then move your hands upwards towards the top of the head. Where your hands meet is Du 20.

Indications: This point **brings the Chi and blood upwards in the body to the head.** It is a good point for **dizziness and vertigo.** It is **also good for prolapses** in the body (where the tissues hang down), such as rectal prolapse and varicose veins.

Du 26 Location: One-third of the way down the philtrum, the shute below the nose that leads to the upper lip.

Indications: **Good for bringing a person back to normal consciousness.** Good for **fainting, epileptic seizure**, etc. Give strong stimulation to the point.

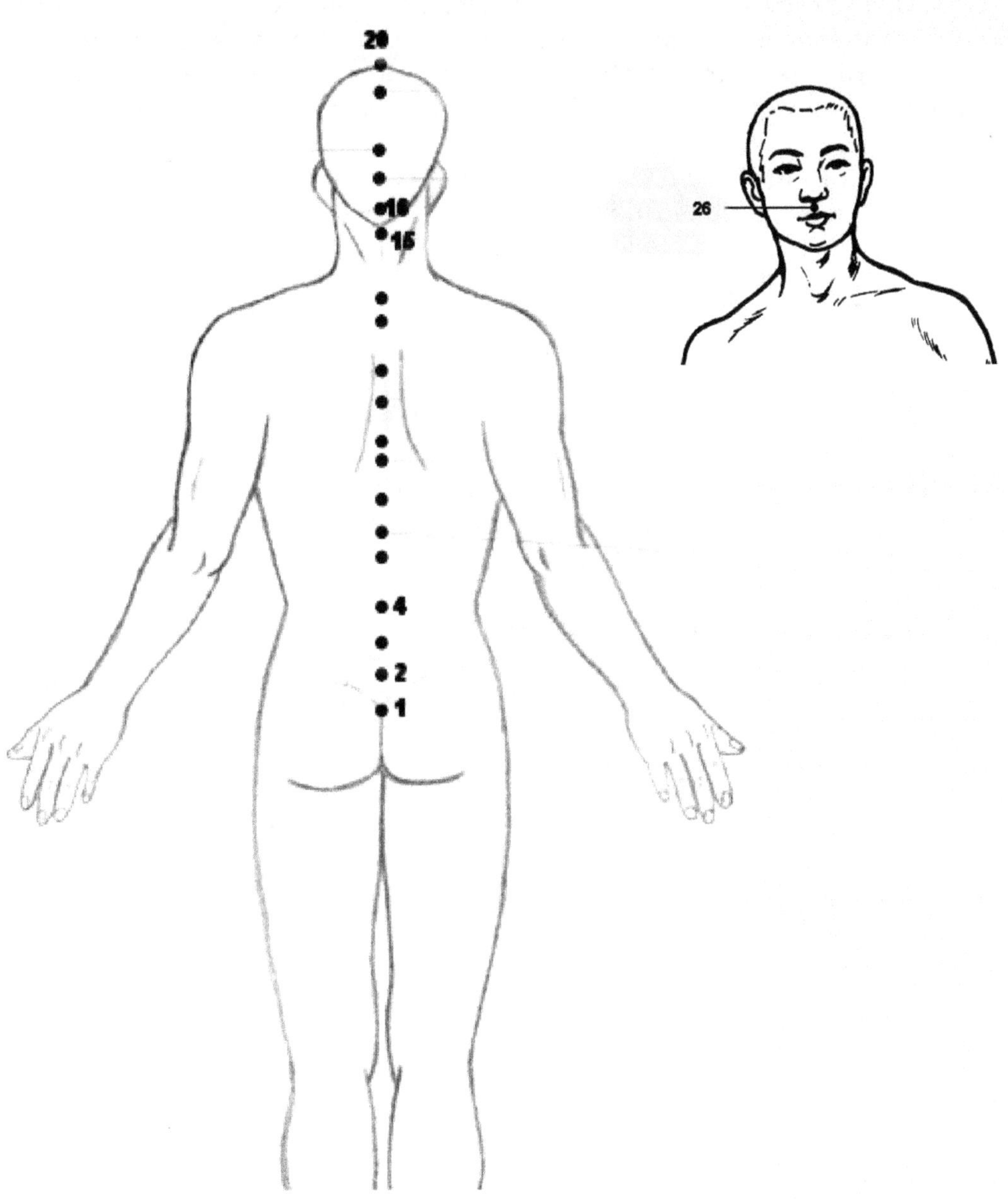
20
18
15
4
2
1
26

Point Combinations

To facilitate the most efficacious acupressure treatment use point combinations. The following are the best point combinations for the given organ imbalances. Note: You can use all the points listed for each organ disharmony every session, or you can start with combination 1 and later use combinations 2, 3, or 4.

For Lung problems: Combination 1 - Lu 1, U.B. 13
Combination 2 – Lu 7, L.I. 4
Combination 3 – Lu 5, U.B. 13

For Spleen/Stomach problems: Combination 1 – St. 36, Spl. 6
Combination 2 – St. 36, Spl. 3
Combination 3 – St. 36, P.6
Combination 3- St. 36, U.B. 21

For Heart problems: Combination 1 – H.7, U.B.15
Combination 2 – Ren 14, U.B.15
Combination 3 – H.7, U.B. 15

For Kidney/Adrenal problems: Combination 1 – K.3, U.B. 23
Combination 2 – Ren 4,6, Du 4
Combination 3 – K.7, U.B. 23

For Liver/Gall Bladder problems: Combination 1 – Liv.3, U.B. 18
Combination 2 - G.B. 36, U.B. 18
Combination 3 – Liv.3, L.I. 4

For Intestinal problems: Combination 1 – L.I. 4, St. 36
Combination 2 – L.I. 4, St. 37
Combination 3 – St. 25, U.B. 25
Combination 4 – St. 25, L.I. 4

Point Combinations for Common Ailments

Colds and Flu: L.I. 4, Lu 7, U.B. 13, Lu.1
Cold with fever: Add U.B. 60
Cold with phlegm: Add St. 40
Cold with cough: Add Lu. 5
Headaches: G.B. 20, Liv. 3, U.B. 18, G.B. 41, L.I. 4
Menstrual Cramps: Spl. 6, Ren 4, 6, G.B. 41, L.I. 4
Low Energy: St. 36, Spl. 6, Ren 4,6, Du 4, S.J. 5, S.I. 3
Tight Shoulders and Neck: G.B. 20, 21, U.B. 10, S.I. 3,11,12, S.J. 15
Diarrhea, Gas, Bloating: L.I. 4, St. 25, 36, 37

Stomachache: Ren 12
Constipation: St. 37, L.I. 4, S.J. 5
Nausea, Vomiting: P.6, St. 36, L.I. 4
Depression: H7, Liv 3, L.I. 4, P. 6, U.B 15

Tips for giving an Acupressure Treatment

Here are a few guidelines for giving an acupressure treatment:

Point manipulation: Use your thumb. Massage the point with your thumb for 10 seconds, pause for a few seconds, then resume for another 10 seconds, etc. It is good to work on a point for 2-5 minutes, but you might need to manipulate a point for more time or you might have to keep coming back to it. If you are massaging the shoulders and neck you will be able to feel how long you need to work. The muscles will begin to relax and loosen up. If you are treating a headache, cramps, a stomachache, etc, keep checking in with the person you are working with. Continue working on the points until your client has begun to feel some relief. Sometimes you may have to give more additional sessions of acupressure if you do not get the desired result in one session. Or, if the condition begins to return, which is sometimes the case with stubborn headaches, consider giving an additional session.

Excess, Deficient conditions: For excessive conditions, such as colds, menstrual cramps, hard shoulders and neck, headaches, excessive emotions, constipation, diarrhea, etc., strongly stimulate the chosen points with your thumb. For deficient conditions, such as chronic illness, very low energy, etc. use a soft manipulation. Also use a soft manipulation for older persons.

Treat both Front and Back points: If possible, when treating an organ imbalance manipulate points that correspond to that organ on both the back and front of the body. Start by having the person lay on his or her back while you manipulate the points on the front of the body, and then have them turn over so you can manipulate the back points.

Use the Four Gates: For any excessive condition, whether it is physical or emotional, consider using the Four Gates. These are the L.I. 4 points on both hands and Liv. 3 on both feet. These points will unblock the Chi in both the lower (Liv. 3) and upper parts of the body (L.I. 4). These are excellent points to use when beginning an acupressure session in order to initially get the Chi moving throughout the body. They also relieve any emotional stress and help the client to relax. For a general relaxation session, use these points with H.7.

Windows to the Sky Acu-Points

Windows to the Sky Acu-Points were first used by Taoist Monks thousands of years ago to awaken the psychic and spiritual centers of perception within each other. Besides providing visionary experience, they also assist one in uniting with their Higher Self and their Guides and Teachers in order to receive guidance regarding how to heal and release the old traumas and difficult feelings and memories that can arise during an acupressure session. Moreover, they can also can give a person a fresh perspective on their personal lives and the directions they have taken.

The Windows to the Sky Acu-Points

These points include both psychic/spiritual points and releasing points.

Psychic/Spiritual Points on the neck: L.I. 18, S.I. 17, S.J. 16, Du 15, U.B. 10.
Massage each of these points for 30 seconds to one minute.

Other Psychic/Spiritual Points

Yintang – This point is an "extra point" and lies directly between the eyebrows. Its helps to activate the Third Eye.

Du 20 – At the apex of the head. This point brings Chi up within the body to activate centers in the head.

H.7 – Calms the mind and spirit and helps one transcend. It also opens the Heart to help one experience divine love.

Liv 3, L.I. 4 – Calms the emotions and activates the Astral Body.

Spl 6 – Promotes production of blood that calms the Heart and spirit and induce meditation.

Windows to the Sky Releasing Points

Always use L.I. 4 and Liv 3 for releasing therapy. They help release blocked emotional residue throughout the body, as well as emotional congestion in the Liver, the seat of the emotional body. For releasing specific emotions, use the following points along with Liv 3 and L.I. 4, and always end a releasing session with H7.

Anger: Liv. 3, U.B. 18
Fear: U.B. 23, K. 1, 3
Grief: Lu 9, U.B. 13
Worry: St. 36, Spl 6
Raucous Joy: H7, U.B. 15.

Points for other emotional/mental issues:

Lack of Willpower: Du 4, U.B. 23, Ren 4, 6, St. 36
Emotional and Mental Confusion: Du 4, St. 36, U.B. 23, Liv 3, H7, K.1
Lack of self-love: H7

Kundalini Activation Points

Special Kundalini activation points can be used by themselves and/or along with Windows to the Sky Acu-Points to activate the alchemical, transformative energies in the body and assist in the activation of the higher spiritual centers. These are the important Kundalini points:

S.I. 3 – This point moves Chi up the Du Meridian. It can help activate Kundalini and move it up the spine.

Note: when combined with Lu 7, S.I. 3 will cause the Chi to rise up the back and down the front of the body, thus creating the Microcosmic Orbit.

U.B. 23, Du 4 – These points direct energy directly to the "Moving Chi between the Kidneys," which is the name for the Mundane Kundalini in Chinese Medicine. With the right vibration or transmission of energy, a higher frequency of this energy, i.e., the Spiritual Kundalini, can be awakened.

Du 20 – This point moves all the energy in the body to the head, including the Mundane Kundalini (normal Chi) and the Spiritual Kundalini.

It is helpful to use these points while also placing Kundalini activating stones in the person's hand and/or along their back. These stones include Meteorites, Black Tourmaline, Obsidian, and Smokey Quartz. Clear Quartz, which has a fiery energy, can also activate Kundalini. These stones should be held in the hands and against the base of the spine. This will help to both activate and ascend Kundalini. If you do not have any stones available, use your body as a magnet to move your client's Kundalini by holding your right, positive hand over his or her base of the spine and place your left, negative hand at the top of his or her head.

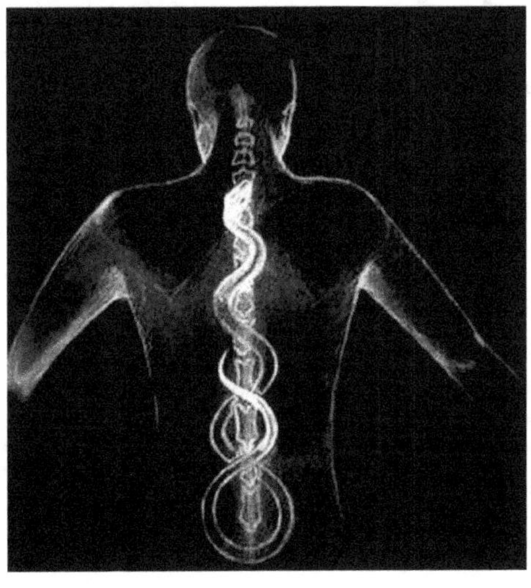

Combine Windows to the Sky and Kundalini Activating Points with Seven Ray Reiki Kundalini Activating Symbols

For a powerful activating and awakening session combine the Window to the Sky points with the other psychic/spiritual points, the releasing points, and the Kundalini points. You can also activate the seven chakras during these sessions by simply placing stones over the chakras, or by shining colored lights on them, or by playing the corresponding note or musical selection.

These symbols, and how to draw them on a client's body, is presented in the following chapter on Seven Ray Reiki.

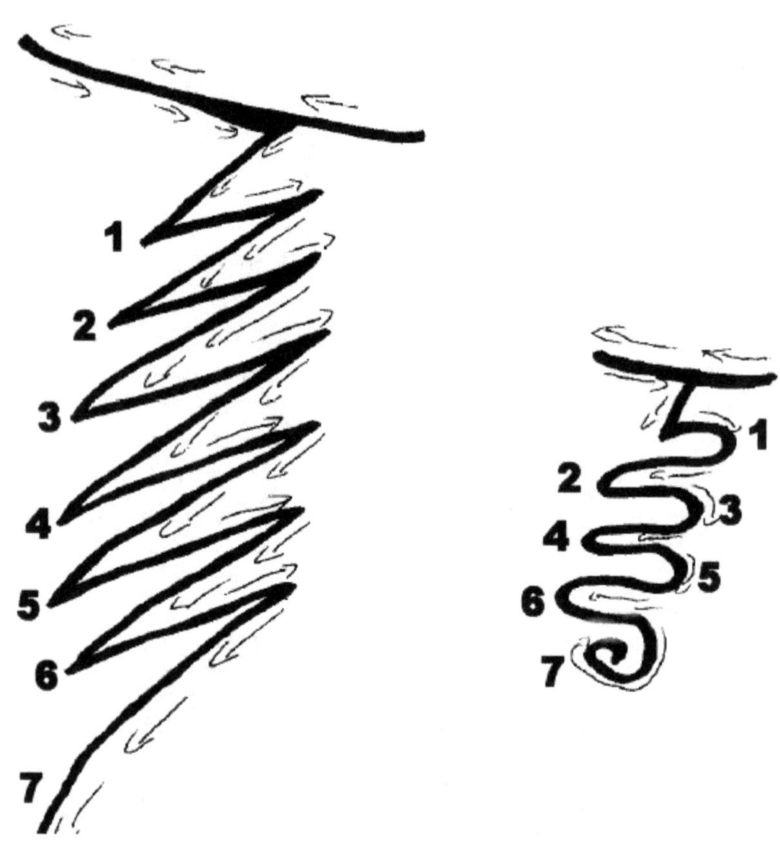

When to use Windows to the Sky Acu-Point Therapy

This form of Acu-Point therapy is excellent to use at any time as long as the client is interested in healing on all levels – physical, emotional, and mental – and they want to progress spiritually. Windows to the Sky acupressure can open a person to parts of themselves that are normally shut down, such as divine love, and it can link them to other dimensions, guides, interdimensional communication, etc. Furthermore, Windows to the Sky Acu-Point Therapy can permanently open the psychic channels which give such experiences. But the most consistent benefit I have seen from the Windows to the Sky Acupressure is that it awakens and unites people to the wisdom and guidance of their Higher Selves. People almost always leave a Windows to the Sky Acu-Point Therapy session feeling clearer about their direction in life and how to confront their current issues and crises.

Combine Windows to the Sky Therapy with IEFs

To empower your Windows to the Sky Acu-Point Therapy combine it with an IEF, an Integrated Energy Field, which is explained in Chapter 7. An IEF will amplify the potential of a Windows to the Sky Acu-Point Therapy session exponentially. An IEF will facilitate an emotional release and psychic activation session with Windows to the Sky, and it will also help catalyze the awakening of Kundalini.

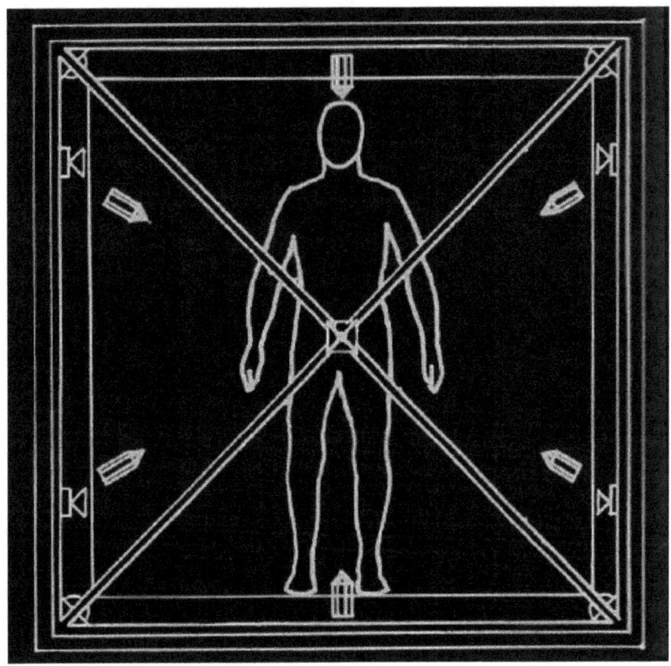

Acu-Point Charts

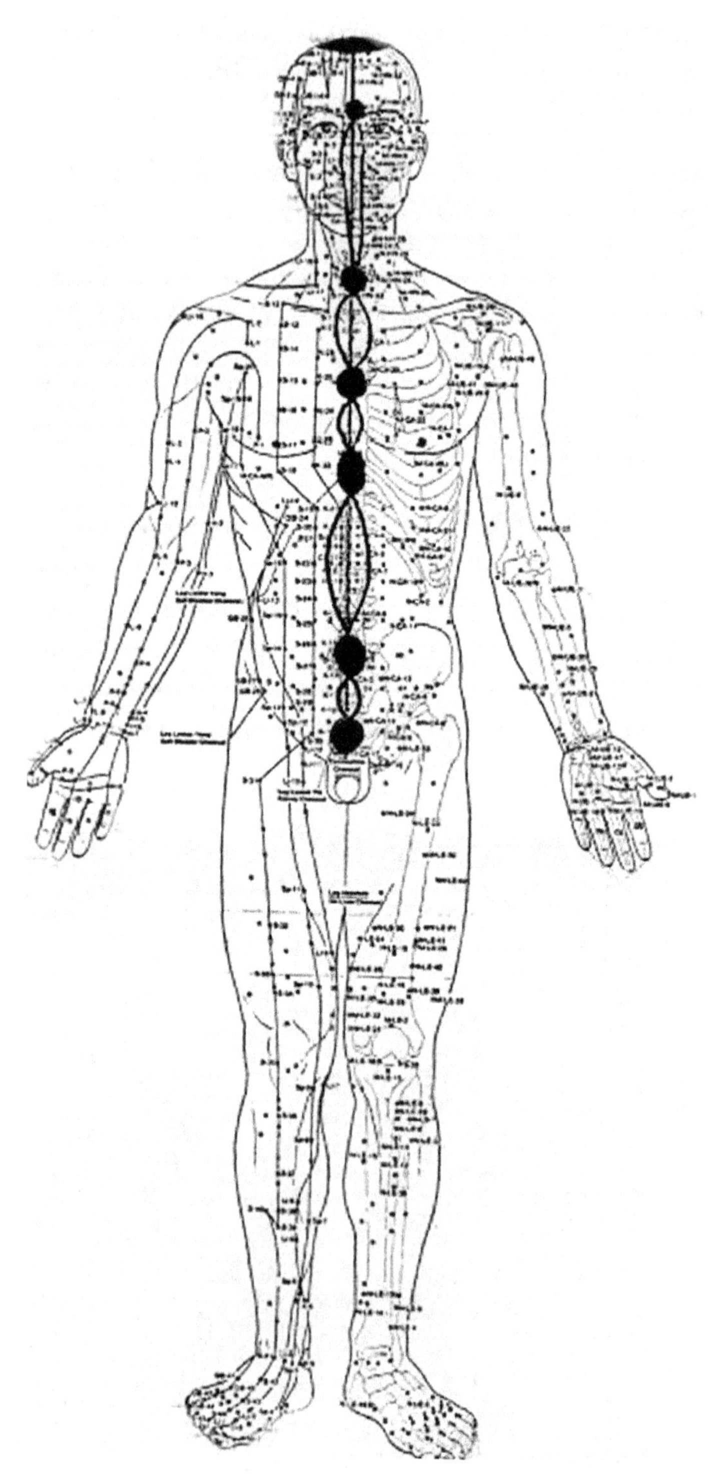

ARM

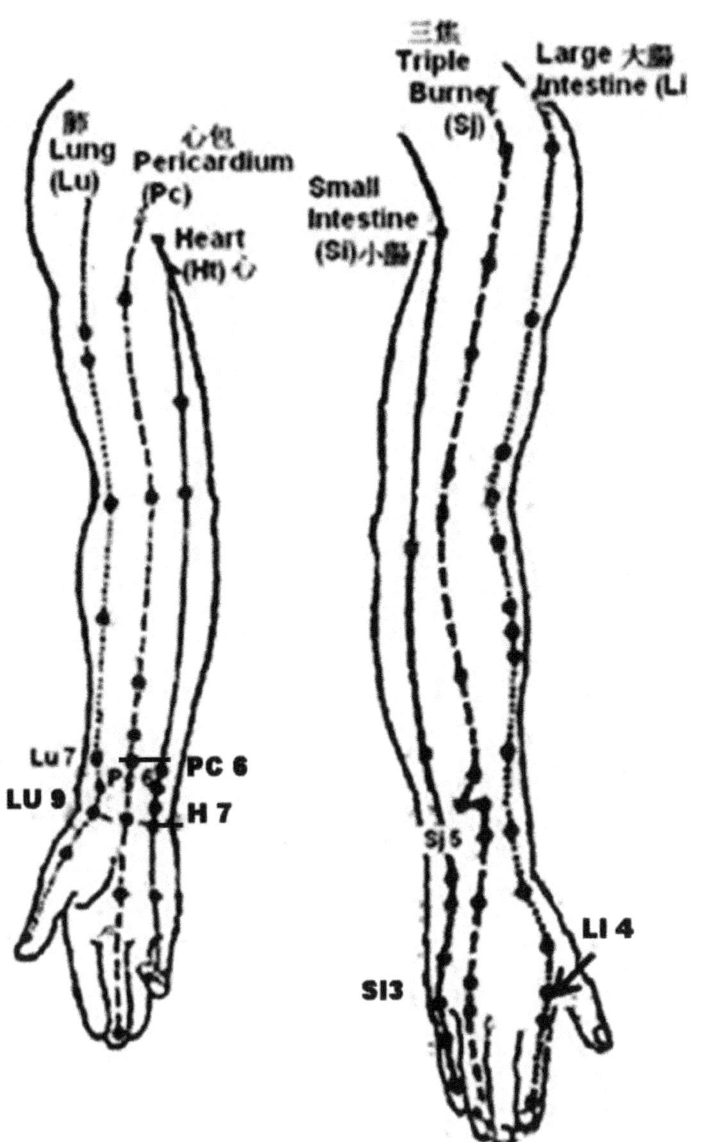

LEG

Gall Bladder Meridian
Gb31
Gb34
Gb43
Bladder Meridian
Bl60
Bl62
Stomach Meridian
St31
St 36
Spleen Meridian
Liver Meridian
Kidney Meridian
Ki1
Sp 6
K3
Liv 2
Liv 3
Sp4

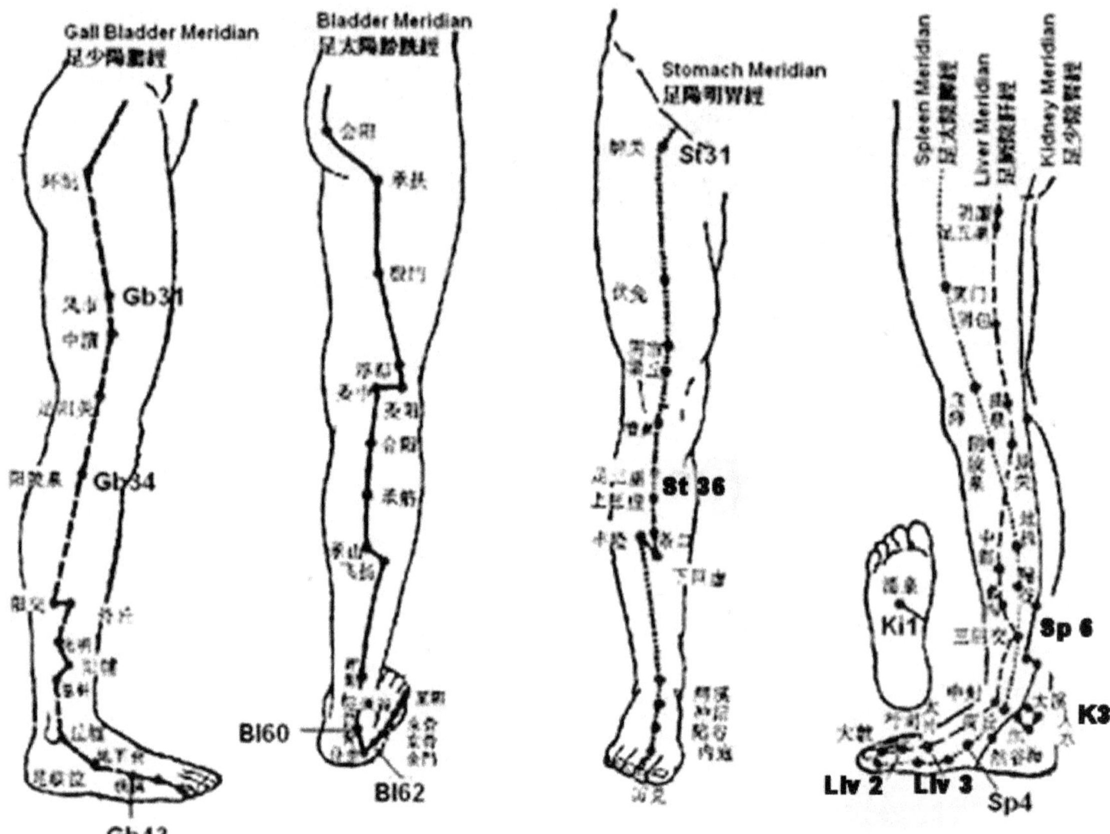

TORSO - FRONT

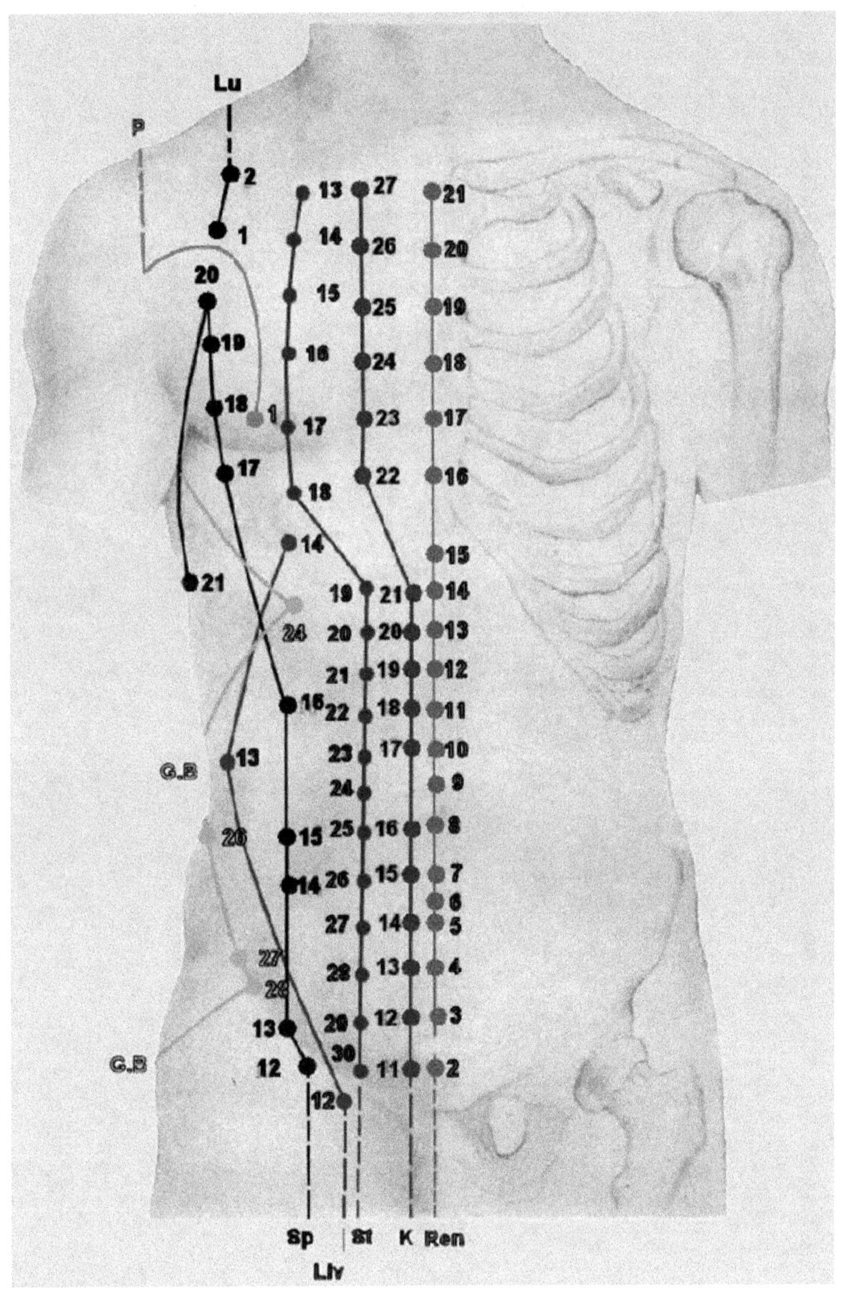

TORSO - BACK

G.B
15
21
L.I
14
13
11
14
15
16
S.J
12
41
13
12
10
12
13
42
11
14
43
11
15
44
9
10
16
45
S.I
9
17
46
8
18
47
7
19
48
6
20
49
21
50
5
22
51
25
G.B
4
23
52
24
3
25
26
31
27
32
28
53
33
29
2
30
54
34
1
35
Du
U.B
U.B

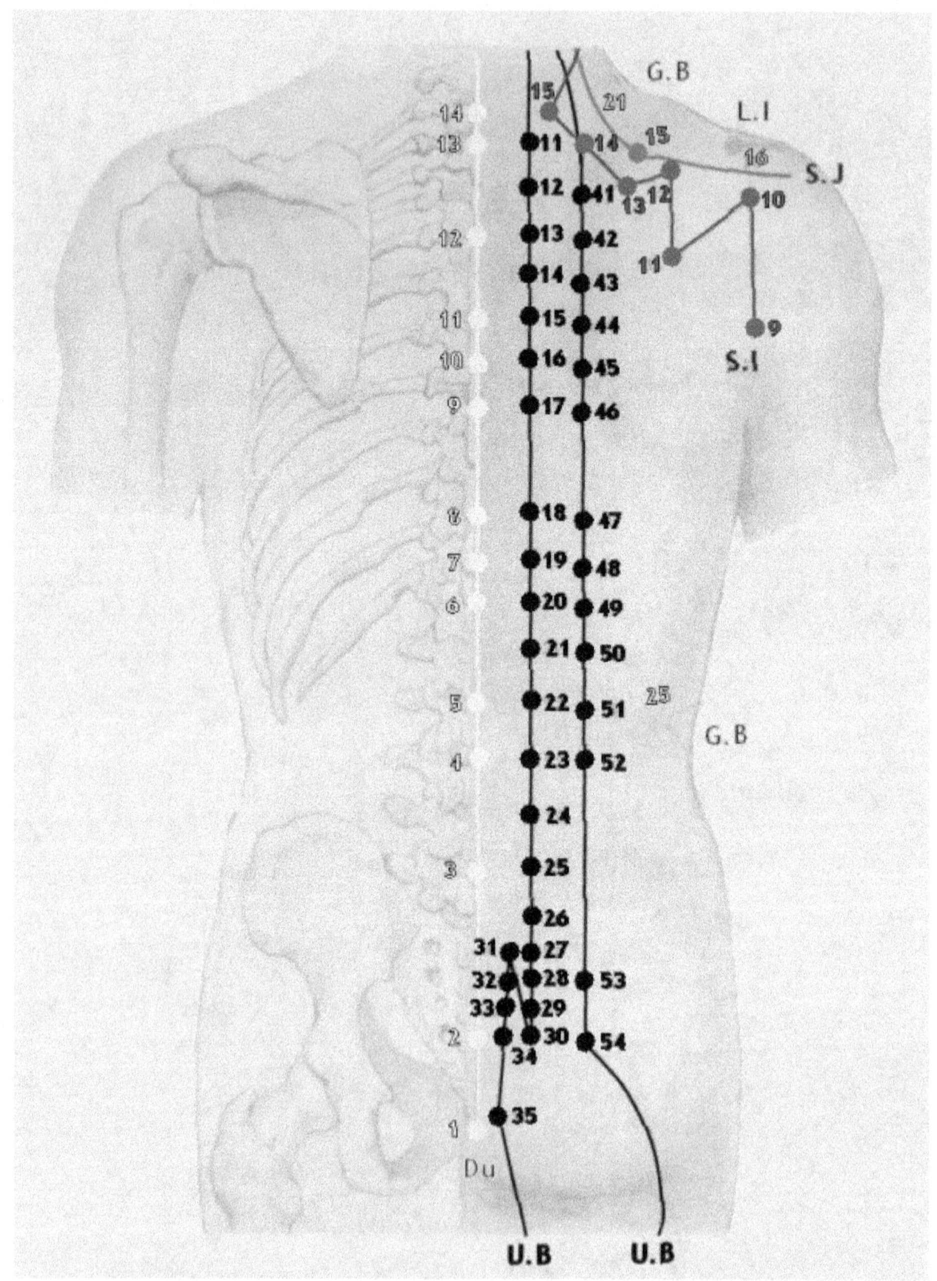

NECK & HEAD

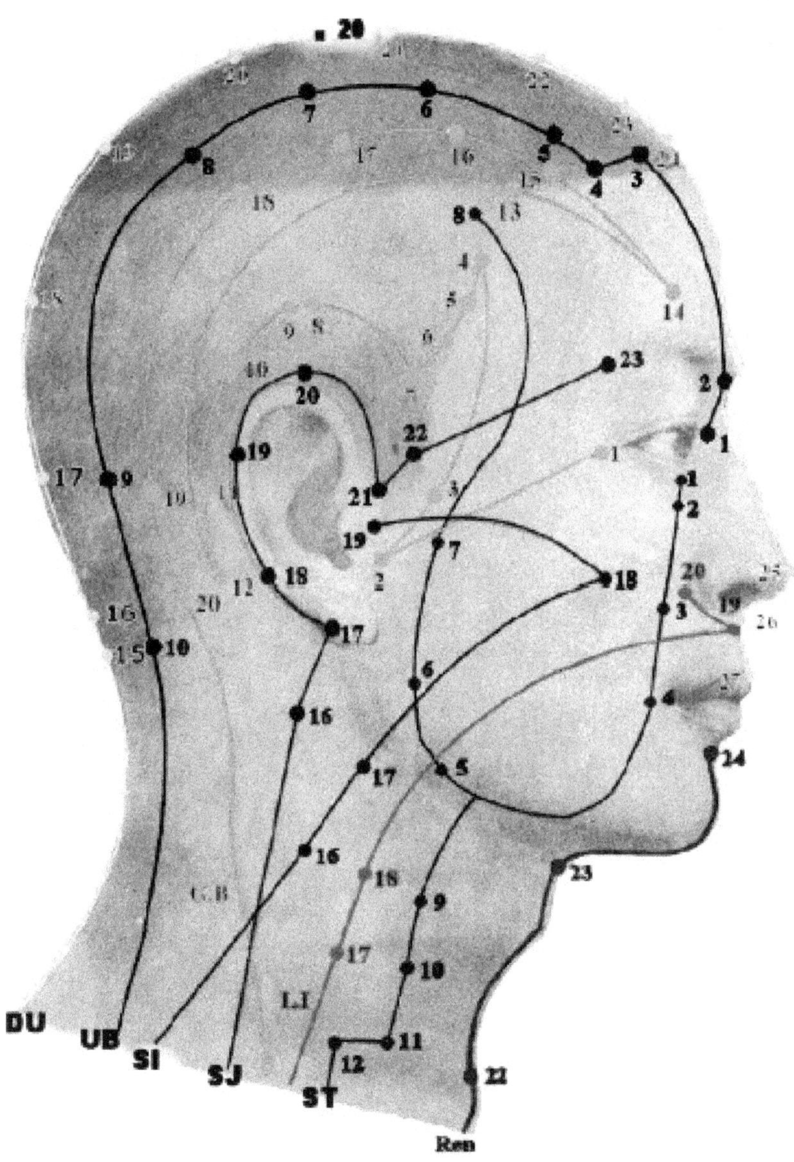

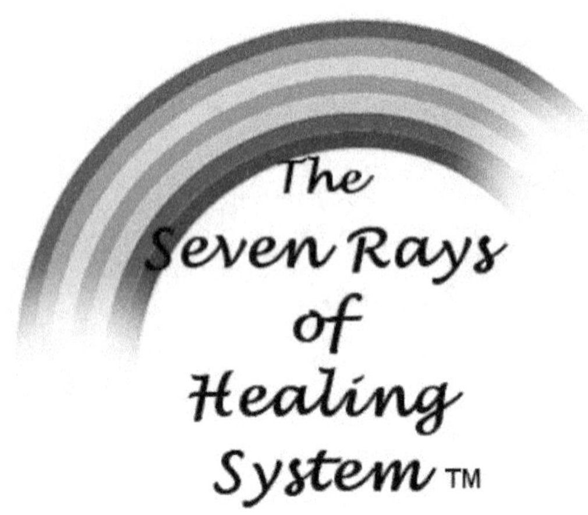

CHAPTER 6
Seven Ray Reiki & Polarity Therapy

Laying-on-hands healing has been an important part of Seven Ray Healing since the time of its inception on ancient Lemuria. Today, it is commonly known by the Japanese name Reiki Dr. Mikaomi (or simply Mikiao) Usui of Japan. Seven Ray Reiki is another "Lemurian" pillar of Seven Ray Healing and should always be considered as an essential part of any Seven Ray Healing treatment.

The History of Reiki

The practice of laying-on-of-hands healing was first taught as part of the Seven Rays of Healing System when it was brought to Earth by the Pleiadian-Venusian missionary Sanat KKumara, the Lord of the Seven Rays. According to the adepts of the Japanese Mikkyo sect of Buddhism, Sanat Kumara, whom they refer to in their tradition as Sonten (a name that is translated as “Universal Life Force”) arrived on our planet as pure life force energy from Venus approximately 6½ million years ago. They maintain that he had three aspects to his nature, each of which corresponds to one of the three powers of the life force: creation, preservation, and destruction. The power of the life force that Sonten is mainly associated with is its destructive/transformative power. This is the frequency of the life force known in other traditions as the transformative Kundalini power. Thus, according to the Japanese Mikkyo sect, the first teacher of Reiki, Sonten, was both an embodiment of the life force as well as its first terrestrial teacher.

After reaching Earth, Sonten or Sanat proceeded to make his home inside the sacred Japanese mountain of Kurama, a name that reflects his other name of Kumara.” At that time Japan was part of Lemuria, the Pacific Continent where today most other esoteric traditions record that Sanat Kumara first landed on Earth from the asterism of the Pleiades via the planet Venus and then became the Spirit of the Earth and the first King of the World. Since his arrival, Sanat Kumara has been pure life force that his mother, the Goddess of Earth, gives birth to each year. His annual life force body condenses and crystallizes into the variegated forms of green vegetation that populate the planet between spring and fall. As the life force, Sanat Kumara is also known as the ubiquitous Green Man, who is known among the Arabs as Khadir, the Greeks as Dionysus, the Egyptians as Osiris, the Yezidis as the Peacock Angel, the Hopis as Masau'u, etc.

It is because of Sanat Kumara’s residence within Mt. Kurama that the Mikkyo Buddhist sect erected a shrine in honor of Sonten and his three powers on the path leading to its summit. This temple was first built in 770 A.D. about half-way up the mountain. The sacred geometrical symbols that currently adorn it are the geometrical form bodies of Sanat Kumara or Sonten as the pure life force.

It was to this temple on Mt. Kurama that Dr. Usui came to worship in the late 1800's. The doctor had traveled the world seeking spiritual wisdom regarding healing and enlightenment but had not yet found the truth that he sought in any existing tradition, although he believed that the laying-on-of-hands healing that Jesus and his disciples practiced was the highest and most spiritual form of healing and he resolved to understand how to perform it. With this goal in mind Dr. Usui came to Mt. Kurama in order to purify himself and open up psychically to the unwritten records of spiritual healing by undergoing a 21 day fast.

On the 21st and final day of his fast Dr. Usui perceived a bright light rushing towards him following the morning sunrise. The light moved into his third eye of wisdom and the doctor temporarily lost consciousness. In that state he saw "millions and millions of rainbow bubbles,"which then coalesced into a group of symbols. Dr. Usui intuitively understood that through the use of these symbols he could perform laying-on-of-hands therapy with the same power that Jesus and his disciples had.

Dr. Usui had his first opportunity to test his new-found knowledge of healing when he descended Mt. Kurama soon after his vision. After painfully stubbing his toe he instinctively placed his hands on it while using the healing symbols, and the toe was instantly healed. The doctor was acutely aware of how quickly his hands heated up as soon as he touched the toe, attributing it to an "attunement" from the spirit of the mountain, whom he had worshiped for years as Sonten or Sanat Kumara.

When Dr. Usui returned to Tokyo he set up a healing clinic and began to daily perform his revived form of laying-on-of-hands healing, which eventually became known as Reiki. His therapy was nothing short of miraculous, and soon many Japanese aspiring healers sought to learn his method. This was the beginning of Reiki training. The power that Dr. Usui had received from Sonten on Mt. Kurama was subsequently passed to his students through a series of "attunements," along with the symbols that had been revealed to him. These symbols are similar to those that decorate the Mikkyo temple on Mt. Kurama and are geometrical renditions of the Lord of Reiki, Sonten or Sanat Kumara.

Before Dr. Usui died he passed the power of the revived Reiki lineage to Chujiro Hayashi, although the doctor also initiated 18 other Reiki Masters with the power to attune others to Reiki. Hayashi passed the grandmastership of the Reiki lineage to Hawaya Takata, who had come to Tokyo from her home in Hawaii for healing from the master. Takata in turn passed the lineage to her granddaughter, Phyllis Furumoto, who brought the art of Reiki to the USA. She became the grandmaster of the *Reiki Alliance*, and continues to serve in that capacity today.

For more information on the ancient history of Reiki, read *Reiki Fire* by Frank Arjava Petter.

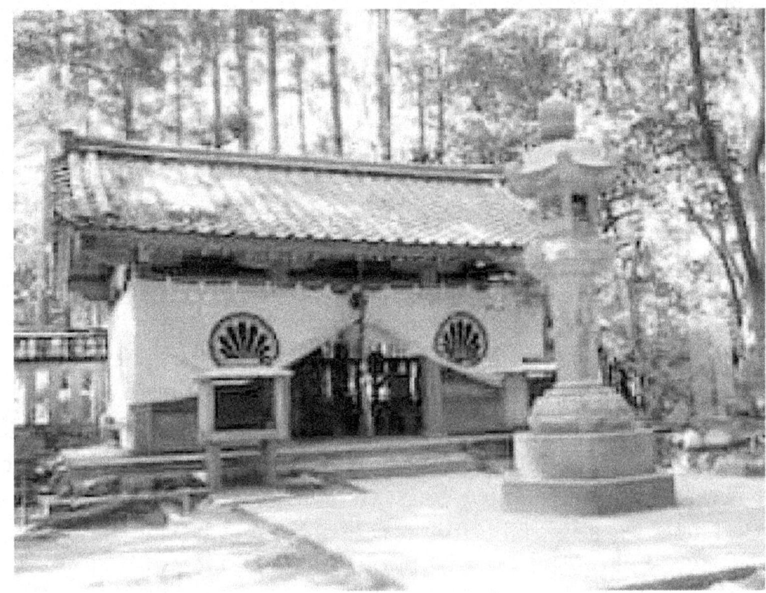

The Temple of Sonten on Mt. Kurama

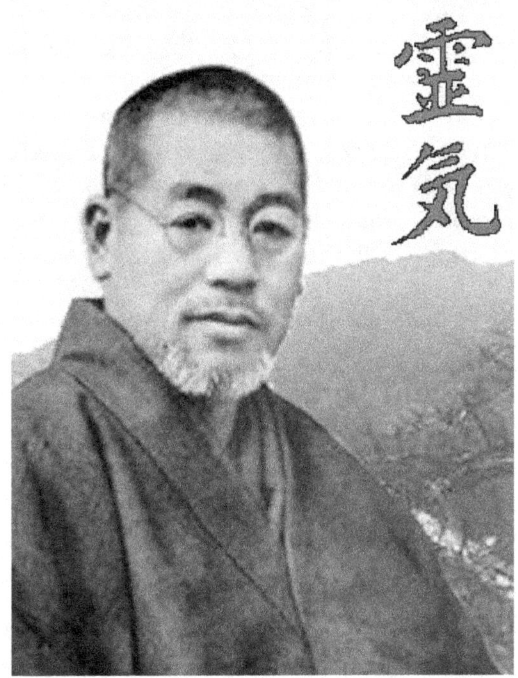

Dr. Mikaomi Usu, the Modern Founder of Reiki

HOW TO PERFORM SEVEN RAY REIKI

How to Channel the Life Force

Everyone has Reiki. All people have life force moving out of their hands that they can direct into themselves or another person or life form for the purpose of healing. The "attunements" given as part of Reiki training are simply initiatory rites designed to open a person's channels and make them a better conductor of the universal life force. These channels are one's Nadis or Meridians that comprise their Dragon Body and can be cleared by various other means as well, including spiritual practices and acupressure. In general, the more evolved and purified a person is the more clear their channels are and the more life force they can channel through them. This explains why Jesus had such abundant life force moving through him. Thus, unless you desire to undergo Reiki training, the best way to become a more proficient channel of the life force is through observing regular spiritual practices, such as yoga, meditation, prayer, as well as living a pure, honest, compassionate and righteous life. It is also recommended that to initially open your channel and then to keep it open you should practice the Dragon Body Activation Technique 1-2x a day. This technique is explained in Appendix 2.

In order to initially get the life force flowing out of your hands just before you give a laying-on-of hands treatment to yourself or someone else, exhale sharply 3x out of your mouth or nose. Then rub you hands briskly together to generate heat. You should then notice some increased energy moving out of your hands. Then, as you work on yourself or another person, place your hands over the body region, organ, or chakra that requires balancing and healing. Leave them in place until there is a new sensation, referred to in Reiki nomenclature as a "pulse." This lets you know your work is complete and you need not continue to transmit anymore life force into the area. Typically this takes 3-5 minutes. Your body will then absorb the received Reiki and move it exactly where it needs to go.

When placing your hands on a body area bring them tightly together in order to keep all the life force in your hands flowing to one specific area. Since it is not always advisable to place your hands directly on an open tissue wound or on a red hot sprain or trauma, place your hands above and/or on both sides of the afflicted area.

To Intensify Reiki - To intensify the amount and force of the Reiki moving from you and into your client, consider wearing bands or material around your wrists under which you place either single terminated quartz crystals laid against the skin with their terminations pointed towards your hands, or better yet, double terminated crystals pointed towards both the elbow and hand so energy can move in both directions. Athletic wrist bands work excellent for this.

Call forth Sanat Kumara, Sophia, or Lord/Lady of the Ray

When you are giving Seven Ray Reiki to another person call forth Sanat Kumara, the Lord of the Seven Rays, or Sophia, Lady of the Seven Rays, and/or one of the lord or ladies of the person's ray to move through you to them. And then while channeling Reiki you can also visualize the color of the needed ray moving down your arm and into them. If you are working on a specific organ or body part, call forth Sanat Kumara, Sophia or a lord or lady of the ray that governs the organ or body part you are working on.

Practice: Place your hands on yourself or another person. Call forth Sanat Kumara, Sophia, and/or a Lord of Lady of a Ray and ask them to move their healing energy through you. Continue to call them forth by name until you experience an inner energy shift. Perhaps you will feel energy pulse in your hands and/or they will heat up. If you or they can feel some distinct increase in the energy coming from your hands, then you will know that your invocation was successful. Thank the Lord or Lady and continue with your treatment.

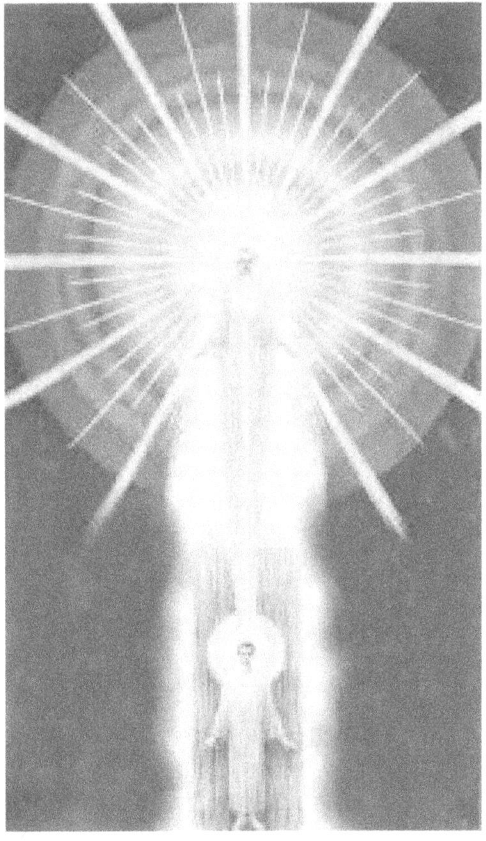

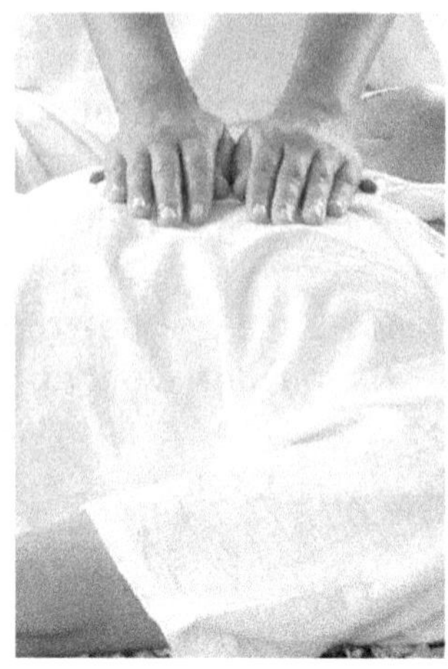

Hold hands close together when giving a
Seven Ray Healing treatment

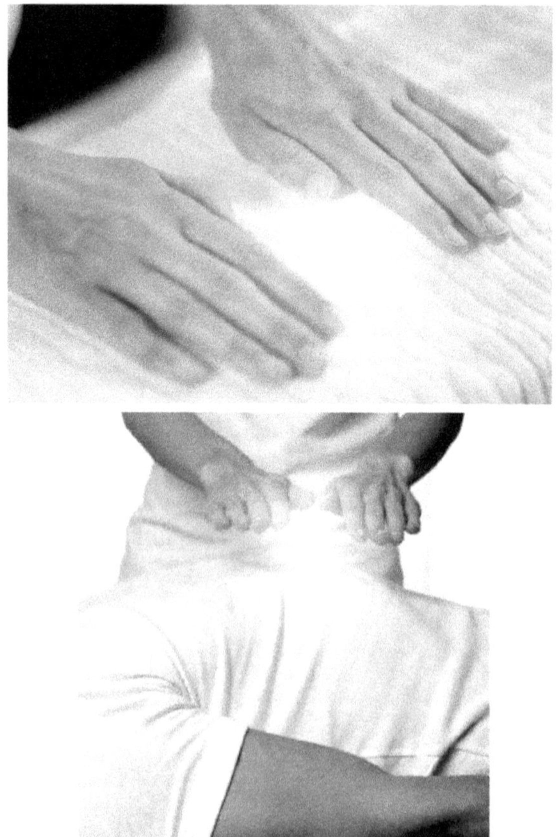

Place your hands above and/or on either side of
of open wounds and very sensitive and inflamed conditions.

The Sacred Reiki Symbols of Sanat Kumara

All the healing symbols of Reiki represent Sanat Kumara. Some represent his seminal yantra or "geometrical form body," while others are the shapes taken by Sanat Kumara in his manifestation as the life force. All these symbols work to move and increase Reiki in the body.

The Yantra of Sanat Kumara

The yantra or geometrical form body of Sanat Kumara is a six-pointed star or Star of David. When you trace this star over the body of a client you are are creating a layer of balanced healing energy around and within them. If you trace the star over a specific body part or organ, you will also re-align the specific subtle currents of life force that surround the area.

With your fingers together and straight, use your right hand to trace first the upward triangle and then the downward triangle over the area you are working on. It is also good to repeat the name of Sanat Kumara while doing this. Or you can repeat one of his other names of Skanda, Murugan or Karttikeya. Trace the star 3x.

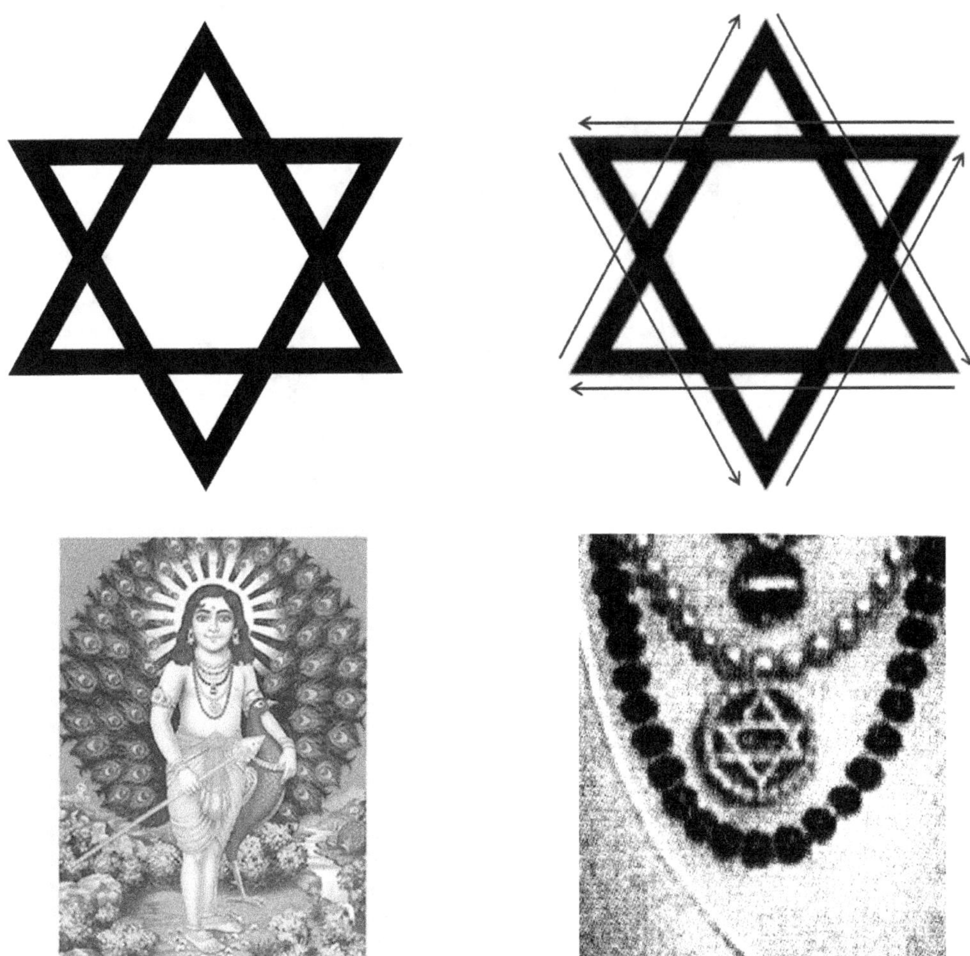

CHO KU REI

Pronounced CHO-KU-RAY

Before laying your hands over and/or directly on top of an area you can draw the Cho Ku Rei symbol over the area in order to increase the amount and intensity of life force that moves into it. Cho Ku Rei means “Placing all the powers of the universe here.” The spiral, which is the foundation of Cho Ku Rei, is the natural movement of life force.

Follow the guide below when drawing the Cho Ku Rei over a body area or chakra. Draw the symbol 1-3x while continually repeating "Cho Ku Rei."

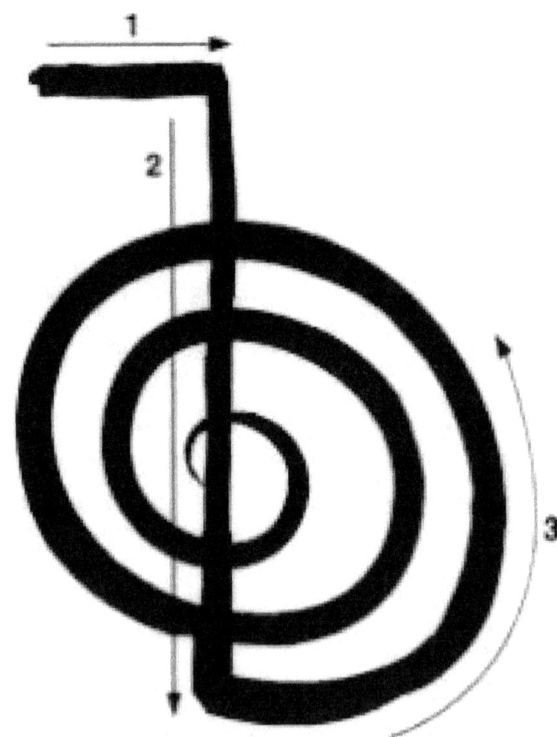

DAI-KO-MYO

Pronounced DIE-KO-MO

The Dai-Ko-Myo symbol has the same influence as the Cho Ku Rei symbol to increase the amount of energy moving into an area, but it also includes other important benefits.

The Dai-Ko-Myo, meaning "Great Bright Light," works on all the bodies and levels of a person to purify and heal. Besides contributing power to the physical and etheric bodies, it also has a very powerful effect in moving and bringing to the surface any corresponding emotional and mental blockages. When used in the healing and balancing of an organ and/or chakra, the Dai-Ko-Myo symbol will not only strengthen Seven Ray Reiki therapy but fully purify all the physical, emotional and mental toxins that have been contributing to the disharmony. The Dai-Ko-Myo generates the frequency of love and is thus good for healing any part of the body, especially the heart and Heart Chakra.

Follow the guide below when drawing the Dai-Ko-Myo over a body area or chakra. Draw the symbol 1-3x with the right hand while continually repeating "Dai-Ko-Myo."

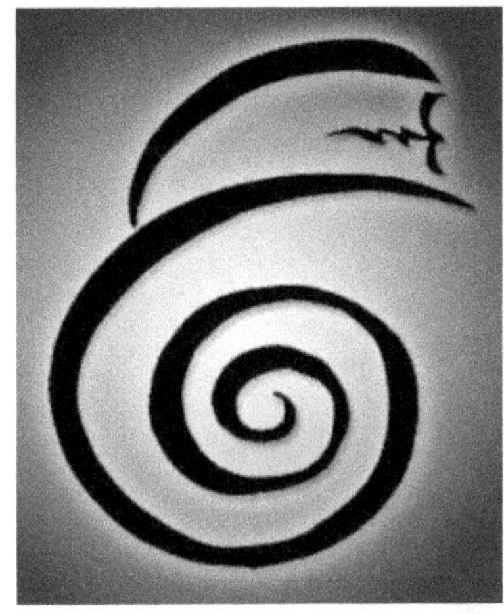

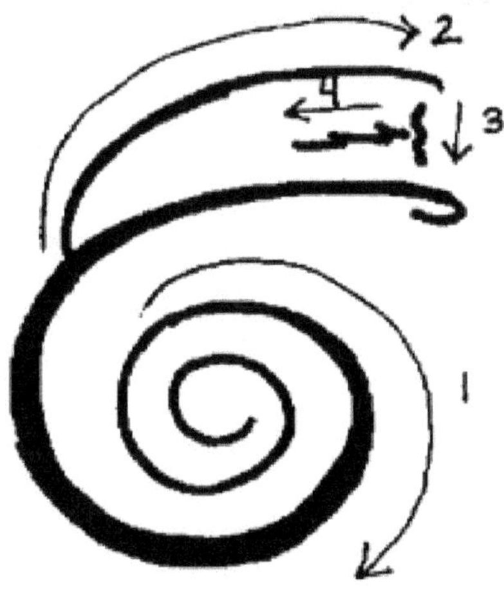

RAKU - Fire Serpent Symbols

The symbols below represent Sanat Kumara in his form of the Fire Serpent or Kundalini. They both have seven points or curves which represent the Seven Rays of Sanat's Kundalini body.

Both symbols below assist the movement of energy from the top of the head to the base of the spine, seat of the Kundalini power. The symbol on the left is yang and electric. It will be more direct and intense in action than the symbol on the right, which is soft, female and magnetic. To draw them on the body begin at the top of the torso on the front and/or back and follow the arrows while gradually moving to below the navel and the base of the spine. Either draw the male or female symbol by itself over the body, or draw both of them, one after the other, to get a more balanced result. You can also use the yang symbol for younger and stronger persons and the yin symbol for older and weaker individuals.

These symbols can be used for Kundalini activation and/or for getting the life force moving more freely throughout the body. They are very effective when a person's energy (and their lives) is bottled up and stagnant. And they are also good for those needing to be more grounded and/or feel the need to work on earth plane, physical issues, such as survival.

Trace the symbols over a person's body 3x while constantly repeating "Raku."

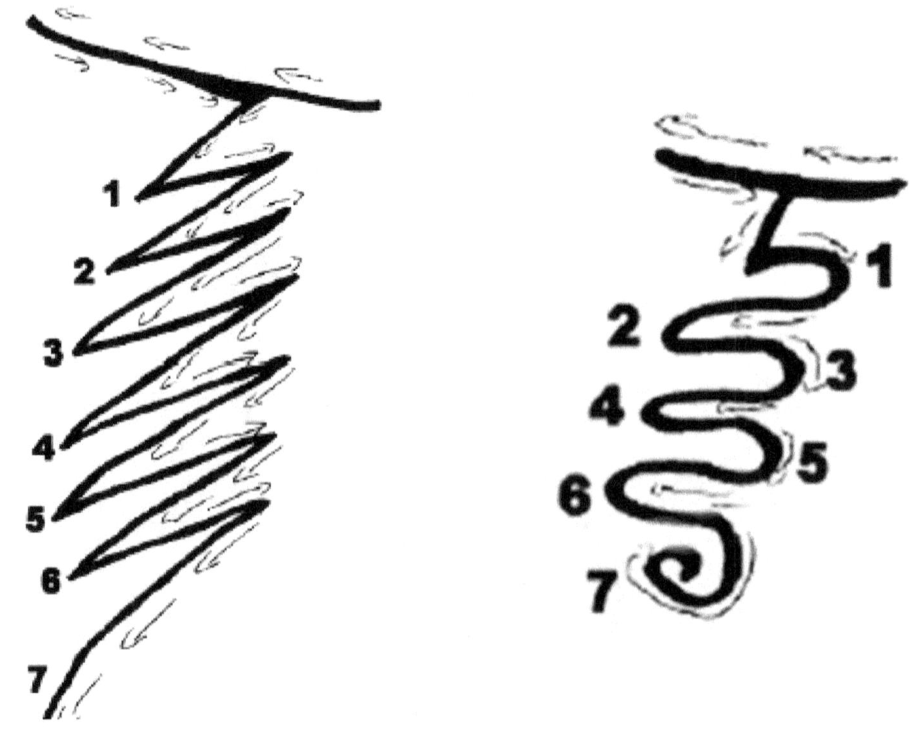

SEVEN RAY POLARITY THERAPY

Closely associated with Seven Ray Reiki, and an important adjunct to it, is Seven Ray Polarity Therapy. Whenever possible, combine Seven Ray Reiki Therapy with Seven Ray Polarity Therapy. This will align both the etheric Dragon Body and the Electromagnetic Body.

Seven Ray Polarity Therapy works to re-establish, re-align and enhance the longitudinal and latitudinal lines of electromagnetism that constitute a person's electromagnetic body. These lines run vertically, horizontally, as well as diagonally while moving between the body's positive and negative poles.

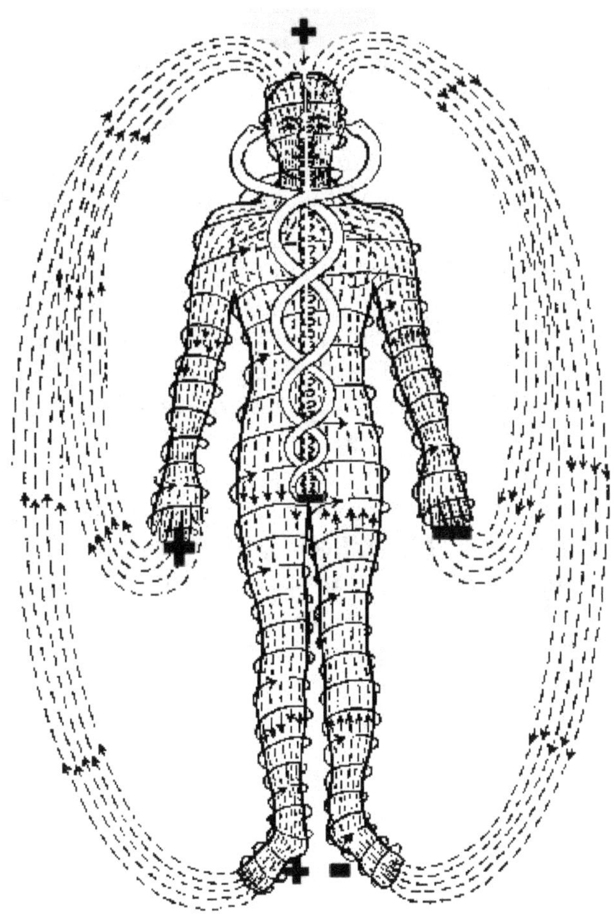

Positive and Negative Charges of the Body: The head and top of the body of a person has a positive charge and the feet and lower part of their body has a negative charge. The left side of the body is negatively charged and the right side has a positive charge.

HOW TO PERFORM SEVEN RAY POLARITY THERAPY

To perform Seven Ray Polarity therapy you will seek to establish or re-establish the currents of electromagnetism that run along a person's electromagnetic body. To do this you will use the charges in your own hands. Your right hand is positively charged and your left hand is negatively charged.

There are two approaches to re-establishing electromagentic currents in a body:

1. **Re-establish the currents of electromagnetism on any part of the body** by placing your right hand above your left hand, and/or your left hand on the person's left side and your right hand on their right side.
   a. **To balance a limb,** place your right hand at their shoulder or hip and your left hand at their hand or foot.
   b. **To balance an organ** place your left hand below it and your right above it and/or your left hand on the left side of the organ (the person's left side) and your right hand on the right side of the organ (the person's right side).

2. **Re-establish the currents of electromagnetism by making yourself part of the renewed circuit.** To do this touch your charged hand to its polarity on the client's body. Example: Join your right hand to their left hand and/or your left hand to their right hand, and vice versa. Then, since opposite charges attract, you will make a current that jumps from your positive or negatively charged hand to the client's positive or negative body part.
   a. **To establish a strong current up the back** touch the top of the person's head with your left hand and the base of their spine with your right.
   b. **To re-establish a strong vertical current** on the right side of the person's body, join their right hand and with your left hand and their right foot with your right hand. Vice-versa on the left side.
   c. **To re-establish strong diagonal currents** touch the person's right foot with your left hand and their left foot with their right hand, and vice versa.
3. **Hold your hands in place for a minimum of 1-2 minutes to establish or re-establish a current.**

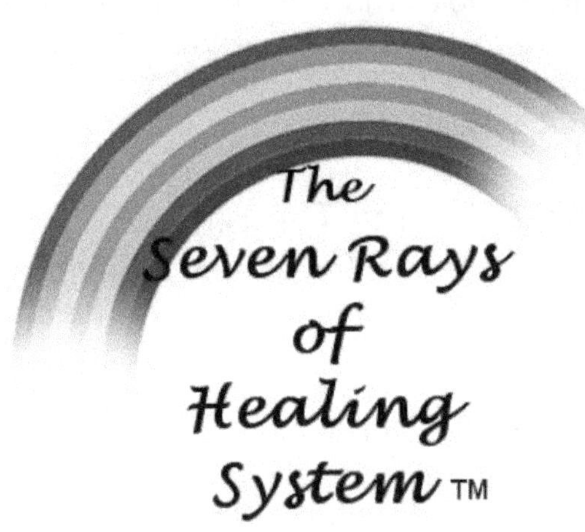

CHAPTER 7
Creating a Seven Ray Healing Temple

When you are ready to greatly empower your Seven Rays of Healing System practice you can construct a Seven Ray Healing Temple. This will create an environment that is highly charged with the healing and transformative life force, and it will give you a convenient place to keep all your healing tools and life force generators. This chapter will give you basic instructions for building a Seven Ray Healing Temple.

Building Your Seven Ray Healing Temple

The first step in creating a Seven Ray Healing Temple is to choose a location for it. The environment you choose should ideally be quiet and used solely for relaxation, healing and spiritual work.

The Shape of your Seven Ray Temple

There are many shapes you can use for your healing temple. Ideally you will want one that is balanced in its dimensions and symmetrical, and one that can easily and quickly facilitate the return of a person to their optimum state of balance. Its shape should be conducive to the accumulation of life force energy and also facilitate the movement of energy within the body of a client to expedite their healing. The best shape is one that naturally unites the male/female polarity to produce the life force in its geometrical form of the Golden Mean Spiral.

If your Seven Ray Temple is inside a pyramidal, circular or geodesic shaped building, then the polarity is being united and healing energy is being naturally produced and efficiently moving within it. There is nothing more you need to do. But in most cases your temple will be inside a common square or cube-shaped building or room. Since energy does not efficiently flow in such environments because its movement is deadened at the corners, you will need to make your room more energy conductive. However, if your square room is rectangular energy will naturally flow within it because its length is twice as long as its width. As shown below, the polarity that exists in a rectangle as the two squares it divides into engenders polarity union and the creation of the Golden Spiral, whose mathematical constant is Phi, 1.618.

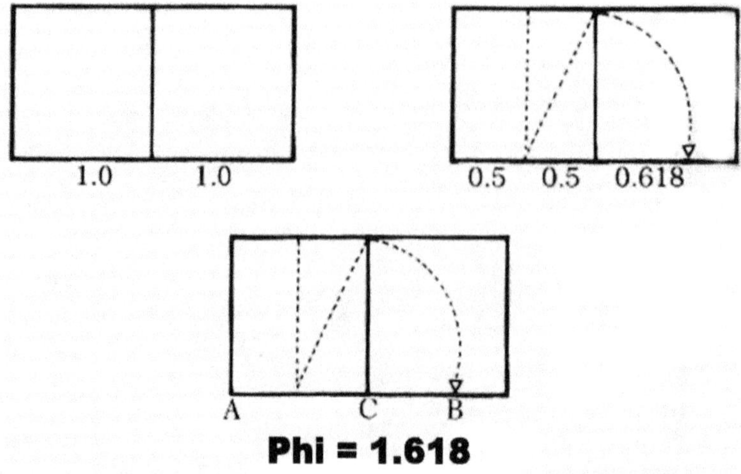

Because of its life force generating property the rectangle was used in the construction of Solomon's Temple, and later it became the shape of the thousands of Freemasonry Lodges modeled after it. It was also the shape of the King's Chamber in the Great Pyramid, which was used for alchemical initiations.

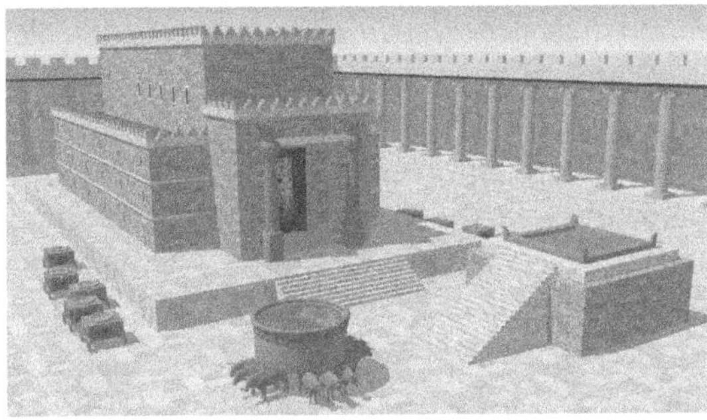

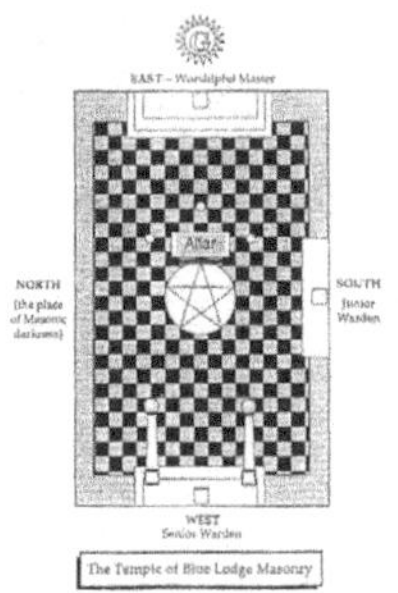

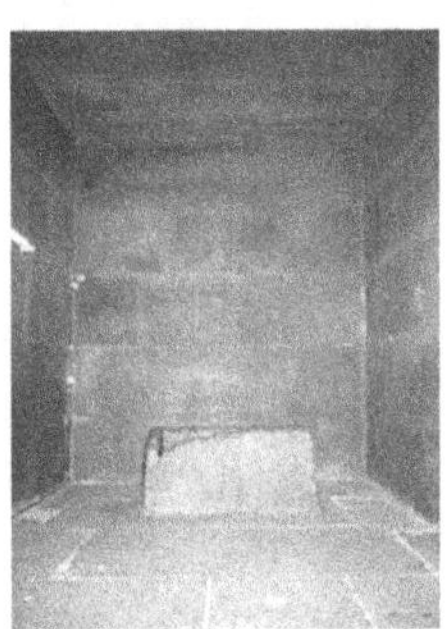

If you do not have a rectangular room you can make your square or cube room more conducive to energy flow by simply placing single or double terminated crystals at the corners with their terminations facing towards the center of the room. This is shown in the image below.

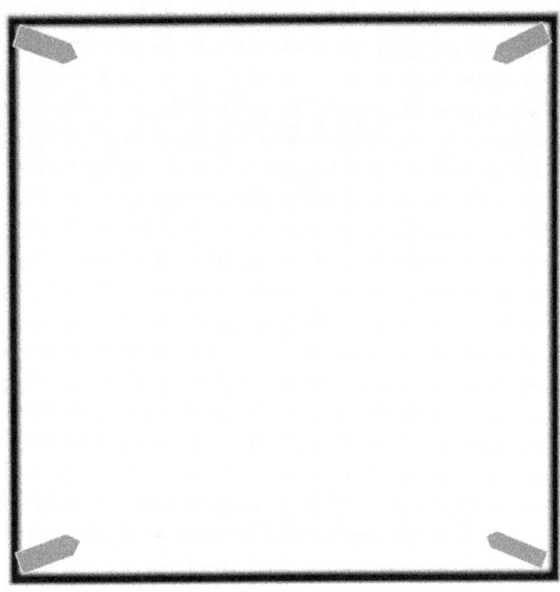

Next: To make your cube or square room even more conductive and empowered, you can place a Sacred Geometrical form, such as a pyramid, in the center of it to generate and move the alchemical life force. If a small or large geometrical shape made out of conductive material, such as metal or crystal, is placed in the center of the room it will radiate its transformative power throughout the room. A geometrical shape large enough for a person to sit or lie down within will serve as the alchemical cauldron and healing chamber of your temple. The inside of a pyramid is very powerful as a healing chamber because of the inner alchemical "fire" it produces. This truth is implicit in the name pyr-a-mid, meaning "fire in the middle."

The Alchemical Properties of a Pyramid

A pyramid naturally unites the universal polarity to produce the alchemical force in a few ways. 1. The structure unites the Sacred Geometrical forms of a Tetrahedron, which is one of the five Platonic Solids associated fire, with its opposing Platonic Solid, the Cube, which is associated with dense Earth. 2. The pyramid is also a polarity uniter through joining Spirit (the apex of the pyramid) to Earth (the square base). 3. And the pyramid unites the polarity by its energy flow, which creates a polarity-uniting octagon. Life force spirals around the outer frame of the pyramid and keeps going downwards after reaching the bottom of the structure until it reaches the apex of a mirror image pyramid below it. It then shoots energy up through the middle of the inverted pyramid and out the top of the upright pyramid. In doing so it produces the Platonic Solid known as the Octahedron, which, as seen below, is the union of the two opposing pyramids. Since the two etheric pyramids unite at the center of the octahedron, a special energetic zone of balance is created. This region corresponds with the floor of your physical pyramid, which is why treating a person who is lying down inside a pyramid will be both very balancing and transformative.

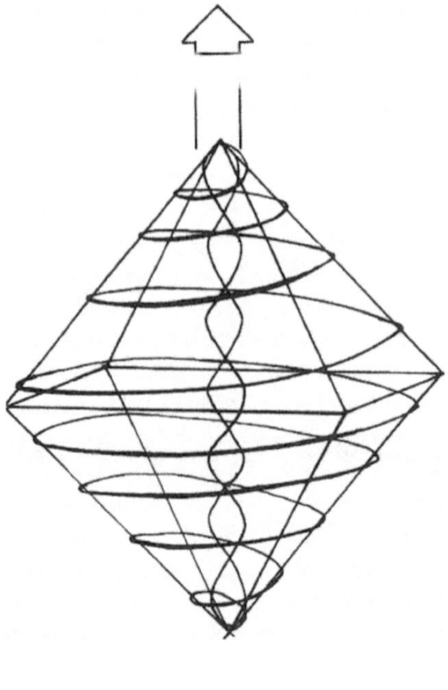

Choosing and Building a Pyramid

The Pyramid you use in your Seven Ray Healing Temple can be made of either metal or wood. A metal pyramid is more energetic and will produce results much faster than a wood pyramid, although a wood pyramid is preferable for long-term relaxation and for sleeping under. **A metal pyramid can be made of platinum, gold, silver, or copper.** Copper is just as effective as the other metals and much less expensive. **A wood pyramid can be made out of any kind of wood, but the harder the wood the more energy conductive it will be.** When set in place, one side of **a metal pyramid should face Magnetic North. By contrast, one side of a wood pyramid should align with True North.**

You can either purchase a pyramid online or construct one yourself. If you do not purchase a complete pyramid consider at least acquiring the corners. Then you can simply cut copper pipe or wooden dowel to the right length and fit them between the corners. **The best alchemical size of a small pyramid is seven feet square at the base. Seven is a number of alchemy and transformation.** You can also make one with a shorter or longer length, but seven feet will not only generate the power you want, it will also provide you enough room to move around a client who is lying down within it. **Whatever size you chose, for every foot of your base the uprights should be cut 11 1/2 inches.** So if your base length is seven feet (84 inches), your upright length will be 80.5 inches.

Using small Pyramids

Although the larger the pyramid you use the stronger will be its effect, **you can also get good results from a very small pyramid, perhaps one that is a foot square or 9" at the base. You** can simply place the small pyramid in the center of your temple and/or attach it to your ceiling so it hangs above the middle of the person you are working on. The best kind of pyramids for this purpose are gold plated, omni-directional pyramids that do not need to be oriented to magnetic north. You should be able to find these on the Internet. Otherwise use a small copper or wood pyramid.

Using rotating Pyramids

To spread the energy generated by the Pyramid around the room of your temple you can place it on a moving surface, like a fan or old record player. If you have suspended one from the ceiling you can attach it to a small motor that keeps it rotating, like the mirrored reflecting balls you find often used at discos. You might be able to find such a motor at an Internet site where such disco balls are sold. Or you can rig up your own continually rotating device.

Quartz Crystal Grids

A Quartz Crystal Grid can be used by itself or in conjunction with a pyramid. If you decide not to use a pyramid, a comparable energy field can be created by placing Quartz Crystals in certain alchemical grid patterns. These can be laid out in the center of your Seven Ray Healing Temple in a size large enough for a person to lie down inside them. **A diameter of seven feet for your crystal grid is recommended if it is not inside a pyramid, six feet if it is.**

The Crystals of a Crystal Grid should be large Generator Crystals. As a rule, these are one pound or more in weight. Or you can simply enlist your largest crystals to serve as Generator Crystals for your grid and reserve your smaller and/or clearer ones to be used as body crystals during the treatment. Place your Generator Crystals so their terminations point to a common center. It is important to use good quality crystals so that energy can move through them efficiently while also gaining both speed and power. They should be clear with few inclusions (imperfections inside the crystal and have terminations that are not chipped or broken. The exception to this rule are rutilated crystals that have numerous hair-sized pieces of metal in them called Titanium Dioxide. These are helpful inclusions because they provide your grid a greater electro-magnetic charge. **To increase the electromagnetism of your temple you can also attach bar magnets to the sides of a crystal by using tape and/or silicon cement. This will amplify the power of a crystal by a factor of three.** You can also wrap them in copper wire.

You can use different kind of Quartz Crystals for your grid to give it a more specific frequency and effect, and to align it more specifically to one ray. You can, for example, use Rose Quartz crystals aligned with the 4th Ray in your grid to create a balanced and emotionally peaceful energy, or you can use Amethyst Quartz aligned with the 6th Ray to make your grid more spiritually uplifting. A grid of Smokey Quartz aligned with the 7th Ray will be more alchemically transformative.

The two principal alchemical formations you can use for your Crystal Grid are a six-pointed star and an eight-sided octahedron. Both are alchemical grids that unite the polarity within your Seven Ray Healing Temple and within the body of those that lie within them. A six-pointed star symbolizes the union of the polarity as two inter-connected triangles. An eight-sided octahedron denotes the union of two "worlds" of four sides, which in this case are the polarity of Heaven and Earth.

If you have many crystals available, you can make a six-pointed star into a twelve-pointed star by equally placing them from a center point and from each other. When perfectly placed in this way they will form a circle. You will then have a double Star of David with double the grid power.

A diameter of 5, 7, or 13 feet will also provide your grid with powerful alchemical properties. In order to easily place your crystals at the corners of your grid and equidistant from each other, you can make a Grid Guide. Simply attach or paint an 11 x 8 figure of a six-pointed star or octagon to a flat piece of wood. Then pound a nail through the center of your star and into the wood below it. Now determine the radius of your crystal grid and cut a piece of string to that length, then tie one end of it to the nail. As you extend the string outwards have it align with and pass directly through one of the corners of your star or octagon. Then, when the string reaches its full extended length, place a crystal on the floor with its termination touching the end of the string. Do that with all the six or eight corners of your geometrical figure. When all the crystals are finally laid out they will mark the corners of your grid. Together they will also lie on the perimeter of a circle.

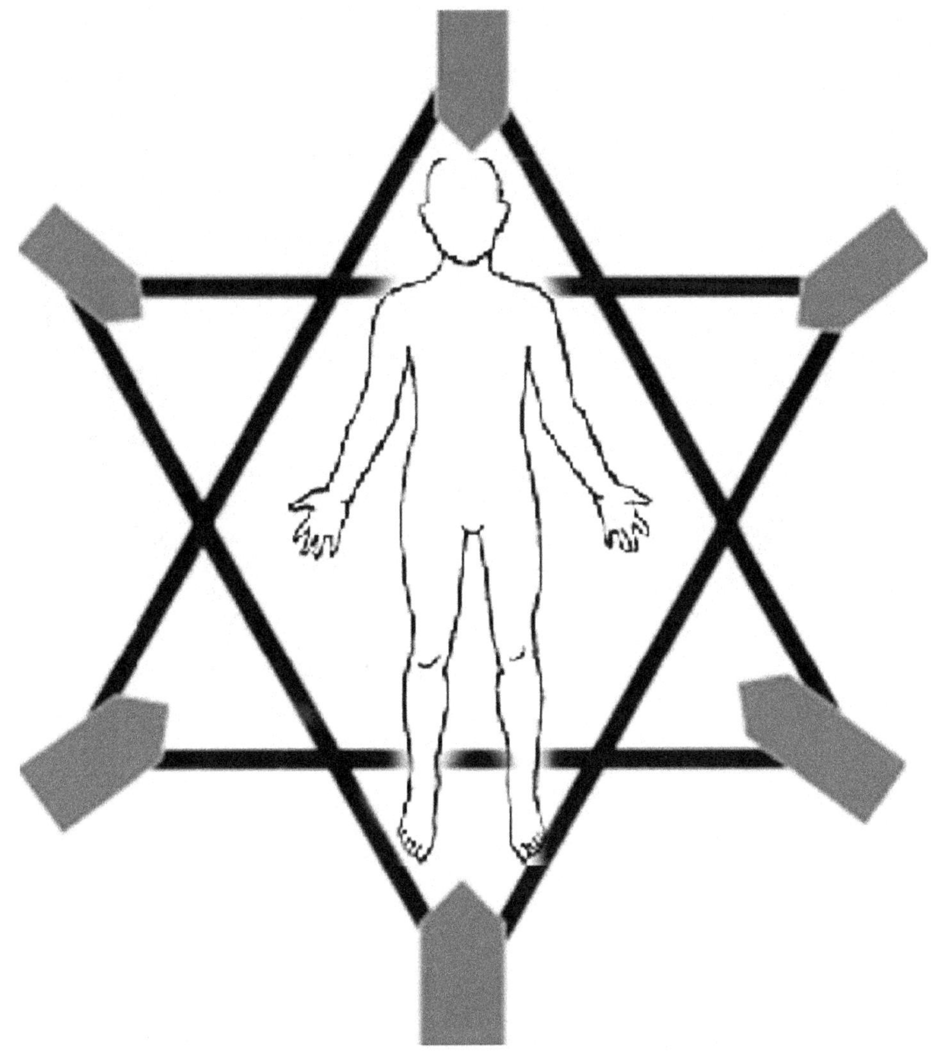

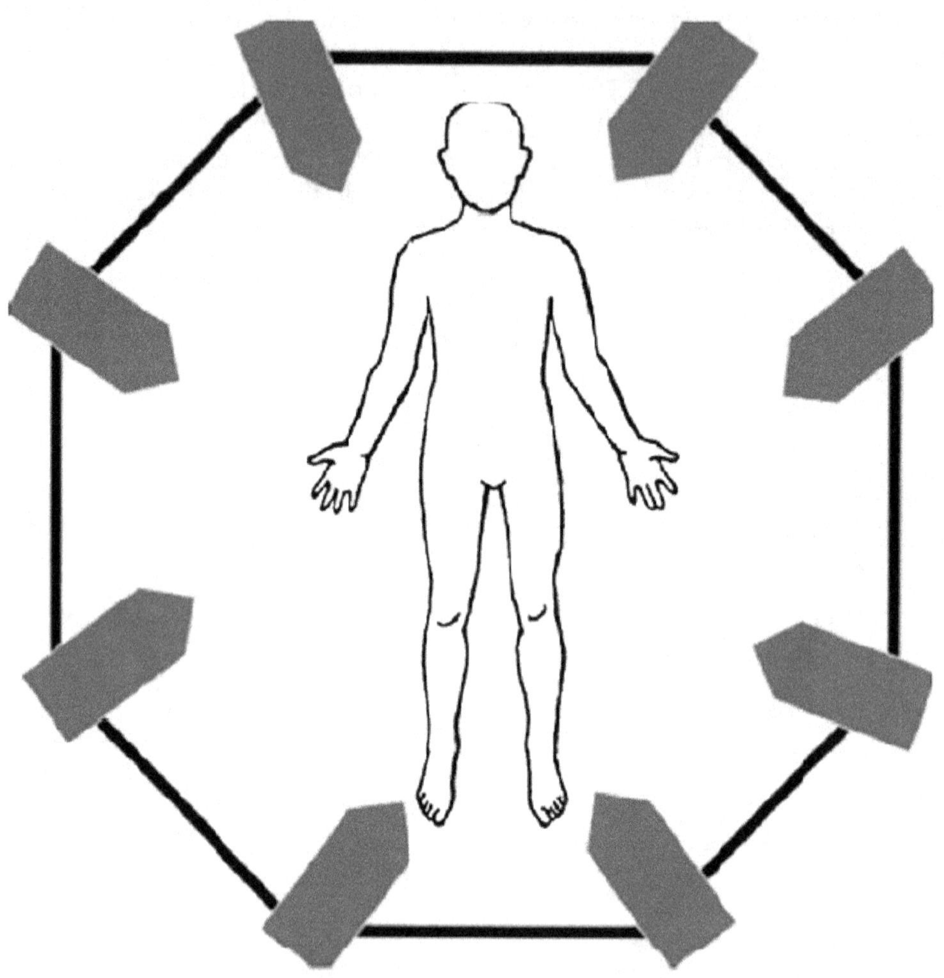

Uniting Pyramids and Quartz Crystal Grids

Pyramids and Quartz Crystals produce complementary alchemical healing forces, and together they produce a perfect synergy for your Seven Ray Healing Temple.

Like a Pyramid, a Quartz Crystal both amplifies and moves life force to produce a spiraling wave of alchemical force. As life force travels through a Crystal's double-helix, tetrahedron lattice it picks up both voltage and amperage (speed and force) and then spirals quickly out of the apex. As it moves through the crystal's apex the life force spiral also becomes altered by the alchemical angle of the termination, which in most cases is the same as that of a pyramid: approximately 52 degrees. This is an important alchemical angle. And like a pyramid, a Quartz Crystal naturally unites the polarity and will do so within anyone affected by its energy. It does this because of its natural hexagonal shape.

Activating and clearing your Seven Ray Healing Temple

To clear the energy in your temple occasionally place a bowl of water with dissolved sea salt in the center of it overnight. This will help clear any dark energy that has accumulated through the release of toxins during your healing treatments. If you toxins are being released heavily on a daily basis consider clearing its energy every day or every other day. If you are using a crystal grid set your bowl of salt water in the center of the grid. If your crystal grid is in a pyramid set the bowl in the center of the pyramid. You can also leave a bowl of salt water permanently in your room to absorb the toxins as soon as they are released. But make sure you regularly change the water.

To activate your temple you can use both sound and light. When either sound of light is broadcast into your temple it will catalyze the dynamic of piezoelectricity, thereby compelling your crystals to release their healing energies. The piezoelectric property of a crystal is stimulated when sound and/or light waves press against the surface of it and thereby stimulates a flow of electrons. When this occurs in your healing temple it will soon be full of healing and balancing crystal emanations. You can also charge your crystals in sunlight before using them or leave them outside during the time of the Full Moon. Placing a crystal inside a pyramid will also charge it, which is why you should keep your crystal grid permanently in place inside your pyramid rather than dis-assembling it after each use. As a rule of thumb, each time you set up a new crystal grid either by itself or inside a pyramid you need to give it at least 20 minutes to become fully activated and ready for use.

Adding an Altar and Sacred Images to your Temple

Once you have created an energy conductive space for your healing temple **you can easily add additional healing power by setting up one or more altars in your temple.** These can be places in the center and/or the sides of our temple.

As a rule of thumb, whenever you place any object on one side of your temple a comparably sized object should be placed on the opposite side of the room. This will help in producing a completely balanced healing energy in your temple. This rule also applies to altars. Thus, if you place an altar on one side of the room it should balanced by an altar or some other object of equal size on the opposite side of the room. And it also applies to how you set up your altar. Any object placed on the right side of the altar should be matched with an object of similar size and directly across from it on the left side of the altar.

An altar will serve as both an energy generator for your temple as well as a table for your healing tools. The pictures and images of saints and deities, as well as your sacred stones and power objects, that you place on your altar will add to the healing power in your temple. The more you honor these images with worship the more power they will emanate. You can also empower your images by waving candles or incense in front of them. Move your candle or incense in a clockwise direction in order to spiral energy into your sacred objects and images.

To generate more even more power and balance in your temple consider attaching sacred images to the walls. Yantras, such as the Sri Yantra, are excellent for this purpose. Like the six-pointed and eight-pointed stars, yantras are the geometrical form bodies of deities that will emanate into your temple the power of their associated deities. The six-pointed star is the pre-eminent yantra of Sanat Kumara, the Lord of the Seven Rays, and the related Sri Yantra and the five-pointed star are yantras of the Goddess. The pentagram is made in accordance with the Golden Mean Proportion so when attached to the walls of your temple they can spin etheric spirals of life force into your temple.

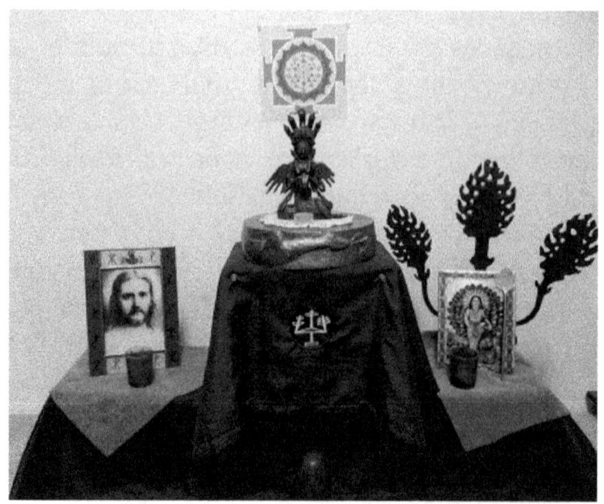

Adding Colored Lights and Sound to your Seven Ray Healing Temple

Once you have set up a crystal grid with or without a pyramid you can add to Light and Sound to them to produce an Integrated Energy Field (IEF). Both Light and Sound are important in an Integrated Energy Field because they will activate many of its component parts, especially your crystals and any crystals or gems you place upon a client's body. Many of the various sources of color and sound that you can add to your temple are presented in Chapter 4.

Adding Colored Lights

Whether you are working on a massage table, or on the floor in the center of your crystal grid, and/or in pyramid, **you can attach your light sources to lamps, poles, tripods or on tables next to your client. If possible, for specific organ treatments your light source should not be more than 18 inches away from its target.** If you are bathing the entire body of your client with colored light you can either raise the light source 3-6 feet above their body and/or onto a table. You can also attach it to tripod set above their feet and pointed towards their head.

AddingSound

As mentioned in Chapter 4 you can generate healing sound in your temple through speakers, live instruments, chanting mantras, etc. When using speakers you can get the most powerful result by placing them above and below the body of the client, and/or to the left and right of him or her. If you place the speakers close to your crystal grid, the sound moving through them will quickly and powerfully activate your temple. For the best results you should focus on creating a synnastry between the colors you use and the sound coming through your speakers. These correspondences are listed in Chapter 3.

When facilitating an emotional, mental and/or spiritual healing treatment with a client you should consider playing special music that synchronizes the brain hemispheres. When speakers playing Hemisphere Synchronization Music are placed on both sides of a client, coded signals generated by the music will enter the ears and travel along the auricular nerves to the brain. There they synchronize the hemispheres and produce Theta frequencies, which are the wave patterns of deep meditation. A person undergoing emotional healing can then better relive the trauma that caused the toxic emotion that arises as well as receive intuitive guidance from their Higher Self regarding how to heal and release the trauma. If using Hemisphere synchronization music interferes with the specific color-related sounds you want played through the speakers, you can play Hemisphere Synchronization Music at the start of a treatment to get you client in a deep meditation state followed by other music But even if you do not use Hemisphere Synchronization Music, the crystals and/or pyramid will work to transport your client into a meditative state.

In the below diagram a person is laying down on their back in the center of the crystal grid located inside a pyramid. There are two small speakers placed at the level of the shoulders and head and two at the level of the knees. This arrangement will completely fill your temple with sound while affecting every part of the person's body. If space is limited, the speakers can be placed just outside of the pyramid.

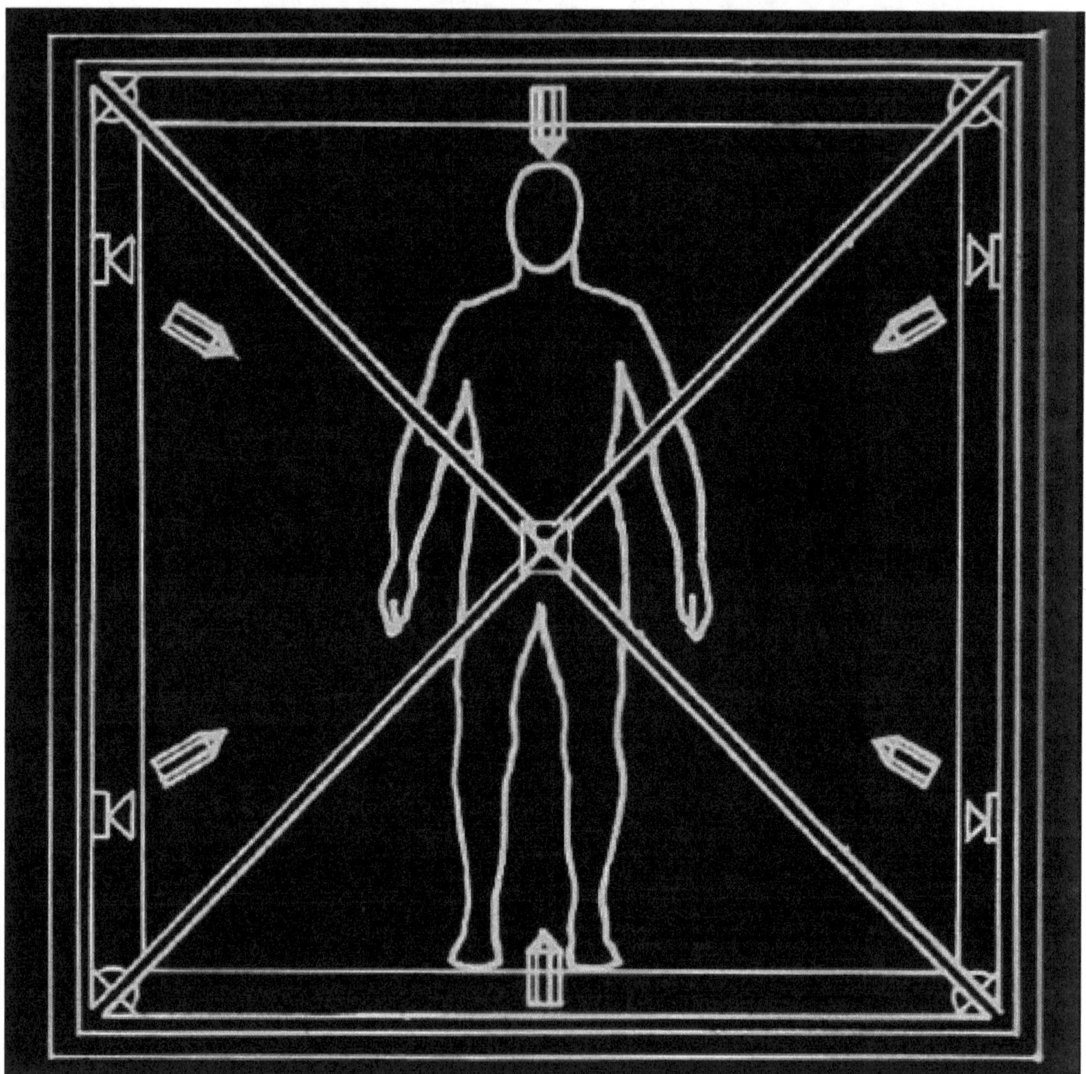

AddingMirrors

In order to reflect back the light rays that are generated in your temple and thereby continue to empower it even further, you can install mirrors upon the temple's walls and ceiling. If possible, try to have them directly across the room from your light source so that they can reflect back the most amount of your generated light. As an additional enhancement to your temple, consider painting or attaching the decal form of a yantra, such as the six-pointed star or the Sri Yantra, on some or all your mirrors. Then the power of the yantra will also be continually reflected back into your temple to further assist in creating balance and generating the alchemical force.

Using Flashing Lights or Strobes

Strobes are very effective in an IEF because their strong pulses of light powerfully activate the crystals and gems. They typically have have dials on them so the speed of their pulses can be modulated to different frequencies. When set at a very fast pulse rate, the strobe will help generate Beta Brain Wave patterns, the patterns that are normally produced in your waking state. Slower frequencies will produce Alpha Brain Waves, and the slowest will generate Theta and Delta Brain Waves. Theta Waves are the waves of deep meditation but Delta Brain Waves are the those of sleep, so be careful you do not turn your strobe down too far. Once you have experimented with a strobe and determined which speed is conducive to the generation of deep meditation, keep it on that frequency. This will assist your client in moving into a deep meditative consciousness where he or she can experience images, visions, memories, and/or the release of blocked emotions. In this state your client can also align with his or her higher self and receive special guidance to help them in their healing process.

You can purchase small light boxes that have a steady colored light and/or a strobe setting. Many are designed to place colored gels over the light, or they have remote controls that can change the radiated light to a variety of colors. Some are specially designed to have crystals set on top of the them. This will powerfully activate the crystal and you will be able to point the crystal termination in the direction of the body part, organ or chakra you are working on. All these products are excellent to use in your temple. Many can be found be found online and at *Spencer Gifts*. The strobe machines on the next page come complete and ready to use. The one on the following page requires some time and ingenuity to put together.

A word of caution: When using strobes it is necessary to first check in with a client to determine if they have a predisposition for epileptic seizures. If they do, then the use of strobes is counter-indicated for them.

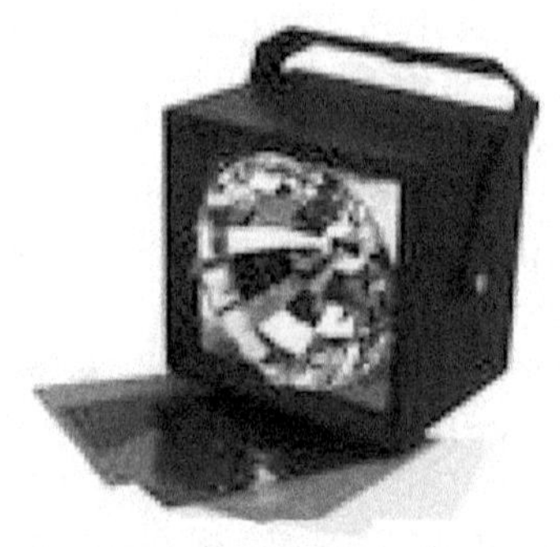

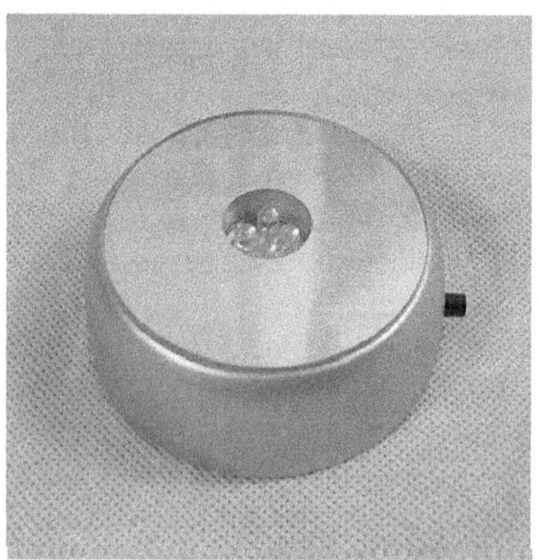

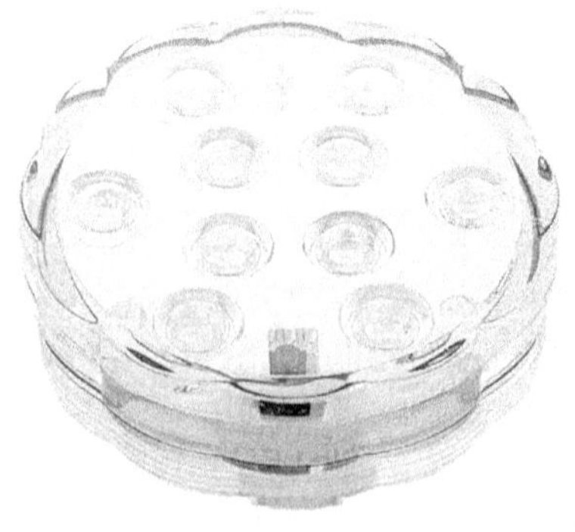

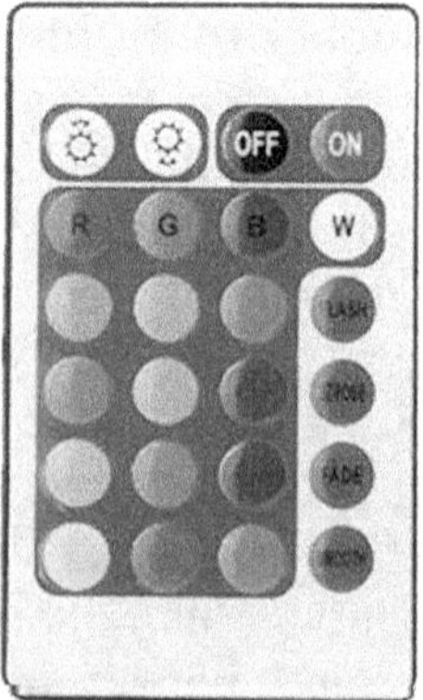
OFF
ON
R
G
B
W
FADE

Making a Seven Ray Light Box

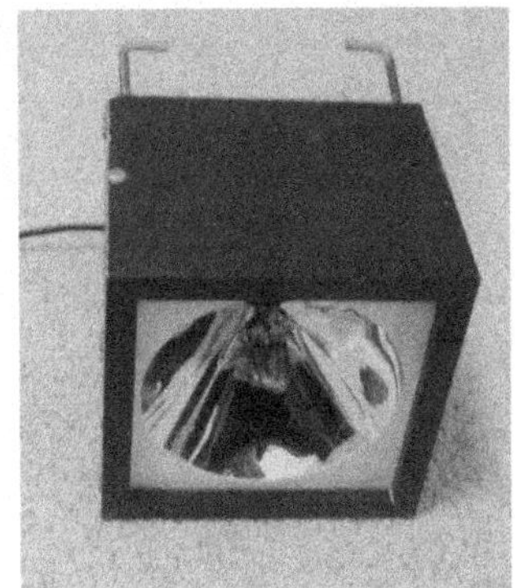

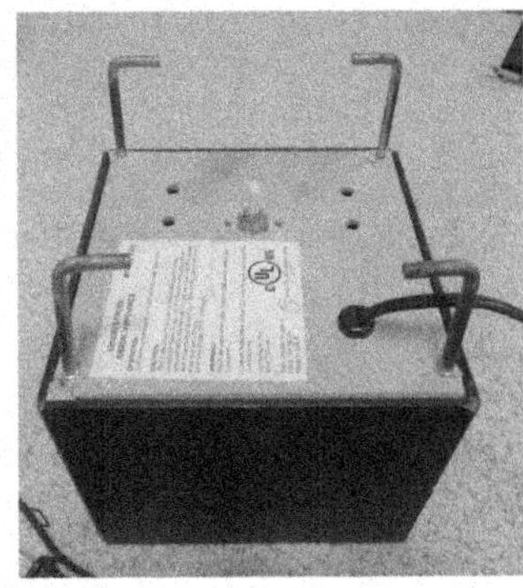

Attach screw-on legs to the bottom of a strobe.

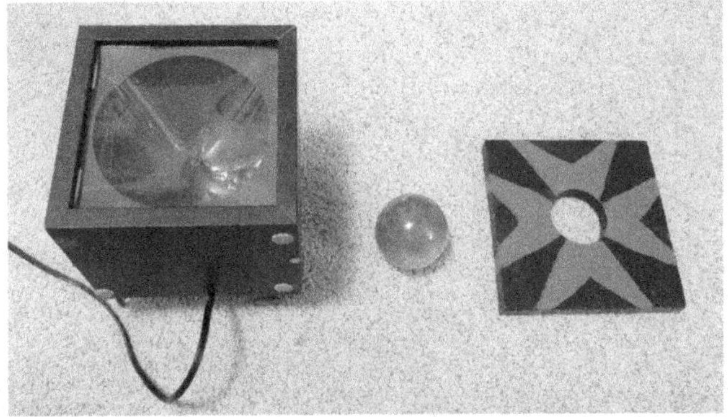

Cut a plywood cover with a hole in it. Put a cut-to-fit color gel over strobe and then place the cover on top.

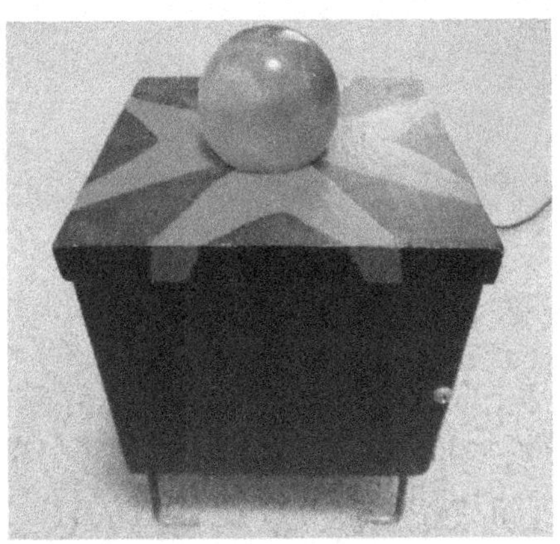

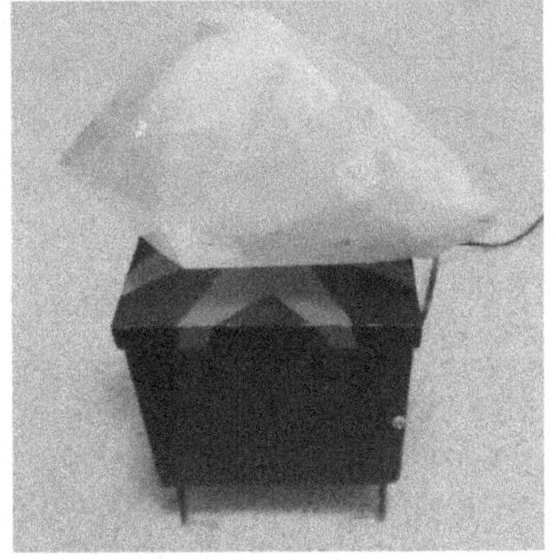

Now place a sphere or regular shaped crystal over the circular opening. Turn the strobe on. Start with maximum speed and experiment with it while slowly dialing it down.

The color emanations from the sphere on the left will move through the entire room you are working in and cover a person's entire body. The termination on the large crystal on the right can be aimed so that the colors moving through it can be directly broadcast, laser-like, onto a specific part of the body you are working on.

Using Lazers

Lazers are excellent tools for activating a crystal or gem both before and during a Seven Ray Healing Treatment. Just direct the beam onto the crystal to active the piezoelectric effect.

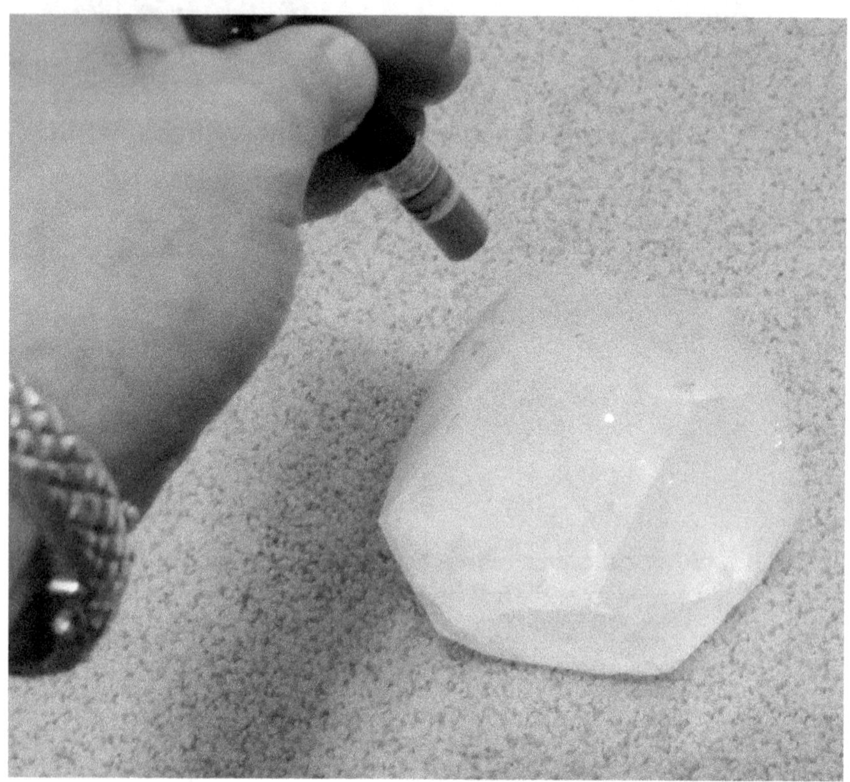

Adding Aroma Therapy

Adding scents in your UEF, thus engendering Aromatherapy, is another way of altering the consciousness of your client and helping him or her relax and sink into meditation. For this you can burn certain kinds of incense in the room. You can also spray a scent over the person during the treatment, and/or you can rub scented oils below their nose, at the third eye, and other strategic places.

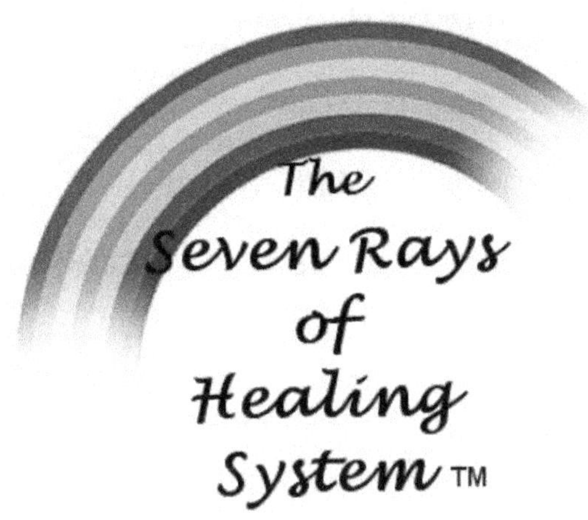

CHAPTER 8

Giving a Seven Ray Balancing Treatment

In this chapter you will synthesize what you have learned in the previous chapters and learn the steps of performing different types of Seven Rays of Healing treatments. **Instructions for administering the following treatments will be presented in detail: Seven Ray Balancing, Chakra Balancing, Third Eye Activation, Kundalini Activation and Opening to Divine Love.**

Important!! It is not necessary to acquire all the equipment and follow all the steps of treatment featured in this chapter. Pick and chose those tools and steps you feel drawn to and find out through experience which ones are the most effective. There are, for example, many modalities listed for use with each chakra, including acupressure, color and sound, Seven Ray Reiki, etc. Choose those that feel and work best for you.

Step 1 for any Treatment: Prepare your healing space/temple

The first step in any Seven Rays of Healing Treatment is to prepare your healing space and/or temple for the treatment. Always clear the energy of the area by smudging with sage or incense, and/or by playing a CD of continuous mantras. Then, unless one is already in place, set out a crystal grid in your pyramid, or around the mat or table your client will be situated upon. Your crystal grid should be in place at least twenty minutes before the session begins. Have your colored lights, sounds, and music in place and ready. Then set out your healing tools near where the person will be lying down.

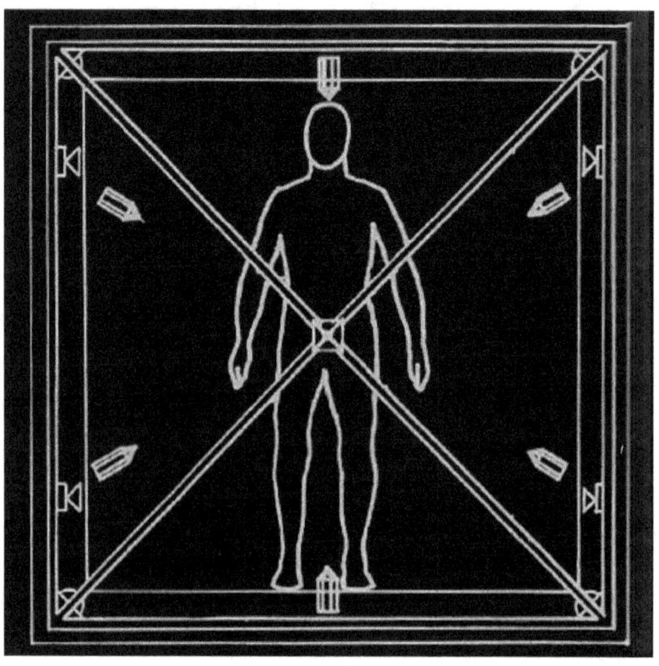

Besides those tools you have in mind for the treatment, below is a grouping of some **Andean Seven Ray Shamanic tools** that you could also use in all your treatments. **Note:** These tools are included because they have been part of Seven Ray Healing in its Andean manifestation. They are still used by the Andean Shamans but they do not need to originate in the Andes. Nor are they absolutely necessary in your treatments. The rattles, feathers, etc. listed in this chapter are general shamanic tools that can be acquired in any country.

Rattle(s): Andean Shamanic Rattles are typically used in pairs, with one of the rattles having a lower tone than the other. Their united sounds will thus be that of the polarity united and help precipitate the same dynamic in your client. Rattles are used principally at the beginning of a treatment. But they can be used anytime during the session that you want to shake up your client's auric field and thereby bring emotional, mental, and physical toxins to the surface to be released. They are especially useful if you or your client are aware of past trauma that needs to be healed and released.

Feathers: Andean Shamanic Feathers are typically Condor Feathers that generate a very cleansing and uplifting vibration, however the feathers of any large bird, such as an eagle or hawk, will work just as well. Feathers are sued to sweep down the body of a client to clear their auric field. This is necessary at the beginning and end of a treatment, as well as any time your client has an strong emotional release during the treatment.

Meteorite(s): Andean Shamanic Meteorites are round and, like Andrea Rattles, typically come in pairs with one a bit larger than the other in order to produce a polarity balancing and uniting effect. The smaller of the two meteorites is considered the female and held in the left hand, and the larger is male and held in the right hand.

Besides uniting the polarity Andean Meteorites will also activate the entire electromagnetic field and assist in removing any blockages contained within it. In addition to activating the EM field, meteorites will also powerfully activate and help clear the more subtle Dragon Body and its chakras and meridians. Moreover, the black color of meteorites will powerfully work in the root chakra to potentially activate the Kundalini in the Dragon Body.

Drums: Andean Shamanic Drums will assist in grounding you or your client and bringing you or them into a sympathetic vibrational harmony with the Earth. They are also excellent when working in the Root Chakra and its associated organs (the Kidneys/Adrenals) to heal, balance and release blockages.

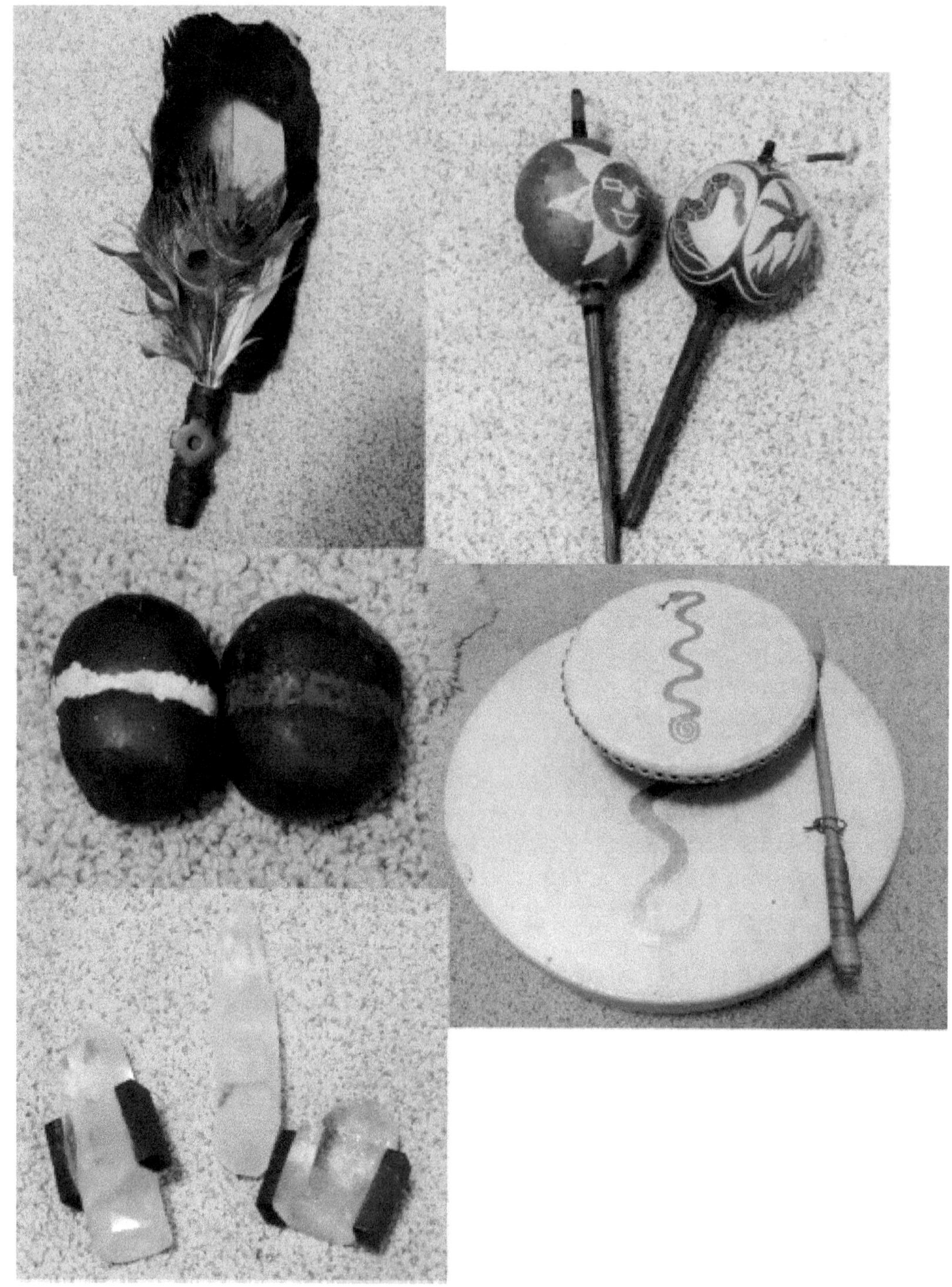

Crystals: Andean Shamanic Crystals can be held in the hands or placed directly over the chakras and organs of a client during therapy. They can also be used as tools by the practitioner to move energy into an area or out of it, and they also open and close a chakra. For all these purposes both terminated crystals and crystal pendulums can be used. Energy will typically be needed in an area or organ that is weak and has exhibited chronic symptoms of dysfunction. In such cases a crystal can be waved in a clockwise direction while slowly spiraling it towards the organ or body part. By contrast, when excess energy needs to be removed in acute illnesses and painful injuries, spiral your crystal in a counterclockwise direction while moving it away from the body of the client. During a therapy session moving energy into the body of the client is also helpful when activating chakras, such as the heart chakra. This is often necessary to remove energy from a chakra when the client is overwhelmed by too much emotion or memories being released from the chakra. For example: too much emotion can be released from the liver and/or heart at one time for a client to process.

Ideally, a Hand-held crystal should be a perfect generator crystal. It should be large in size (one pound or more), and it should have good clarity and a well-defined and non-chipped termination. To increase the strength of your crystal, you can attach bar magnets to two of its opposing sides with tape or silicon glue.

Another excellent crystal tool to use is a crystal pyramid that has as 1-3" square base. A crystal pyramid can be set over a disharmonious organ or chakra to deeply cleanse and purify it with its octagonal pyramidal energy flow.

Crowns: Crowns are excellent tools for moving energy in the head of a person and for activating their 6th and 7th Chakras. Crowns can used during times when it is efficacious to activate the 6th and 7th Chakras. And they can also be used in any treatment to order to assist a person in establishing contact with their Higher Selves. With their support a person can receive inner guidance related to the emotional and mental issues that arise during a session.

Make Your Own Wand, Hand-held Crystal, or Staff

Both a Hand-held Crystal or Crystal Wand can be used to spiral life force energy into or out of a specific area of the body, such as a chakra or a sore arm or leg. For infusing energy into an area, move the wand or crystal in a clockwise direction, and to remove an excess of energy out of an area move it counter-clockwise.

Crystal Wands can be purchased or self-made. To make your own, use a conductive hard wood or metal (1/2 and 3/4 inch copper pipe works well) and then attach crystals and gems to its shaft and at least one of its ends. You can attach stones along the side with any or all the colors of the spectrum. To attach stones to your wand you can use silicon glue. You can also wind copper wire around your wand to give it added conductivity, but make sure that the rings of wire do not overlap. This will cause a block in the energy flow.

Seven Ray Staffs are very practical and useful healing tools. Instead of placing many individual stones and gems on a person at the beginning of a session, you can use a staff (either bought or self-made) that has stones of the seven different colors attached to it. The stones should be arranged with the seven colors in succession, beginning with red stones at the bottom and ending with violet, gold, or clear ones at the top. The staff should be made of an energy conductive material, either a hard wood, such as oak, or a metal, such as copper, brass, or silver or gold. The staff should be approx. 1 1/2 – 2 feet in size. If you are making it yourself, you can attach the stones to the staff with silicon glue. Seven Ray Staffs can remain on the body of a person through a treatment to continue balancing their chakras, EM and Dragon Body fields.

A Hand-held Crystal should be a generator crystal, i.e., large in size (one pound or more), and it should have good clarity and a well-defined and non-chipped termination. To increase the strength of your crystal, you can attach bar magnets to two of its opposing sides with silicon glue.

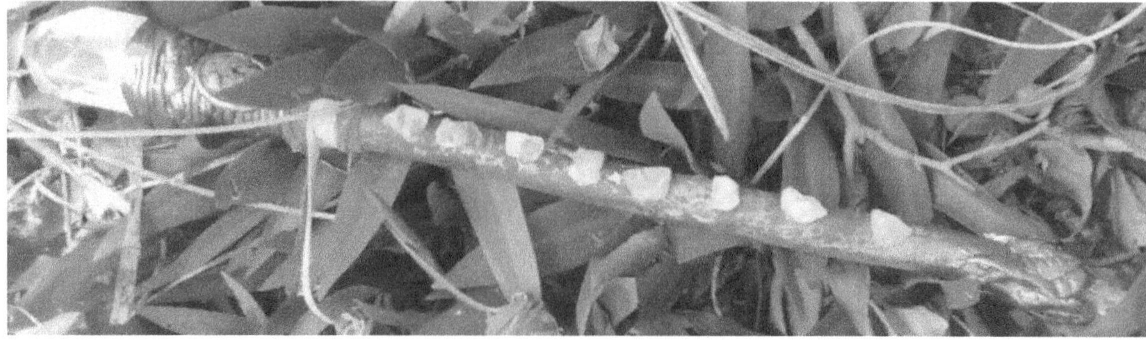

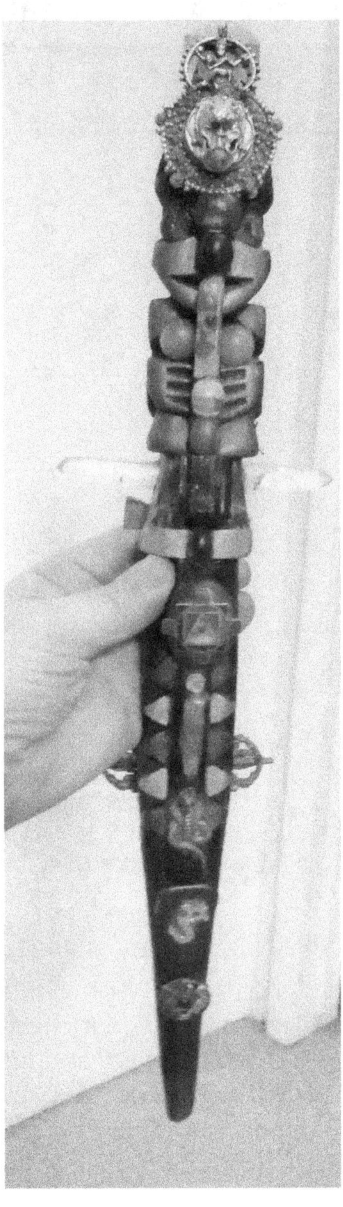

The Seven Ray Staff above is large enough to lay on the body of a client so that it extends most of the way from the breast bone to just above the sexual organs. The base is a hard wood and along its length are attached stones that correspond to each of the 7 chakras, beginning with red stones at the bottom, followed by orange carnelian, citrine quartz, green tourmaline, rose quartz, aquamarine, turquoise, azurite, and ending with a violet amethyst pyramid at the top. In between the stones are symbols that have a special meaning to the author, as well as crosses and crystals, such as those in the center of the staff. These assist in balancing the vertical and horizontal lines of energy in the client.

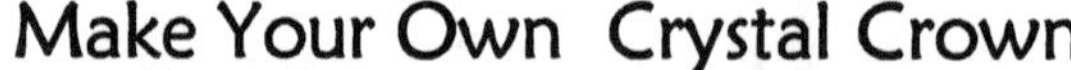

Make Your Own Crystal Crown

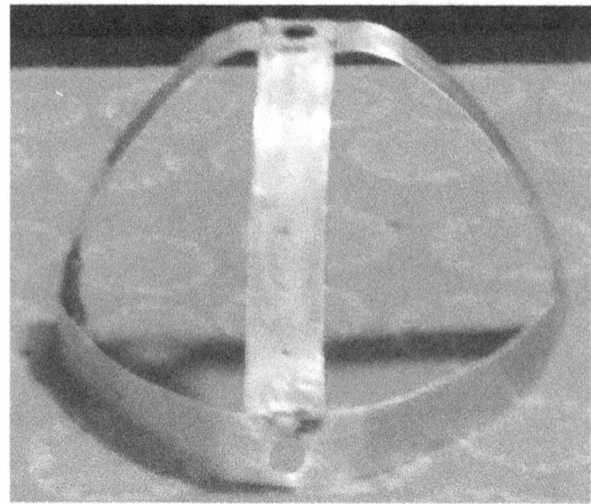

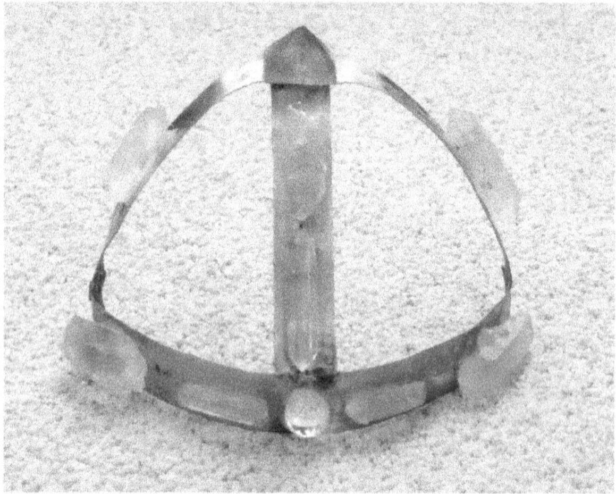

The above crown is designed to be worn with a person lying on their backs. It will move any energy blockages within their heads while also activating the 6th and 7th Chakras associated with psychic activity and interdimensional experience.

To make the above crown begin with a frame like the one at the top of the page. The frame is made of copper, but it can be made from any conductive material. Holes are drilled at the area of the crown that will lie directly over the 6th and 7th chakras. Crystals are then added to activate the underlying chakras. An Amethyst pyramid is attached to the 7th Chakra and a clear quartz sphere is attached to the region above the 6th Chakra. You can place whatever stones or gems you desire over these portals as long as they are specific for the underlying chakras. The other crystals on the crown are all clear quartz double terminated crystals that will move energy both up and down the head. All the crystals are attached with silicon adhesive.

Make an Inexpensive "Crown": Rather than making a costly and time-consuming crown design, consider putting an athletic head band over your client's head at the level of the Third Eye. Now place crystals and/or gems under the sweat band over the Third Eye and some single or double terminated crystals at the temples to move energy up and down the head and body.

Gems: Gems and Stones are excellent tools for emanating the various colors for Seven Ray Healing. They also both move and amplify energy. Gems and their color and chakra associations can be found in Chapter 4. In order to amplify the power of a gem - and to make sure that it does not fall off during the course of a Seven Ray treatment - you can place it on top of a crystal, such as a flat "Tabular Crystal." And if you want to permanently unite your gem with a crystal you can glue them together with silicon glue.

Chakra/Organ Clusters: You can also make permanent Chakra or Organ Clusters of gems and crystals that work together on specific chakras and organs. An example of this would be to permanently unite gems and crystals onto a Chakra/ Organ Cluster that is specific to the physical heart and the Heart Chakra. These could include a combination of heart stones such as rose quartz, pink tourmaline, rhodachrosite, and perhaps green tourmaline and emerald. Another Chakra/ Organ Cluster could be designed specifically for the third chakra and the stomach and liver. They could feature a combination of yellow-gold stones, such as citrine quartz, yellow topaz, yellow sapphire, and amber. And a third Chakra/Organ Cluster for the Third Eye and Pineal Gland could include: azurite, lapis, amethyst, sugilite, purple tourmaline, etc. Herkimer diamonds are also very good to use as they have powerful Third Eye activation properties. Besides a Tubular Crystal, a crystal pyramid could form the base of Chakra/Organ Cluster. When gems and stones are attached to a crystal pyramid their frequencies will accompany the downward pyramidal energy flow into the chakra and/or organ below them. This can be facilitated by activating the pyramid with color and sound, and or waving in a clockwise motion a handheld crystal held over the apex.

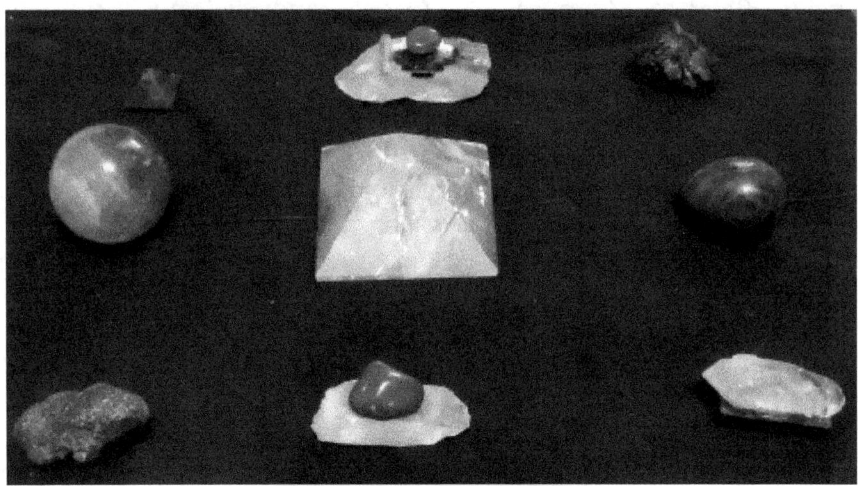

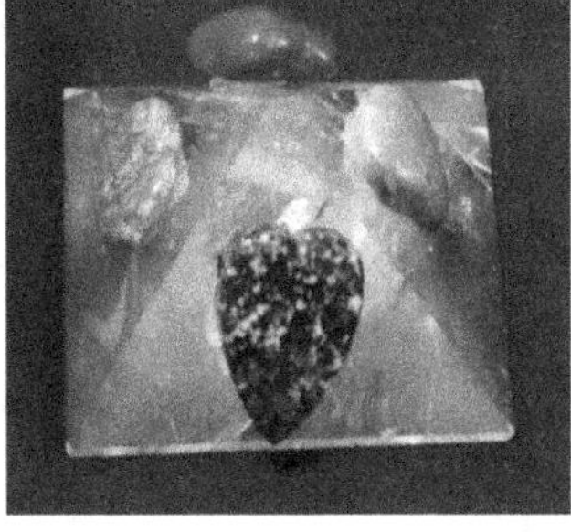

Step 2: Activating your Temple

Begin activating your temple 20 minutes before giving a treatment. Play music and/or shine lights into your crystal grid and the crystals and gems you will place upon the client's body. Playing mantra music will both charge your temple and purify it. You can also burn sage or incense to assist the purification and to add aroma therapy to your treatment.

Step 3: Diagnosis

Before your client enters your temple you should already known their Ray(s) and have some idea of their predispositions regarding potential physical, emotional and mental health issues. You should know their Ray-ruled organs and the chakras that correspond to those organs, and you should plan to balance them during the treatment. Initially inform your client about their ray, its attributes, its Lords/Ladies, etc. and determine if they are in alignment with with the goals, desires, etc. of their ray. Such imbalances could be detrimentally influencing their health.

After determining your client's Ray and ray organs/chakras determine if there are other areas of the body, inner organs and/or chakras, that need re-balancing so you can also give special attention to them during the session. Also inquire what predominant excessive emotions the client has been experiencing and plan to address the associated organs accordingly. Refer to Chapter 4 (basic) and 8 (advanced) for organ diagnosis.

Step 4: Activating your Client's Energy Field

Once your client has entered your healing temple and become comfortable place the tools (crystals, gems, sounds, colored lights, etc) you intend to use during the ensuing Seven Rays of Healing treatment, you are ready to begin the session. Advise your client that you are there for them at all times during the session if they need you. Explain what they could expect during the session as their blocked energy is released, including as sudden jerking movements, spontaneous emotions, and the recall of stored memories. Because you will be activating the higher psychic centers in your client, they could also have visions, astral travel, or any number of possible psychic experiences. Lines of communication between your client and his or her Higher Self will be opened during the treatment, so advise your client that the session is an excellent time to get questions answered and receive helpful guidance for both the present and future.

Just as you did with your temple, now focus on activating the person's energy field. If you have a crown, place it over the person's head now. And if you have a shamanic staff place it over their chakras to align both the chakras and the longitudinal lines of the person's electro-magnetic field. If you have meteorites, place them in the person's hands. Otherwise give them clear quartz crystals to hold. If you are using a strobe light place a green color gel over it and set it on a speed that will induce meditation. You can place a strobe on either side of the person and/or at their feet. Do not place it at their head. Besides moving energy, the strobe will assist in uniting the brain hemispheres and moving the person into a deep meditative state wherein they can connect with the guidance of their Higher Self. Such guidance will assist them when the emotions and memories of past traumas arise.

Now have your client begin **Connected Breath**. This is a pranayama - i.e., a controlled breathing technique - designed to stimulate the movement of the life force in the Dragon Body. Also known as **Circular Breath**, while engaged in it a person can envision it as a circuit of energy that moves from the lungs to the nose on the in-breath and then moves from the nose to the base of the lungs on the out-breath. Advise the person to try and perform Connected/Circular Breath for at least a few minutes at the beginning of the treatment, and if they feel inspired they can continue to perform it throughout most or all of the session. As long as they are performing this form of breathing their energy will be moving and toxins will be released.

If you have **rattles**, shake them above the client's entire body as they are preforming Connected Breath to release of blocked energy. If you don't have rattles you can vibrate a **crystal bowl or a Tibetan bowl that is tuned to Note C** while moving it above the client's entire body. This will have a similar effect as the rattles. You can also use rattles and bowls in conjunction with each other, one after the other, for an even more comprehensive cleansing.

Next step: Trace the Star of David and one or more of the Dragon Force-Kundalini Activating symbols over the front and/or back of the body. Trace the symbols 3x. The center of the Star of David should be the person's heart chakra. Call forth Sanat Kumara while tracing the symbols.

Now move to the head region of the client. Massage their neck in order to get energy movement into the head to activate the psychic centers. Massage the Windows to the Sky Acu-Points. This massage will help the client to align with their inner guidance.

Now move to the sides of the body and activate the Four Gates (LI4, Liv3 Acu-Points). This will help move blocked anywhere in the body and stimulate the release of physical, emotional and mental toxins.

You are now ready to commence your treatment.

A Ray Balancing Treatment

For both the Birth and Dasa Ray(s)

Step 5: Broadcast Birth and Dasa Ray Color; Invoke Ray Lords/Ladies

Now bathe the person in the color of their Birth Ray while you summon the Lord and/or Lady of Seven Ray Healing, Sanat Kumara or Sophia. Their presence will endow your temple with the frequencies of all the Seven Rays. Then, call in the Lords and Ladies associated with the person's Ray(s). Afterwards, if you know the person's current Dasa Ray you can broadcast its associated color on the person while summoning its Lords and Ladies.

Step 6: Treat the Ray Organs

Now move to the Birth and Dasa Ray organs and balance them by broadcasting the appropriate tonation and corresponding sounds upon them. Do this while simultaneously moving chi by stimulating their local (nearby) and distal (distant) Acu-Points on the meridians associated with the ray organs. If there has been long term or chronic problems with these organs give a shorter and milder acupressure massage, and give a longer massage for acute or short term issues. Also consider placing appropriate gems over over the organ or a pyramidal crystal and using your hand-held crystal to spiral energy either into or out of the organ. Spiral energy into the organ for weak and chronic problems, and draw energy out of it for acute and painful conditions. If you know what chakra feeds the organs you can also work to balance those chakras with gems, crystals, color tonations and sound therapy. Try to make all your tonations at least 20 minutes in length. Also: whatever organ or chakra you work on administer Seven Ray Reiki and leave your hands in place 3-5 minutes or until you feel a "pulse."

Step 7: Completion

At the completion of a session, sweep down the body of the client one final time with your feathers.

You should end your treatment by systemically tonating your client's entire body with the color Green while playing that color's corresponding note and music. All tonations should end with Green, the most balancing color. As you broadcast green you can be injecting energy into the Heart Chakra and lightly massaging some important heart points, such as H7. Complete by tracing the Star of David over the person's heart 3x.

Step 8: After the Treatment

Make sure to give your client plenty of time to assimilate their session before they leave the mat or table. Check in with them to see if they need to continue releasing through counseling before they leave, and/or if they just want to share their experience in order to gain more clarity regarding it. At this time try to determine whether future sessions will be of benefit to the client and, if time allows, give them some prophylactic measures that they can observe on their own to remain in balance. Such measures, which are determined by their Birth and Dasa Rays, as well as the organ(s) you have just balanced, could include gems, yoga, diet, color therapy, herbs, etc.

Further counsel your client regarding their Birth and Dasa Ray(s) if you believe it will be helpful for them. Inquire whether any feeling, emotions, visions, etc. associated with their Ray(s) emerged during the session. Then make suggestions regarding how the person can stay healthy and aligned with their Ray(s). Determine if they are living a life aligned with their Ray(s) and make suggestions if they are not. And also suggest gems, and mantras to align with their Ray(s), as well as how they can give themselves regular light therapy at home to remain aligned.

During the week following their treatment advise your client to broadcast a light of the color needed by their afflicted organ/chakra at least once a day for a minimum of 45 minutes while playing the associated music. They can also ongoingly broadcast the colors of their Birth and Dasa Rays upon themselves. Colored lights (60-75 Watt) can usually be purchased at local discount stores. They can also make and regularly drink the appropriate colored water.

If the person has a difficult time grounding after the session give them some tea and/or gently massage K.1 at the bottom of their feet. Also give them a black colored stone, such as Smokey Quartz or Obsidian, to hold for a few minutes. If they still remain ungrounded, have them walk barefoot on the ground outside while breathing deeply the fresh air.

Thank the Sanat Kumara, Sophia, and/or the Lords and Ladies you have invited into your session. Ask them to continue working with the client once they leave if you believe he or she needs ongoing healing assistance.

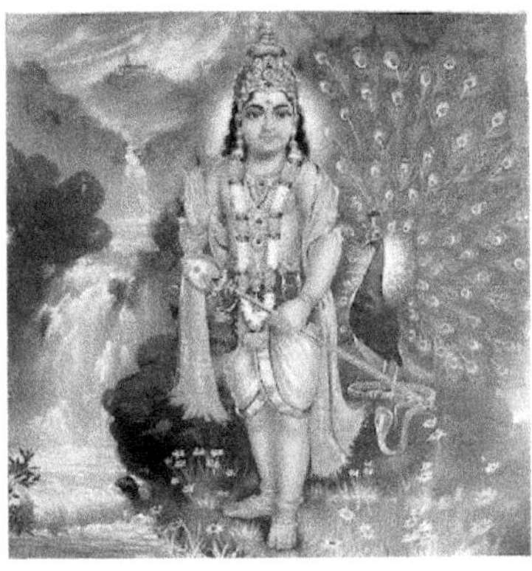

A General Chakra Balancing Treatment

Balancing all the 7 Chakras

Step 5: Move down to the Root Chakra

Following Steps 1-4 to initiate a general balancing of the person's chakra system. Review Chakra section in Chapter 5, if necessary, and then begin.

If you are working with sound you will now begin playing deep bass sounds that work within the Root Chakra. You can use a live instrument, such as a drum, or you can play a musical CD with continual rhythmic drumming on it. Broadcast a red light over the lower part of the body and place red/black and/or clear crystal gems and stones over the Root Chakra area (front of body: just above sexual organs; back of body: base of spine.). Meteorites and clear crystal pyramids are good, effective stones to use. If you have a pendulum, a hand-held crystal, or a crystal wand, wave it in a clockwise direction while spiraling downwards towards the Root Chakra. This will fuel any emotional blockages associated with this chakra and its associated issues (fear, survival, spacey-ness, etc.). It could, for example, cause fear issues around survival to emerge into consciousness in a very tangible and powerful way. If this happens, and if the client needs to talk about their issues, counsel him or her through them. Or, if it feels right to you, suggest that the client call upon the guidance of his or her Higher Self to assist the healing and release of the emotion. Initiating rapid Circular Breath at this time will also assist the subject in moving through the blockage.

If the client becomes overwhelmed by the issues that are emerging, stop moving energy into the chakra. Instead, move your hand-held crystal, pendulum or wand in a counter-clockwise direction above the chakra. This will help to close the chakra down and sedate it for the moment. The client can continue working with the issues that correspond to the chakra at a future session. Then, at the end of any emotional release connected to the Root Chakra, or any other chakra, use your feathers to make broad sweeps over the client's body. This will clear the client's energy field of any residual toxic energies, and it will also clear the area around them of any toxic energies they may have just released. If you don't have feathers, sweep the person's body with your own hands, and always move from head to foot.

When you are working with the Root Chakra it is also important to keep in mind that if the client is prepared spiritually he or she could have a spontaneous activation of the Kundalini, the alchemical force that resides in the lowest chakra. An awakening could manifest as the feeling of energy being suddenly released and/or pressure at the base of the spine, the vision of a snake or serpent, a sudden and powerful movement of energy in the body, etc. There are many possible manifestations of this phenomenon. The one consistent manifestation of Kundalini awakening is, however, a pulse, throb, pressure and/or a feeling of heat at the base of the spine.

While you are working with the Root Chakra also address the organs it governs, such as the kidney/adrenals, especially if your initial diagnosis has revealed some problems related to those organs and/or if the person's Ray(s) are intimately connected to these organs. As a rule of thumb, it is always a good idea to channel some energy into the kidneys during any treatment because they are the root of all the inner organs. The gems, colored lights and music will help to nourish the kidneys, but you can also channel energy into them through Seven Ray Reiki by placing your hands on the area of your client's body that is just below his or her navel after first tracing a Star of David and Cho Ku Rei over the region. You can also perform a mild stimulation to Ren 4 & 6. Remember to also call in one of the Lords of the 1st Ray governing the kidneys, such as Sanat Kumara, and ask them to channel their healing force through you.

You should continue working on the Root Chakra and its associated organs for at least 5-10 minutes.

Step6: Moving up the Chakras

When you complete work on the Root Chakra area move up the client's body. You will next work on the 2nd chakra and the area just below the navel followed by the 3rd chakra at the solar plexus, the 4th chakra at the heart, etc. **For each chakra and its associated body region observe the following steps:**

1. Play the appropriate music and broadcast the appropriate colored light
2. Place stones associated with the chakra over that chakra, and place similar chakra stones in the hands of the client. For any chakra you can, if you desire, simply use clear quartz because its white light vibration is inclusive of all color and chakra frequencies. You can also simply place your shamanic staff on the torso if it has gems for all the chakras. And you can also keep meteorites in the hands of your client throughout the session. By moving the electromagnetic field they will continue to influence all the chakras.
3. Vibrate a Crystal Bowl or Tuning Fork over the chakra that is set to the chakra's specific note frequency
4. Spiral energy into the chakra by rotating a wand, hand-held generator crystal (large crystal), or pendulum in a clockwise direction to bring up any blocked issues. Once emotions and issues related to the chakra arise you can intensify the experience by continuing to rotate energy into the chakra. Or, if the experience gets too intense for the person, you can stop rotating your wand and/or rotate counter-clockwise to remove some of the energy from the chakra.
5. Each time If the person has a major energy release sweep their body with your feathers.

   Finish your Chakra Balancing Treatment with Step 8

Note: For all clients and all treatments it is good to address the Heart, Kidneys and Liver, three very important organs that are associated with Shen/mind, Jing/physical energy, and Emotion. Do this by spiraling energy into or out of the organs and/or by using Seven Ray Reiki. The Kidneys will always benefit with an infusion of energy from your hands. The Liver, since it is the seat of the emotional body and the filter for physical toxins, can get congested and it is often requires the removal of excess energy. If this is the case of your client who is displaying Liver excess symptoms, such as a lot of anger or a stress or migraine headache, remove energy. Otherwise infuse energy into the Liver in order to bring to the surface emotions blocked within the organ. The Heart almost always responds favorably to an infusion of energy. Seven Ray Reiki over the Heart not only energizes the organ but also calms the mind and spirit.

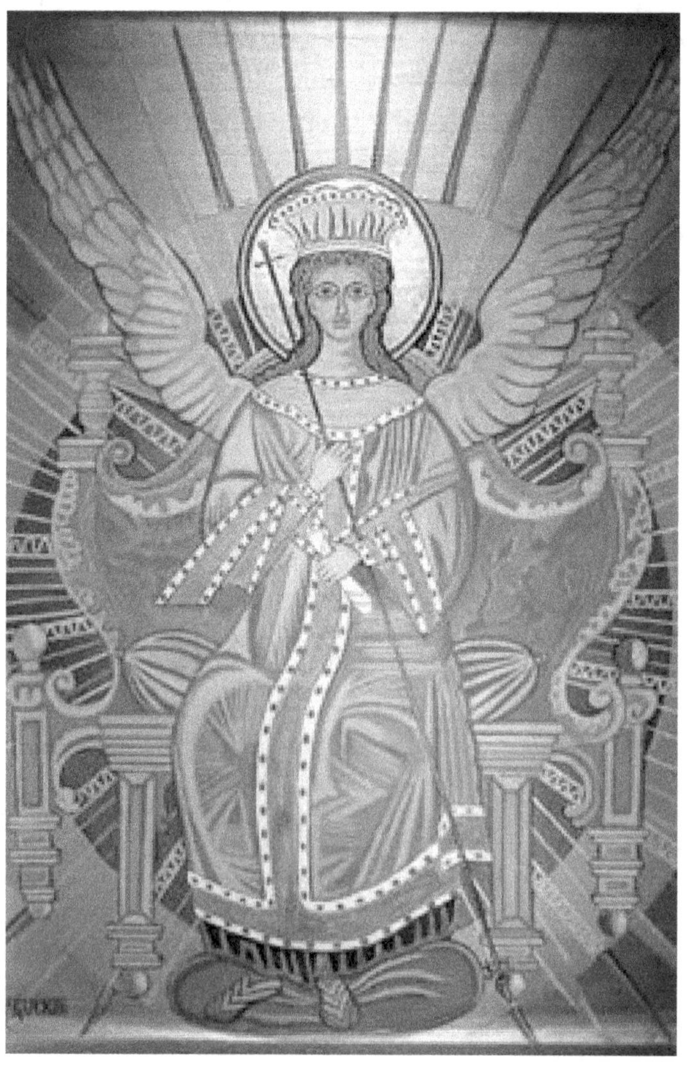

A Short Treatment for One Specific Organ or Chakra

1. Begin by calling in the person's Ray Lord or Lady, and/or Sophia or Sanat Kumara.
2. Observe Steps 1- 4.
3. Move directly to the afflicted organ or chakra. Determine the Ray and/or Chakra color and beam a colored light while generating the associated notes and sounds over the area.
4. Use acupressure to massage the acu-points associated with the organ/chakra.
5. If the organ is weak, and/or the chakra is not functioning properly, rotate energy into it and perform soft acupressure on the associated organs and meridians. If the organ or chakra is generally strong but suffering from an acute issue or trauma, rotate energy out of it. Give the organ's meridians, and the chakra's associated organ, a strong and sustained acupressure massage.
6. Call forth a Lord of Lady associated with the organ/chakra's ray and ask them to move their healing energies through you and into the organ/chakra.
7. Perform Seven Ray Reiki on the organ/chakra for 3-5 minutes. If it suffers from an excessive and acute condition, place your hands 2-3 inches above the organ/chakra. If chronic and weak, place your hands directly on it.
8. Add Seven Ray Polarity Therapy with your hands placed above/below and on each side of the afflicted organ.
9. End with broadcasting a green color systemically over the entire body while playing the Note C and music associated with the color green. See Chapter 3.

During the week following a Short Treatment for a Specific Organ advise your client to broadcast a light of the color needed by the afflicted organ/chakra at least once a day for a minimum of 45 minutes while playing the associated music. Colored lights (60-75 Watt) can usually be purchased at local discount stores. They can also make and regularly drink the appropriate colored water.

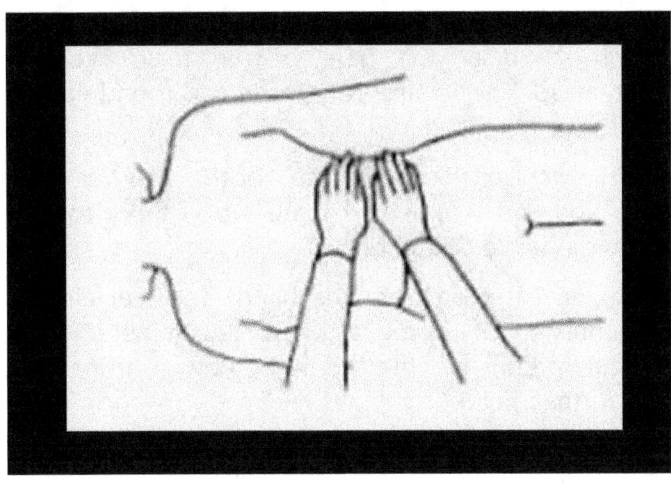

Alchemical Treatments

In the following pages are specialized alchemical treatments for those ready to purify and evolve spiritually. They include treatments for Kundalini Activation, Opening to Divine Live, and Third Eye Activation.

Kundalini Activation Treatment

1. Begin by calling in the person's Ray Lord or Lady, and/or Sophia or Sanat Kumara, the Lady and Lord of the Seven Rays.

2. Have your client sit straight up inside your Crystal Grid and/or Pyramid Temple. Have them hold meteorites or clear quartz crystals in their hands and begin Connected Breath Pranayama. Shine a red color light over their back with or without a strobe & play Root Chakra music (drumming, didjeridoo, etc.). While sitting on the left side of your client first trace trace one or both Raku symbols (on following page) over the back. Now trace Cho Ku Rei over the Third Eye and base of spine and then place your left hand over their Third Eye and your right hand over the base of their spine. Hold your hands in place for 2-5 minutes while your client continues to observe Connected Breath pranayama. Then have them stop the pranayama and recline onto their backs while they continue to hold the stones in their hands.

3. Move to the head and stimulate the Windows to the Sky Acu-Points. Afterwards, if you have a Crystal Crown, place it on your client's head.

4. Have your client resume Circular Breath. During the remaining Kundalini Activation Session Circular Breath should be engaged in as much as possible. A red light should be broadcast over the body at the same time while you play its associated note and music (Drumming, Djeridoo).

5. While at your client's side perform Seven Ray Polarity with your left hand at the head and right hand at the base of the torso while stimulating Du 20 at the top of the head. Then shake your rattle and sound your Tibetan or Crystal Bowl over their entire torso.

6. Starting at the collar bone, trace both of the Raku symbols over the torso, 3x each, and end at the base of the torso. Continue to repeat the name of "Skanda" while doing this.

7. Stimulate the Four Gates on both the hands and feet along with S.I. 3 at the side of the hand. Stimulate S.I. 3 for at least 2-3 minutes while leading the person in a guided visualization of the Serpent Power rising from the base of the spine to the top of their head.

8. Have the person observe 2-5 more minutes of Connected Breath, then relax. Complete session with systemic green toning with associated music.

RAKU ACTIVATION SYMBOLS

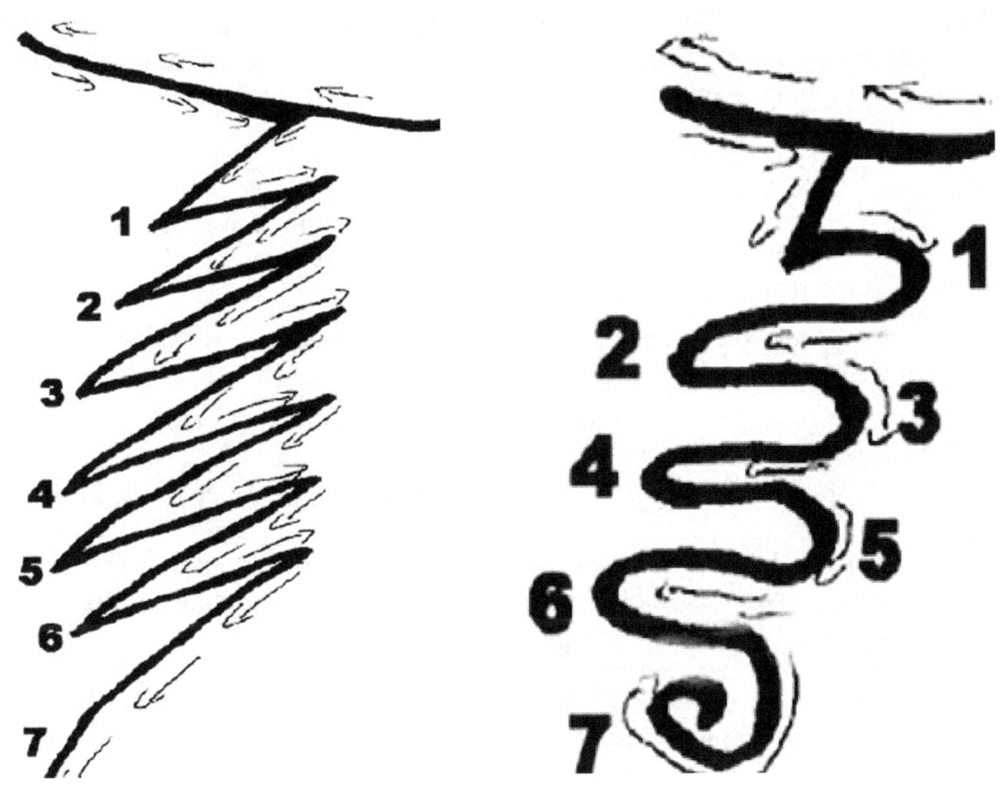

During the week following a Kundalini Activation Session advise your client to perform the Dragon Body Activation Technique in Appendix 2 once in the morning and once at night. Instruct them in what to expect if the Kundalini awakens, including a serge of energy in the body: pressure and heat at the base of the spine; unique dreams, visions, deep meditations, and/or periods of deep peace. If the Kundalini Activation results are overwhelming and/or they decide they would like the activity of the Kundalini to abate, they can simply discontinue any spiritual work they have been doing and/or summon their deity, guide or spiritual teacher to assist them. The best teachers to summon in order to control the Kundalini are the Siddhas and Satgurus, who are enlightened adepts that have achieved God-Realization and become Masters of the force. Currently, one of the best on the planet is Mata Amritanandamayi, aka Amma, meaning "MOther." . If your client does not have a spiritual teacher he or she can pray to Amma for assistance.

Opening to Divine Love Treatment

During this Alchemical Treatment you will be overseeing the alchemical release of blocked emotions and traumas that are preventing the person from completely opening their heart. You will also feed the Heart Chakra with expansive and loving energy to assist in its purification and evolution.

There are two parts to this treatment.

Part I - During this first half of the session you will be stimulating your client's Liver and Third Chakra to release toxins that create blockages in the Liver. The Liver filters the blood and serves as the seat of the emotional body.

Part II - During the second half of the session you will be stimulating and balancing the Heart and Heart Chakra.

Start Treatment:

1. Call in the person's Ray Lord or Lady, and/or Sophia or Sanat Kumara.
2. **Begin Part I:** Perform Step 4 to activate the person's energy field. While stimulating the Four Gates also massage the Heart 7 and Spleen 6 Acu-Points.
3. Systemically tonate the body with a green light while playing the corresponding music. See Chapter 3.
4. Trace the Dai-Ko-Myo symbol over the solar plexus.
5. Place green stones over the solar plexus and in the hands of the client.
6. Have your client resume Connecting Breath if they have previously discontinued it.
7. Rotate energy clockwise into the solar plexus with a hand-held crystal or wand.
8. If issues arise that overpower the client, discontinue inserting energy into the area.
9. **Begin Part II:** Tonate the body with a pink light and play the corresponding music.
10. Place pink stones over the Heart Chakra while also placing them in the person's hands. Use Pink or Watermelon Tourmaline stones, if possible.
11. Have your client resume Connecting Breath if they have previously discontinued it.
12. Trace the Dai-Ko-Myo symbol over the heart 3x. Rotate energy clockwise into the heart with a hand-held crystal or wand. Stop this practice if emotional issues arise that overwhelm the client.
13. Call forth the Universal Goddess to move through you and then perform Reiki on the heart for 5-10 minutes. Then place both hands together over the heart if client is male; and place the left hand above breasts and right hand between them if your client is female.
14. End with a systemic tonation of the green light with its corresponding music.

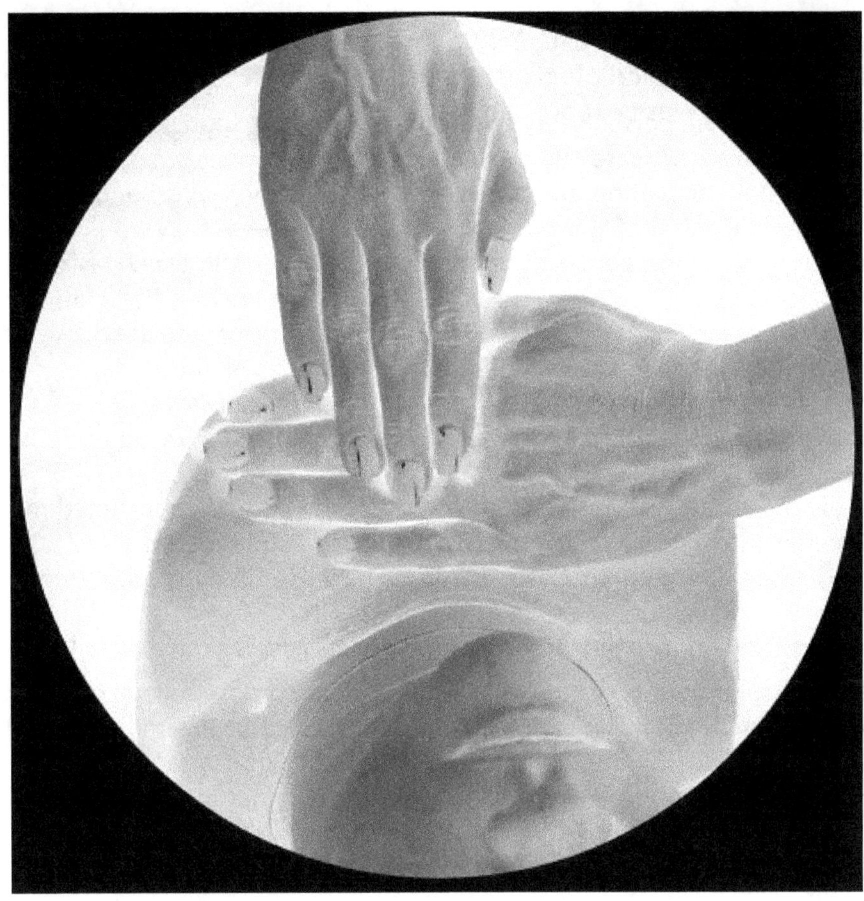

During the week following a Divine Love Session advise your client to perform the Dragon Body Activation Technique in Appendix 2 once in the morning and again at night. 1x each day they should bathe themselves in a green and/or pink light for at least 45 minutes while repeating the Heart Mantra of Kumara and placing their hands over their Heart Chakra. Green and Pink Colored lights (60-75 Watt) can usually be purchased at local discount stores. They can also make and regularly drink green-colored water as instructed in Chapter 3.

Third Eye Activation Treatment

During this Alchemical Treatment you will be overseeing the release of blockages in the head and the alchemical opening of a person's Third Eye of Wisdom.

1. Begin by calling in the person's Ray Lord or Lady, and/or Sophia or Sanat Kumara
2. Perform Step 4b to activate the person's energy field while they are laying down. Spend extra time activating the Windows to the Sky Points and Du 20. When stimulating the 4 Gates add SI 3 point.
3. While standing or sitting above the person's head, trace the Dai-Ko-Myo or Cho Ku Rei symbol over the Third Eye and then perform Seven Ray Reiki on the area for 2-5 minutes. Use Seven Ray Polarity Therapy: Place your left hand over the Third Eye and your right hand under their head at the base of the skull. Remove crown during this process then replace it.
4. Place Blue/Indigo stones in the person's hands. Replace crown or place Blue/Indigo stones over the Third Eye.
5. Systemically broadcast a Dark Blue/ Indigo color while playing associated music.
6. Rotate energy into the Third Eye with a wand or terminated crystal. Stimulate the stones and/or crown gem that is over the Third Eye. Repeat this step every five minutes.
7. Complete session with systemic toning of the green light with associated music.

During the week following a Third Eye Activation Session advise your client to perform the Dragon Body Activation Technique in Appendix once in the morning and again at night followed by 10-15 minutes of meditation. Once each day they should bathe themselves in an indigo light for at least 45 minutes while lying down and playing the associated music. Also place an indigo gem over the Third Eye during this period. They can also make and regularly drink indigo colored water as instructed in Chapter 3

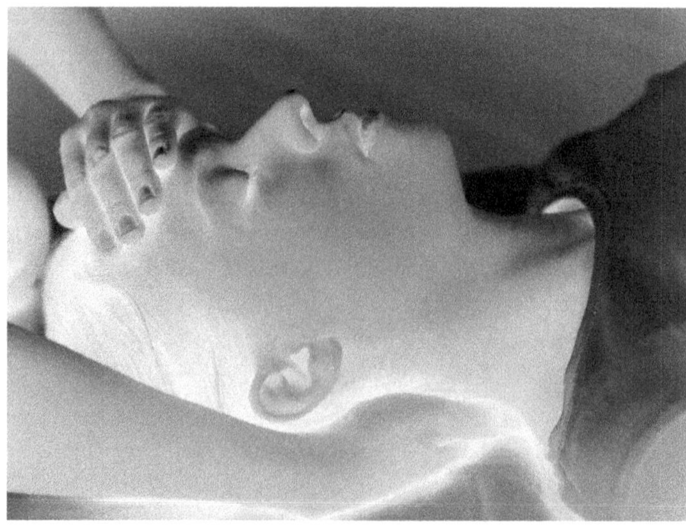

Additional Instructions for all Seven Ray Treatments

1. Do not use the same treatment for more than five sessions unless you perceive continued improvement of the condition. If you are using acupressure, after five sessions vary your choice of points; you can use some of the original ones you chose if you want but add some new ones. If you are using music therapy, change the music you are broadcasting during the session.

2. Important: Know you limitations. If you don't trust yourself to be able to give your client a beneficial session – perhaps because they exhibit symptoms that you cannot identify - then consider referring him or her to another therapist. Or, if you have worked on a person over a series of sessions and have not gained the hoped-for results, again consider referring the person out. Because of pre-arranged karmic contracts we have with people, we are able to always able to help many persons who require our assistance. And often times people are just not ready to be healed no matter what treatment they receive, or who the therapist is, because it would involve transforming a deep inner part of themselves they are not quite ready to change.

3. It is always recommended that you give your client some suggestions of things they can do on their own when you are not treating them. In general, getting an hour of therapy once a week is not enough. The healing energies need to be working on an organ or chakra every day. Encourage your clients to observe certain dietary recommendations, consume daily herbs, practice yoga and meditation, etc. You can also suggest that they give themselves daily Seven Ray Reiki treatments and/ or buy a colored light bulb to administer regular color therapy on themselves while simultaneously playing the appropriate note and/or healing music in the background.

4. In order to become proficient and quick in your diagnosis, practice performing the Seven Rays of Healing diagnosis techniques on yourself, friends and family. And also practice the treatment modalities on them. Only through continual administration of these modalities on yourself and others will you know how effective they can be. And once you get confidence in them, they will be more powerful when you use them on clients.

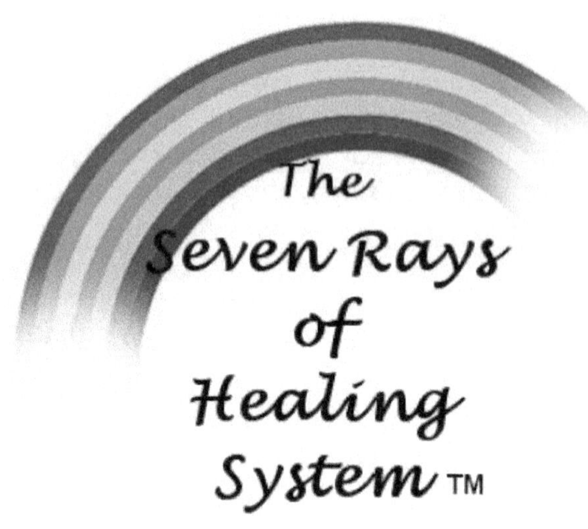

Chapter 9

Advanced Diagnosis Techniques and Treatment of the Inner Organs

In this chapter you will learn Advanced Diagnostic Techniques that you can add to the basic techniques presented in Chapter 4. Pick and choose the ones that suit you best, then determine which ones give you the most consistently accurate results. This section will also offer additional treatment suggestions for each inner organ.

Advanced Diagnosis Techniques

The 8 Principles, Tongue and Pulse, and the Palpation techniques that will be presented in this chapter are Advanced Diagnostic Techniques that work together and mutually confirm each other. Together they determine whether a person is more Yin (female, cold, wet) or Yang (male, hot, dry) and how to bring the body back into a state of balance.

Part I

The 8 Principles

All disease is caused from either an imbalance of the Yin/Yang polarity. The 8 Principles is especially designed to determine which polarity is out of harmony. This diagnostic technique is based on the concept that there are two primary energies or principles within the universe, Yin and Yang, which comprise all form and need to be kept in a state of balance if harmony and health are to be maintained. In the human body the balance or imbalance of these opposing principles determines the health or dis-ease of the body. When either Yin or Yang becomes deficient or excessive, their balance is lost and physical, emotional, or mental dis-ease can result. Only when the balance of Yin and Yang is re-established through either decreasing or increasing one or the other, can a return to balance and health be re-established.

The 8 Principles

Yin	Yang
Deficient	Excess
Cold	Hot
Internal	External

The 8 Principles are divided into two columns. One is headed Yin and the other Yang. The principles listed under Yin are divisions or characteristics of the Yin Principle and those under Yang are divisions or characteristics of the Yang Principle. When someone exhibits the Yin characteristics of deficiency, coldness or internal disharmony, they are exhibiting a Yin condition and a Yin imbalance; when their body is excessive, hot, or disharmonious on a superficial level, they are exhibiting a Yang condition and a Yang imbalance. If any of these Yin or Yang manifestations reveal themselves to you during your diagnosis, you can conclude that the person has become predominantly Yin or Yang. Treatment then requires you to correct the imbalanced principle and return the body to its normal harmony. An understanding of each of the 8 Principles and how to identify and balance them will be covered in the following pages.

Tongue and Pulse

Tongue and Pulse diagnostic techniques give unique information to help you confirm your pathological assessments based upon the 8 Principles. All three forms of examination - Tongue, Pulse and 8 Principles - should occur before making your final diagnosis and treatment plan.

Tongue Diagnosis: When examining the tongue look at the body of the tongue, its color and its coating. Each will give you information relating to imbalances of Yin or Yang. In general, a tongue that is pale, flabby and/or with a whitish coating is a Yin tongue, and it points to a Yin imbalance in the body. One that is reddish in color, has a firm body and/or a yellowish coating is a Yang tongue and points to a Yang imbalance.

Pulse Diagnosis: Put you index, middle and ring fingers together and gently place them just below the crease on the wrist on the thumb or radial side of the wrist. The radial artery is just inside the radius bone. Feel whether the pulse is thin and weak or wide and strong. A Yin pulse is a thin and weak pulse. It is often as thin as a thread, hard to find, and becomes nearly imperceptible when you place thumb pressure on it. A Yang pulse is a wide and strong pulse. It is easy to find and may even become stronger when you press down on it. Such a pulse can denote a Yang condition, but it can also be a normal pulse in a healthy individual. So you need to look for other confirming symptoms of Yang excess before making a diagnosis. Also, check whether the pulse is too fast (over 80 beats per minute) or too slow (less than 60 beats a minute). Count the beats for 6 seconds and then multiply by 10. Fast pulse denotes Yang condition and a slow one denotes a Yin condition in the body. Also, if the pulse is very tight and rebounds against your fingers like a guitar string - a "Wiry Pulse" - it often denotes tightness and stress in the body, and can be a sign of Liver disharmony.

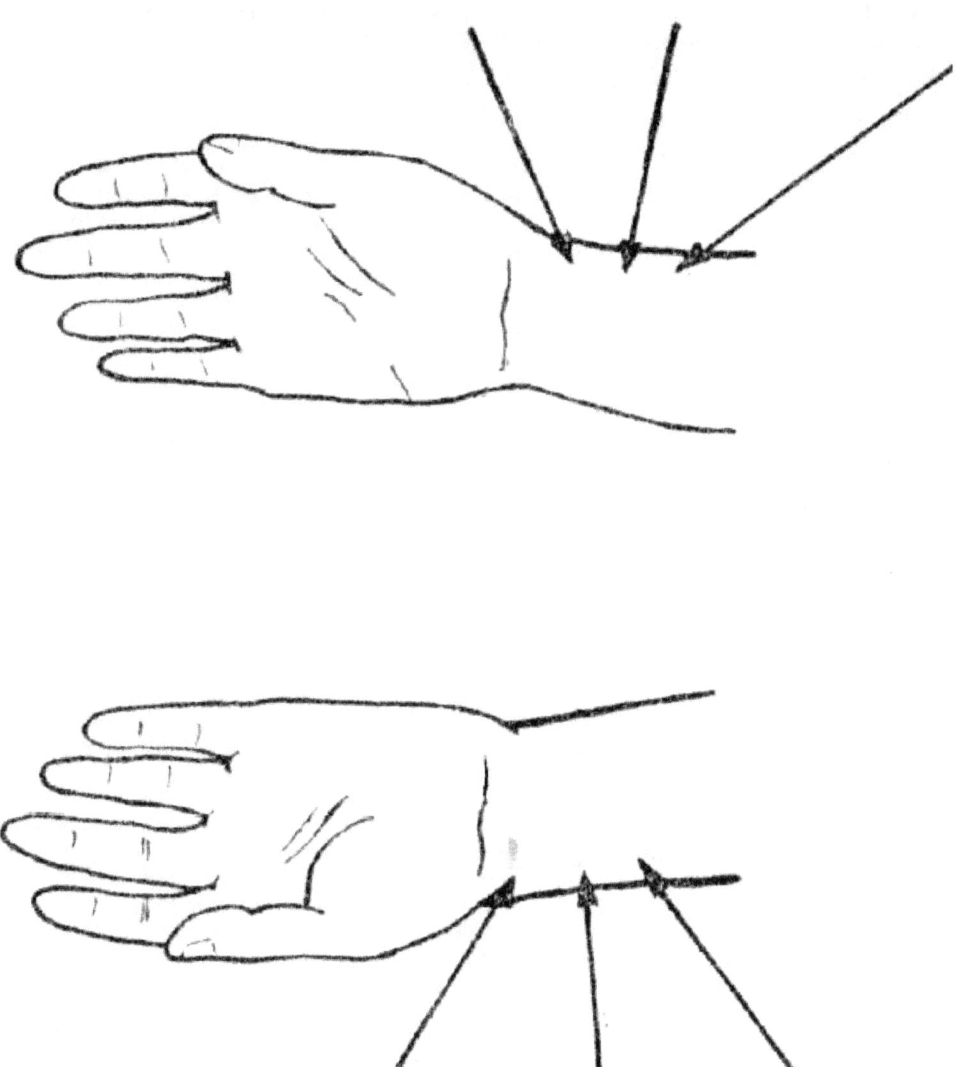

Pulse Positions

Palpation

Palpation or touch diagnosis supports and confirms the 8 Principle and Tongue and Pulse diagnoses. A patient's reaction to the warmth or coldness of applied touch, as well as its depth and pressure, tells a lot about whether the person's condition is more Yin or Yang. In general, persons who have become more Yin are weak and cold and prefer a light warm touch, while Yang persons prefer a cool but deep touch. Yin persons also tend towards chronic aches and pains, while the aches and pains of a Yang natured person are usually acute and quickly healed.

Palpation diagnosis also includes palpating or massaging acupressure points associated with certain organs and along the channels specifically associated with those organs. If there is inordinate pain when depressing points on a channel, then there is likely to be a disharmony in the organ that the channel is associated with.

Part II

Combining Tongue and Pulse, and Palpation Symptoms

You have now learned Tongue, Pulse and Palpation techniques that will help you determine whether Yin or Yang is out of balance. You can stop here, if you desire. Or, if you desire to learn how to use tongue, pulse and palpation to determine if a Yang condition specifically points to an Excess or Heat or External condition of the body, and if a Yin condition specifically points Deficiency or Cold or an Internal disharmony, please read on. Once you learn how to detect if the person's condition is principally Excessive, Hot, External, or Deficient, Cold, internal, you will have a better idea of how to treat them. Modalities and techniques to correct these Yin/Yang imbalances are presented later in this chapter.

Deficiency/Excess

Yin Deficiency

In general, deficient persons usually have frail and thin bodies. They chronically lack energy, and usually exhibit a pale, whitish complexion. They tend towards chronic illnesses because their immune systems are too weak to combat pathological conditions.

Tongue: The tongue of a deficient person is usually pale in color. It may also lack definition and be somewhat flabby, a sign of chi deficiency. There is usually a whitish coating that may be pasty, mixed with a lot of mucous.

Pulse: The pulse of a deficient Yin person is thin and weak and may disappear when pressure is applied to it. It is also often slow.

Palpation: Deficient persons usually like a warm touch with light pressure. And they often like a long, prolonged touch. Touch provides them with the energy they lack.

Yang Excess

Excessive persons are Yang in nature. Yang conditions result from an excess of something in the body while Yin conditions usually result from too little of some necessary nutrient. A Yang person tends towards being overweight. They don't like wearing a lot of clothing because they have an abundance of heat in their bodies. And they can be aggressive, angry, stressed-out and have chronic high blood pressure. Normally excessive persons suffer from acute rather than chronic illnesses.

Tongue: The tongue of an excessive person tends to be reddish in color with a light to heavy yellow coating.

Pulse: The Pulse of an excessive person is usually fast, wide and forceful. It can also be "Wiry" and feel tight like a tightly stretched guitar string or wire, especially if the person is under a lot of stress.

Palpation: Because of their excess heat, excessive persons usually like a cool touch for a short period of time. They also like a deep touch, because a lot of pressure helps to release some of their excess energy and tightness. These persons tend to have very tight shoulders and necks.

Cold/Hot

Yin Cold

Persons who are chronically cold are lacking in warmth because their bodies are too frail and weak to generate enough heat. They are Yin in nature. They resist being in cold climates and often sleep curled up in the fetus position with a lot of blankets covering them. This is unless the cold condition is caused by a virus; then the feelings of cold are intense and acute, and sometimes alternate with sensations of excessive heat. In this case there will be excessive symptoms, such as excessive phlegm and coughing.

Tongue: The tongue of a cold person is pale and the coating is usually white. If the person has a virus, or acute cold, the white coating can be excessive.

Pulse: The pulse of a cold person is normally slow and less than 60 beats per minute. If the person has chronic cold, then the pulse may also be weak, but if their cold is acute their pulse will be both slow and forceful.

Palpation: A cold person likes a warm touch. A chronically cold person will like a soft, warm touch, while an acutely cold person will like a deep and warm touch.

Yang Hot

Hot conditions are generally classified as Yang. A Yang person often feels excessively warm; they wear scant clothing and sleep with few blankets covering them. They do not curl up when the lie down to hold in heat, but extend their arms and legs to release excess warmth. Some Yang persons also have a ruddy complexion and a reddish skin color caused from their internally generated heat. They may also have an angry temperament and a tendency towards headaches, which are caused by heat and stress affecting the liver.

Tongue: Heat conditions usually manifest as a reddish colored tongue. If the heat is acute and caused by a virus, there may also be a thick yellow coating covering the tongue.

Pulse: Just as cold manifests as a slow pulse, heat conditions are reflected in a rapid pulse; one that is 80 or more beats per minute.

Palpation: Heat conditions seek relief through a cool touch for short duration. Heat conditions caused by a virus respond to both a cool and deep touch, in order to breakup and move the underlying excessive buildup of blocked energy.

Internal/External

Yin Internal

Symptoms of internal illness are chronic or long-term illnesses, especially to one or more of the important internal organs, such as the Heart or the Kidneys. These are the organs that become afflicted when an illness hangs on for a long period of time and becomes "internal." Liver disharmony can be a symptom of either internal or external illness.

Tongue: A tongue that reflects an internal condition can be either pale or red. Since internal conditions consume the body and its fluids, the tongue may also be lacking a coating. A general rule regarding the coating is that if the coating is abundant there is usually an excessive Yang condition in the body, but if it is deficient there is usually a deficient Yin condition afflicting the body.

Pulse: The depth of the pulse can tell you a lot about the depth of a dis-ease. If the pulse is easy to find and seems to lie "on the surface" of the wrist (known as a "superficial pulse") then the imbalance is external, but if you have to press your fingers hard to locate a pulse that seems to be well "below the surface," then chances are that the illness is internal.

Palpation: For an internal Yin condition you might have to push deeply into the body before pressure is felt.

Yang External

External Yang conditions are normally caused by acute illnesses that have not existed long enough to effect the internal environment of the body. Such conditions generally attack the Lungs, Stomach and Intestines, organs that consistently serve as the first line of defense for external pathogens entering the body. Included in the list of eternal illnesses are viral and bacterial infections, colds and flues, stomach and intestinal problems. External problems usually run their course and clear up within a few of days.

Tongue: External conditions generally reveal themselves as either a pale or red tongue, but there is usually an abundance of tongue coating and phlegm.

Pulse: An external pulse is one that seems to lie on the surface of the body, just like the disharmony itself. It takes very little pressure to feel it, and when you press down deep enough it often seems to disappear.

Palpation: Little pressure is needed to diagnose external conditions. Since the disharmony is on the surface, just a slight amount of pressure can be tangibly felt by the client.

Quick Diagnosis Chart

Now that you have learned pulse, tongue, palpation and the 8 Principles, you canarrive at a quick diagnosis of a client by using a Quick Diagnosis Chart like the one below and on on the following page. This will keep all your diagnosis information in one place and make it easier to both diagnose a client and to come up with a treatment plan for them.

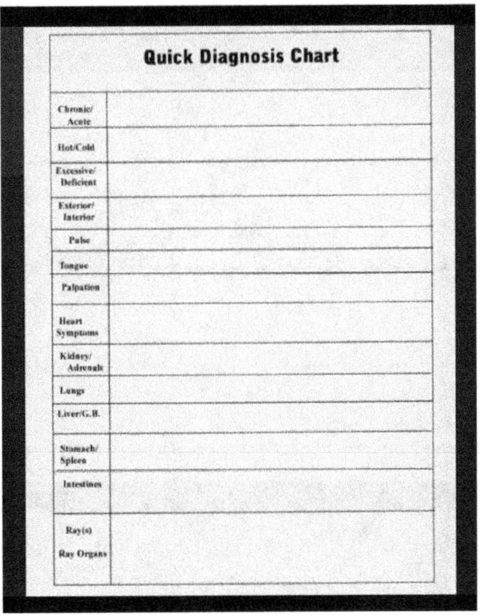

Quick Diagnosis Chart

Chronic/ Acute	
Hot/Cold	
Excessive/ Deficient	
Exterior/ Interior	
Pulse	
Tongue	
Palpation	
Heart Symptoms	
Kidney/ Adrenals	
Lungs	
Liver/G.B.	
Stomach/ Spleen	
Intestines	
Ray(s) Ray Organs	

Quick Diagnosis Chart	
Chronic/ Acute	
Hot/ Cold	
Excessive/ Deficient	
Exterior/ Interior	
Pulse	
Tongue	
Palpation	
Heart Syptoms	
Kidney/ Adrenals	
Lungs	
Liver/ G.B	
Stomach/ Spleen	
Intestines	
Ray (s) Ray Organs	

Treatments for Balancing
Yin/Yang Conditions

Once you have determined whether Yin or Yang has gone out of balance, you need to know how to correct the imbalance. Treatment usually involves either warming and tonifying a Yin deficient condition, or cooling and dispersing a Yang excessive condition. This can be accomplished through a variety of therapies, including herbs, diet, color therapy, and gems.

Balancing with Herbs

All herbs have certain properties that determine how they are to be used. Some herbs are, for example, naturally heating while others are cooling. Some are tonifying and many have a dispersing and releasing effect. One way to identify the properties of an herb (or a food) is through its taste. The following corresponds one of the five tastes to its inherent property:

Taste	Associated Property
Spicy	Heating, Dispersing
Bitter	Cooling, Dispersing, Detoxifying
Sour	Cooling, Astringent*
Sweet	Tonifying, Warming
Salty	Heating, Astringent

*The Astringent property holds in fluids.

Another way to differentiate the property of an herb is in accordance with the part of the plant it comes from. In general, the higher up on the plant it grows, the higher in the body will an herb work. And its height and softness also make an herb more dispersing in effect. In general, the soft flowers of a plant are the most dispersing, the leaves and stems are both dispersing and building, and the hard roots are the most tonifying.

Herbs for Deficiency/Excess Conditions

For deficient Yin conditions your therapy should be to tonify and build-up the body. The best all-around tonifying herb is Ginseng Root. There are a few kinds of Ginseng; the one you chose should be in accordance to the severity of the deficiency, as well as the constitution of the client. Red Chinese and Red Korean are the strongest kinds of Ginseng, but also the most stimulating. If you client has difficulty with strong stimulants you need to give them a milder form of Ginseng, such as American or Siberian Ginseng. For tonifying the blood, such as after a heavy menstrual period, the best herb is Tang Kuei (or Dang Quai).

For excessive conditions you should prescribe cooling, bitter herbs, unless the excessive condition is the common cold. In that case you would prescribe an herb that is both warming and dispersing, such as fresh Ginger Root. The bitter dispersing herbs include Chamomile (both dispersing and relaxing) and Honeysuckle. If the excessive person is constipated, give cooling Cascara Sagrada, and if they exhibit toxic symptoms (boils, rashes, etc) give cooling and dispersing Echinacea or Dandelion Root. For excessive stress and/or nervousness, prescribe Valerian Root, Chamomile, Skullcap, and/or Lobelia. For excessive cramping use Lobelia, and for menstrual cramps use Cramp Bark.

Herbs for Cold/Hot Conditions

For chronic cold conditions, give tonifying herbs such as Ginseng and Licorice, as well as Ginger Root. An excellent warming tea is made of equal parts of Licorice and Ginger Root. Acute cold symptoms that are the result of overexposure to wind and cold, or the common cold, require the heating influence of Ginger Root or Ephedra but without the tonifying influence of Ginseng or Licorice. Never tonify an excessive condition. This will just create more phlegm and may make the condition worse.

For chronic hot conditions give cooling herbs, such as chamomile. If the hot condition is acute, and perhaps infectious, and/or caused by toxins, give Echinacea or Dandelion Root. For hot, infectious diarrhea, cooling Rhubarb Root is a good herb to use. A beneficial herb for hot fevers is Boneset. For hot conditions that accompany a cold, give the cooling and dispersing Peppermint.

Herbs for Internal/External Conditions

Certain herbs work mostly on the external regions of the body, while some work principally deep in the interior. External herbs are given when the illness is a common virus or bacterial infection and the illness is mainly affecting the lungs, stomach and intestines. The best of these herbs is fresh Ginger Root, which helps the body throw off a common illness while benefiting both the lungs and stomach. Other good external herbs include all dried flowers, such as Elder Flower, and all herbs in the mint family (Peppermint, Spearmint, etc.). Internal herbs work specifically on the important inner organs, such as the Kidneys, Heart and Liver. They include well-dried leaves and roots. When Ginger Root is fresh it works externally, but when it is dried it works internally.

Diets to Balance Ying/Yang Conditions

Persons with a Yang excessive body or exhibiting hot or excessive symptoms should eat a light, cooling diet, full of fruits, vegetables and grains. A diet with plenty of roughage is important to move the excess out of the body. Persons with a Yin deficient constitution, or those exhibiting a cold, deficient symptoms should eat warm building foods with ample protein and fat. If their illness has become internal and they are chronically weak, they should consume easy to digest foods, preferably in a soup of broth. Someone whose body is naturally balanced - not too Yin or too Yang - should consume a diet modeled after the Japanese Macrobiotic diet. The foods constituting this diet are generally neither Yin nor Yang but fall somewhere in between, such as grains, beans and cooked fruits.

Color Therapy for Yin/Yang Conditions

There are three principal colors that are used in color therapy to bring the body back into its proper Yin/Yang balance. These are blue, green and red. Blue has a Yin, cooling effect; green, the color of balance, promotes the perfect balance of Yin/Yang; and the color red has a Yang, heating influence.

For a body that is excessive and hot: bathe the entire body in a blue light.

For a deficient and cold body: bathe the body in red light. In both cases, you should bathe the body for at least twenty minutes. At the end of any session always bathe the body in green in order to bring back to a perfect Yin/Yang balance.

Color Therapy can also be approached through diet. The red frequency can also enter the body through warming and spicy foods and red colored food, such as apples, cherries, strawberries red peppers, red meat, red seafood, etc. The blue frequency can enter the body through cooling and blue colored foods, such as blue berries, black cherries, blue plums, mushrooms, blue seaweed, blue figs, etc. The green frequency can enter the body through temperate and green colored foods, such as leafy vegetables, broccoli, lettuce, peas, green beans, green bell peppers, green olives, kiwi fruit, lines, green grapes, etc.

Gem Therapy

Use Gem Therapy like Color Therapy. For hot, excessive conditions have the client wear Yin colored stones – blue, violet, indigo, etc. For cold, deficient symptoms have the client wear Yang colored stones – red, orange, and yellow.

Advanced Diagnosis and Treatment using Pendulums and Kinesiology

Pendulum diagnosis is very simple and a great tool for further confirming your other Yin/Yang diagnostic indications. First take your pendulum and program it. Swing it clockwise while affirming that this indicates a Yin condition. Then swing it counterclockwise while stating that when the pendulum turns in that direction it indicates a Yang condition. Now move the pendulum across the surface of the body while your client is lying face-up. Wherever the pendulum begins swinging counterclockwise you know you have a Yin imbalance, and when it moves clockwise you have a Yang condition. When you have finished the front, do the person's back. You might want to start by waving it over organs you suspect are in disharmony and then progress to other areas of uncertainty.

If you are not sure that you are prescribing the right herbs, foods or gems to a client you can try a couple of confirmation techniques. If you have a pendulum, try waving it above the substance in question. Ask the question "Is this the right cure for ____". If the pendulum swings in a clockwise direction above the substance then you know it will help them. If the pendulum swings to the left and in a counter-clockwise direction then avoid the cure. It is not in your client's best interest. Also swing your pendulum above the dosage you are prescribing while asking if it is a good one for your client. Another easy approach to confirming the efficacy of a substance is to let the person's body tell you whether it wants it or not. This information can be acquired through the technique of kinesiology. Simply have your client hold the substance in question in their right hand, and then move the hand close against the body. Have the client hold their left arm straight out at their side. Ask the client's body if the substance is best for him or her and then lightly press down on your client's arm. If the arm strongly resists your pressure, then the substance is beneficial for your client. But if the arm is easily pushed down to your client's side and gives very little resistance, then the substance is not the best for him or her.

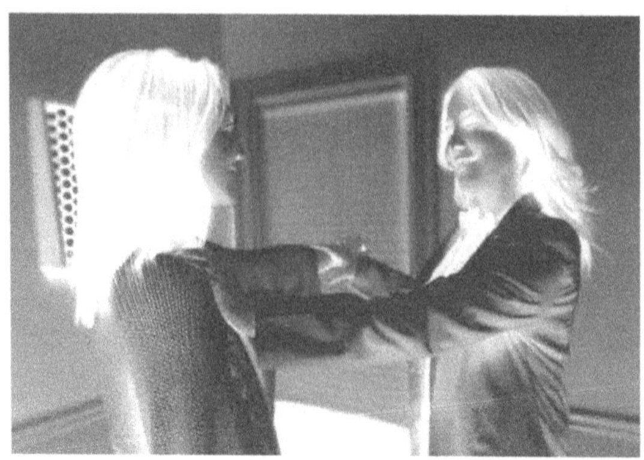

Advanced Diagnosis and Treatment for Individual Organs

Heart

People with a pre-disposition to Heart dysfunction:
Typically Ray 3 Individuals

This Ray gives a tendency for Heart problems, especially if the person being considered has Leo Rising.

Physical Symptoms:
Pulse: Overly Fast, Slow, or Irregular (not regular rhythm)
Tongue: Red, Pale or Purple (purple color indicates blood is not moving smoothly)
Blue or purple lips
Pain: Pain in chest and/or pain radiates down left arm.
Heart Palpitations
Shortness of breath
Pain along course of Heart Meridian
Pain at Heart points
Chronic fatigue

Mental and Emotional Symptoms:
Over-active mind
Inability to feel or give love
Little or no joy in life
No spontaneity
Mental Illness; psychosis

Treatment of Heart dysfunction:
Invoke Sanat Kumara or Sophia, Lord and Lady of the Seven Rays, and/or the Lords and deities of the 3rd Ray.
Invoke Sophia and Sananda Kumara, the Lord of the 4th Ray of Love and Balance, for emotional Heart problems.
Perform 7 Ray Reiki over Heart. Do both back and front of body.

Broadcast red light for physical ailment; green and/or pink light over Heart for mental/emotional issues.
Place red stones for physical problems and green and pink stones on Heart area for mental/emotional issues.
Play Note G for physical Heart problems; Note C for emotional and mental problems.
Use Acupressure points, such as H7, UB15. Use 4 Gates (LI 4 & Liv3), especially for emotional and mental problems
Give medium stimulation to the points
Use herbs, such as Hawthorn Berry, Garlic, Licorice and Ginseng Root for physically weak Heart, and Camomile, Valerian to calm the mind, spirit and emotions.
Bitter foods
Balance Heart Chakra with Reiki, colored light, stones

Liver/Gall Bladder

People with a pre-disposition to Liver dysfunction:
Typically Ray 2, 3 and 7 Individuals
All these Ray natives have some tendency to Liver problems, especially those with Sagittarius and Scorpio Rising Signs

Physical Symptoms:
Hypochondriac pain (side pain, especially right side)
Headache
Jaundice
Difficulty digesting fats and oils
Chronic tightness in shoulders and neck
Tightness all over body
Not flexible tendons and muscles
Tendency to tendinitis
Cracked, ridged and/or broken nails
Pulse: Fast, full and strong, tight (like pressing on tight guitar string)
Tongue: Usually red with yellow coating
Tenderness along Liver and Gall Bladder Channels
Tenderness at Liver and Gall Bladder points
Eye problems

Mental and Emotional Symptoms
Chronic Anger
Over emotional; easily stressed
Explosive
Judgmental
Controlling
Difficulty planning for future

Treatment for Liver/Gall Bladder dysfunction
Invoke Sanat Kumara or Sophia, Lord and Lady of the Seven Rays, and/or Call in Lords and Ladies of the 2nd Ray.
Perform 7 Ray Reiki over Liver area
Acupressure: Liver and Gall Bladder points,: Liv3, UB 18, GB 20, 21 - (for headache and tight neck and shoulder)
Also use 4 Gates. Give strong stimulation to points.
Herbs: Buplerum (Chinese), Milk Thistle, and Dandelion Root to cleanse Liver; use Valerian and Chamomile to calm emotions.
Broadcast yellow, lemon and/or green light over Liver
Place yellow and/or green stones on body
Play Note B with yellow light; Note C with Green light.
Play soothing music if person is emotionally distraught.
Give Massage, especially to neck and shoulders
Administer Lemon juice to cleanse the Liver
Observe Juice fast with apples and/or carrots to cleanse Liver.
Sour foods; Non-fatty foods

Kidneys/Adrenals

People with a predisposition to Kidney dysfunction:
Typically Ray 1, 4, 6 Individuals
Tendency to Kidney problems are often seen especially in persons with Capricorn Rising, Libra Rising, and Pisces Rising

Physical Symptoms:
Chronic low back pain
Pain in Kidney region of torso
Chronic low energy
Difficulty breathing deeply; asthma
Weak knees
Low libido
Chronic Urinary Bladder problems
Chronic cold hands and feet
Need to get up a lot at night to urinate
Black color around eyes
Head hair falls out
Hearing problems
Chronic dizziness
Pulse: weak, thin, slow
Tongue: pale, white
Weak immune system

Mental and Emotional Symptoms
Chronic fears/paranoia
Spaceyness
Forgetful
Ungrounded
Difficulty focusing on mental work
Lack of willpower
Difficulty making up mind; tendency to vacillate

Treatment for Dysfunctional Kidneys/Adrenals
Invoke Sanat Kumara or Sophia, Lord and Lady of the Seven Rays, and/or Call on Lords and Ladies of the 1st Ray.
Perform 7 Ray Reiki over Kidney region, both front and back.
Acupressure: Kidney points K3, UB 23, Ren 4 & 6
Use mild stimulation on points
Broadcast black, dark blue, and red light. Red light is especially helpful for lack of energy.
Place black or red stones over Kidney region
Play Note E for Blue light; Note G for Red light.
Balance 1st & 2nd Chakras
Herbs: Rehmannia (Chinese), Ginseng
Foods: Salty, black beans, red or orange colored foods

Stomach/Spleen

People with a predisposition to Spleen/Stomach dysfunction: Typically Ray 4, 5 Individuals
Especially 4,5 Ray persons with Cancer Rising, Virgo Rising

Physical Symptoms
Stomachache
Indigestion
Gas, abdominal distension after eating
Heartburn
Chronic Diarrhea
No appetite
Pain along Stomach and Spleen channels
Pain at Stomach/Spleen points
Pulse: Usually full, strong, fast
Tongue: Usually thick white or yellow coating

Mental and Emotional Symptoms
Chronic worry
Over-active mind

Treatment for dysfunctional Stomach/Spleen
Invoke Sanat Kumara or Sophia, Lord and Lady of the Seven Rays, and/or Call in the Lords and Ladies of the 2nd and 4th Rays
7 Ray Reiki over Stomach area
Acupressure: Stomach/Spleen points St. 36, Spl 6, Ren 12
Can also use LI 4
Herbs: Ginger root (poor digestion and indigestion), Peppermint (indigestion), Ginseng (for chronic low appetite & poor digestion)
Sweet foods
Broadcast yellow/lemon light over Stomach area a
Place yellow/gold stones on body
Play Note B for yellow/lemon light
Balance 3rd Chakra

Lung

People with a predisposition to Lung issues
Typically Ray 4,5 Individuals
Especially those with Gemini Rising

Physical Symptoms:
Cough
Difficulty breathing
Abundant phlegm
Body hair (arm and legs) falls out
Tendency to get colds easily
Pain along Lung Meridian
Pain at Lung points
Tightness of upper back

Mental and Emotional Symptoms
Chronic grief

Treatment for dysfunctional Lung
Invoke Sanat Kumara or Sophia, Lord and Lady of the Seven Rays, and/or call in the Lords and Ladies of the 4th and 5th Rays

7 Ray Reiki over Lung region front and back
Acupressure on Lung points UB 13, Lu5, 9
Massage upper back and shoulders
Perform Diaphoresis (See Appendix 1)
Broadcast red light for cold in lungs, blue light for heat in Lungs
Same for colored stones. White colored stones on lungs to balance chronic weak lungs.
Pulse: Usually full, excessive. Slow for cold, fast for heat in lungs
Tongue: Red and yellow coating for heat in lungs, pale and white coating for cold in lungs.
Herbs: Ginger Root (esp for cold lungs and abundant phlegm), Ginseng (for chronic Lung weakness)
Foods: Spicy foods

Intestines

People with dysfunctional Intestines
Typically Ray 5 Individuals
Especially Virgo Rising

Physical Symptoms
Constipation
Both acute and chronic diarrhea
Feeling hot (infectious or bacterial diarrhea) and feverish or cold
Pulse: Fast (heat) or slow (slow)
Tongue: Red and yellow coat (heat) or pale and white coat (cold)
Pain along Large Intestine Meridian and Large Intestine Points
Gas, distension
Abdominal pain
Nervousness

Mental and Emotional Symptoms
Over-active mind
Assimilating too much information
Fear

Treatment for dysfunctional Intestines:
Invoke Sanat Kumara or Sophia, Lord and Lady of the Seven Rays, and/or call in Lords and Ladies of the 2nd and 5th Rays
7 Ray Reiki over the abdomen and lower back Acupressure: LI 4, St. 25, 36, 37

Broadcast yellow light over abdomen. Esp. for chronic diarrhea. Can also use red light for acute cold diarrhea and blue for diarrhea with heat symptoms. Blue has astringent properties
Herbs: Cascara Sagrada (constipation)
Blackberry Root Bark (diarrhea)
Astringent herbs
Foods: Dry toast, black tea, ripe bananas (diarrhea) Whole grains, fruits (constipation)

Organ Relationships

According to the Chinese Medicine System, the organs are interrelated. When one organ is dysfunction its sister organ is also often in a state of disharmony. So if your diagnosis reveals an imbalance in an organ also check its paired organ for problems. Of course, when there are chronic problems with the Kidneys all the organs are likely to suffer, because the Jing and chi of the Kidneys drive all the organs. Here are two important inter-relationships of organs that can negatively affect each other:

Liver and Stomach/Spleen: Issues with Liver can "invade" Stomach/Spleen
Kidneys and Lungs: Weak Lungs can adversely affect and weaken Kidneys, and vicer-versa.

If you decide to do a deeper study of Chinese Diagnosis you will want to study the Five Elements. The chart below shows which element is associated with which organ and how the elements and their assocaited organs are inter-related.

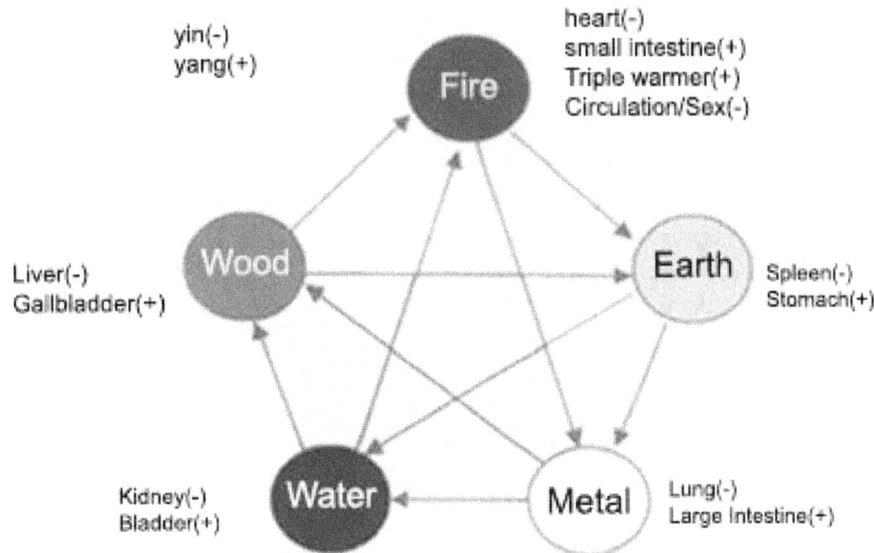

Appendix 1
Additional Seven Rays of Healing Modalities

Purging

Purging therapy is for persons with excessive symptoms. Purging clears the body of its unwanted toxic waste. The principal purging approach is through cleaning the Large Intestine with colonics and laxatives, such as Cascara Sagrada, Senna, Fennel seed, and Rhubarb Root. But Purging also involves cleaning the blood stream with blood purifiers, such as Echinacea, Chaparral, Red Clover, and Dandelion Root. Fasting falls within the category of Purging, but this approach to deep cleansing should be approached with caution. Someone who has never fasted before should never fast more than three days, and those who have fast before should not fast more than seven days. Seven days constitutes a very powerful and cleansing fast, because after the third day of a fast the body starts living off of and consuming its own toxins. No fast should be exclusively a water fast. A person should consume solid fruits and vegetables for a moderate fast; for a strong fast they should only drink fruit and vegetable juices, and for the strongest and most effective fast they should have only fresh fruit juices. The fast should occur either in the spring or summer. A fast undergone in the Fall and Winter can make one ill because a fast naturally cools the body, and a fasting person will have difficulty handling the chilly weather.

Diaphoresis

Diaphoresis is sweating therapy used to treat a Yang excessive condition that is still on the exterior. A person in need of diaphoresis may have a cold or flu with a mild fever that they need to sweat out. Give these persons either Ginger Root tea (a cold or flu with cold symptoms) or Peppermint tea (a cold or flu with heat symptoms) and then have them wrap up in blankets and sweat out their toxins. If you give a person anything cool or cold to eat or drink when they have a cold or flu it could make it harder for the body to throw off the illness, and it will produce more mucus. Diaphoresis is also necessary for high fever caused by other excessive conditions, in which case you would make a tea of Boneset and then have them sweat it out. A low grade and chronic fever signals that the person is very weak and/or the illness has gone well into the interior. Do not give herbs for sweating in this case because a strong sweat will further weaken the body. These people have fever not because they have an excess of Yang, but because they have a deficiency of Yin. They require a Yin tonic, such as Rehmannia 6 formula.

Diuresis

Diuresis is eliminating excess water in the body through urination. Excess water can manifest as excess water in the tissues (edema), and/or bloating in the abdomen that is often accompanied by poor digestion. There are many diuretic herbs that can be prescribed, including Horsetail, Uva Ursi, Parsley, Nettles, Cleavers, etc. Diuretic herbs cool the body, so some of them are also used for hot, infectious conditions, like Uva Ursi, an herb commonly used in Bladder infections.

Astringent Therapy

Astringent Therapy is used when too many fluids are exiting the body, such as with chronic diarrhea. Astringent herbs normally have tannins, the active component that precipitates an astringent effect. For diarrhea, Bayberry Bark is an excellent herb to use to hold in fluids, as is black tea, which is full of tannins. To help hold in the fetus during pregnancy, the astringent herb Squaw vine has been used among the Native American tribes for thousands of years with great results.

Appendix 2

The Dragon Body Activation Technique

The Dragon Body Activation Technique is a very effective alchemical technique that combines pranayama and meditation to purify and activate your Etheric or Dragon Body. This technique will both awaken and move the Dragon Force of Kundalini at the base of the spine, and it can fully awaken the seat of Dragon Wisdom, the Third Eye. It will also help a Dragon-in-Training to open his or her heart and assist them in connecting with the Spirit inside, ultimately endowing him or her with true Self-Knowledge, the highest Dragon Wisdom.

During this technique you will be stimulating the three principle gnostic centers: the Root Chakra, the Third Eye and the Heart Chakra. The Root Chakra is home to the Kundalini, which alchemically takes one to gnostic awareness. The Third Eye is the seat of your gnostic intuition. And the Heart is the home of your inner Spirit and your true identity. When you fully unite with it you know yourself as the embodiment of the Infinite Spirit that created the universe and has existed forever.

To awaken the Kundalini and Ajna Chakra during this technique you will be placing your right hand over the base of your spine and your left hand over your Third Eye. This will create an electrical circuit. The base of the spine has a negative charge and the right hand has a positive charge. Thus, when they unite a flow of electrons is created. Similarly, your left hand possesses a negative charge and the head possesses a positive charge. When these connections are made a complete circuit is created that moves from the base of the spine to the top of the spine and Third Eye, and then down through the two arms and back to its base. This circuit will assist in the awakening and upward movement of Kundalini to the Third Eye. During the sec-ond part of the technique the two hands are placed over the heart. This will nourish and activate the Heart Chakra, and it will assist in the development of Divine Love and the awareness of one's true identity.

Step 1:
Sit down on a floor with legs crossed or cross your legs while seated in a chair.
Place your left hand on your forehead over the Third Eye.
Place your right hand over the lower spine (region of the Kundalini). This creates a circuit.
Breathe in through the nose and out through the mouth, fairly quickly. Do not pause between the in-breath and out-breath.
Repeat these in and out breaths 15 times.
While breathing, visualize energy coming up the spine on the in-breath.
On the 15th breath, inhale and hold your breath for a few seconds and then slowly exhale.
Now keep your hands over Third Eye and base of the spine for 15-20 seconds while inwardly repeating to yourself "Arise Serpent Fire" or "Arise Dragon Force."
Repeat Step 1

Step 2:
Place your right hand over your heart.
Place your left hand on top of your right hand.
Breathe in through the nose and out through the mouth, fairly quickly. Do not pause between the in-breath and out-breath.
Breathe into the heart. Repeat these breaths 10 times.
On the 10th breath inhale, hold a few seconds, then slowly exhale.
Keep hands on heart for 15-20 seconds while inwardly repeating "Awaken Gnosis," "Awaken Divine Love," or "Awaken Dragon Wisdom."
Repeat Step 2

Step 3:
Keep your hands on your heart. After you have finished repeating "Awaken Gnosis" (or Divine Love) slowly repeat "Ma Om" to yourself (mentally) while breathing in through the nose on the syllable Ma and out through your nose on Om. Ma activates the heart and Om activates the Third Eye.

Continue silent mantra repetitions for 5-15 minutes. Your breathing will become gradually slower and you will drift into a meditative state.

This entire practice should be observed 1-3 times daily for best results. Early morning is best, then sunrise & sunset. But any time or place is beneficial.

THE AUTHOR

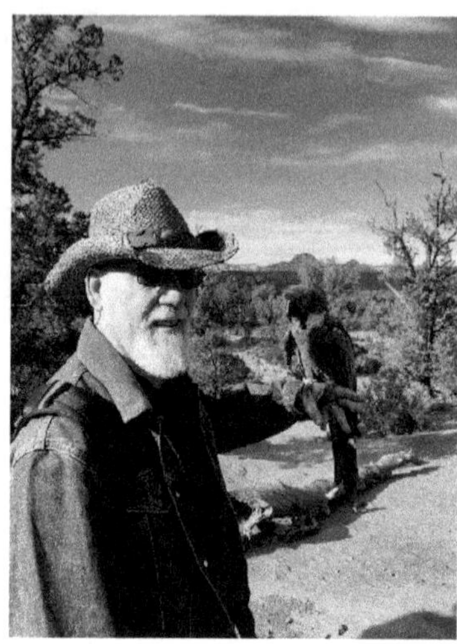

Mark Amaru Pinkham is an internationally known author, teacher, and guide to the world's sacred sites. During the past 30 years Mark has traveled extensively around the globe while leading spiritual tours for Sacred Sites Journeys (www.SacredSitesJourneys.com). During this time he has written eight books that cover the world's mystery traditions since the dawn of the human race. Mark is currently Director of *The Order and Mystery School of the Seven Rays* and *The Path of the Dragon Mystery School* (www.sevenrayorder.com) located in Sedona, Arizona. Recently, in Sedona's largest vortex, Mark discovered the remains of the ancient court of the legendary monarch known by the Hopis as Masau'u, by the Hindus as Karttikeya, by the Sumerians as Enki, by the Egyptians as Ptah-Osiris, etc. His 30 years of research is presented in his book *Sedona: City of the Star People.*

Other Books by Mark Amaru Pinkham
Purchase books at www.SevenRayOrder.com/books-courses-tours

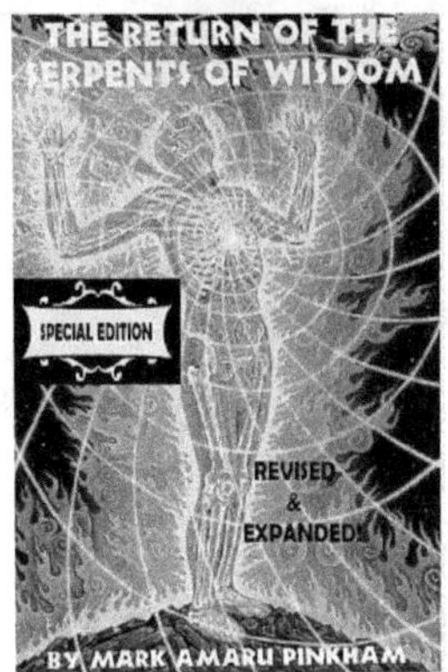

The Return of the Serpents of Wisdom - Special Edition brings together the lineages and teachings of the spiritual masters around the world whose symbol has been the serpent or dragon. The book traces the fabled beginnings of these adepts from the legendary continents in the Atlantic and Pacific Oceans, to their later occurrences as the pyramid builders, priest kings and hierophants of pre-Christian cultures around the globe, and finally to their clandestine manifestation as the Secret Societies of Europe. Learn the history and teachings of the Nagas of India

*The Lung Dragons of China *The Djedhi of Egypt *The Amaru of Peru *The Druid Adders of Britain *The Levites of Palestine *The Ashipu priests of Mesopotamia *The Quetzlcoatls of Mexico *The Snake Clan of North America *The Templars, Freemasons, and Rosicrucians 400 pgs, richly illustrated. $19.95

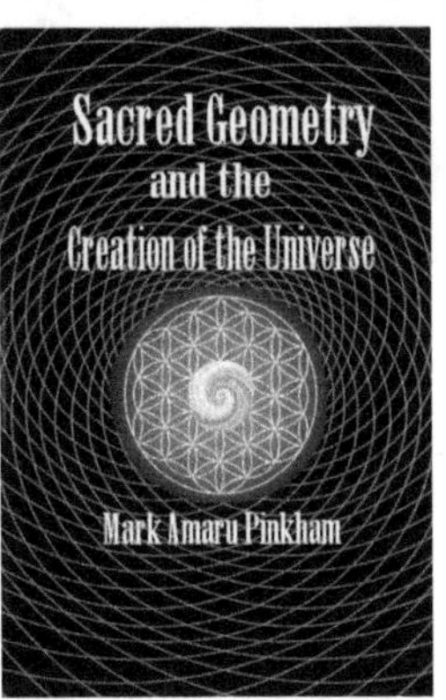

In *Sacred Geometry and the Creation of the Universe* the intricate shapes of Sacred Geometry are explained as representations of the successive stages in the creation of the universe. Beginning with the Big Bang, each Sacred Geometrical shape is shown to correspond to an important step in the creation of the cosmos. With large print and illustrations covering each page, this book clearly and easily gives an deep understanding of both Sacred Geometry and the cosmology of the universe. 140 pgs. richly illustrated. $12.95

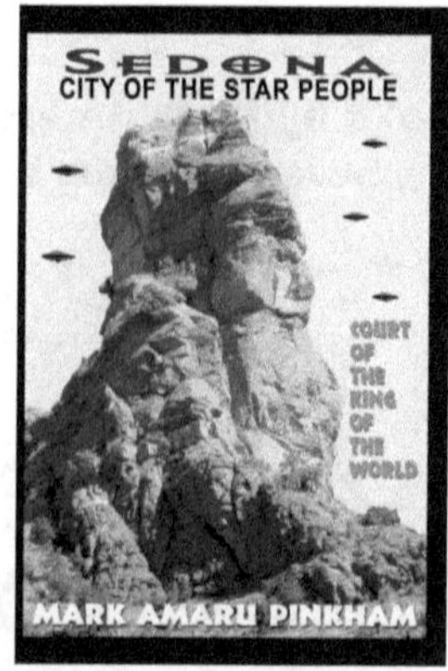

Sedona: City of the Star People is full of radically new information and discoveries about the ancient mysteries of Sedona uncovered and experienced by Mark Amaru over a 30 year period that could rewrite history. Topics covered: * The one million year history of Sedona *Mark's 30 years of interdimensional experiences of Sedona when it was Palatkwapi *The Hopi legend of Palatkwapi, the City of the Star People * The red rock temples of Palatkwapi that still exist physically in Sedona *The ancient court of Masau'u-Sanat Kumara-Tawsi Melek, the universal King of the World * Sedona, Root Chakra of Earth * The Sedona Grid and Chakra Points* 300 pgs. richly illustrated. color plates. $19.95

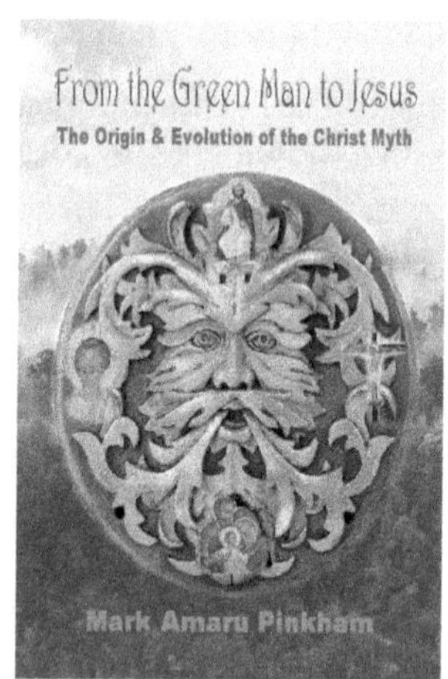

From the Green Man to Jesus: The Origin and Evolution of the Christ Myth reveals that the story of the life of Jesus Christ was based on a much older Christ Myth that began with the Neolithic Green Man who was born to a virgin and a father in the heavens in December and later resurrected in the spring. The Green Man Christ Myth evolved into the Christ Myths of many Near Eastern and Far Eastern Divine Sons of God, including the Hindu Murugan, the Mesopotamian Tammuz, the Egyptian Osiris and the Greek Dionysus. It also evolved into the Persian Christ Myth of the Divine Son of God, Mithras, and in this form it was taken west by by Magi Priests to Tarsus of Cilicia and into the hands of the city's most famous resident, St. Paul. When the future Apostle traveled to Palestine with the Roman Legions and heard the life story of Jesus, he recognized the Jewish Messiah to be Mithras. Later, St. Paul amalgamated most of the important events in the life of Mithras onto the life of Jesus. 150 pgs. richly illustrated $14.95

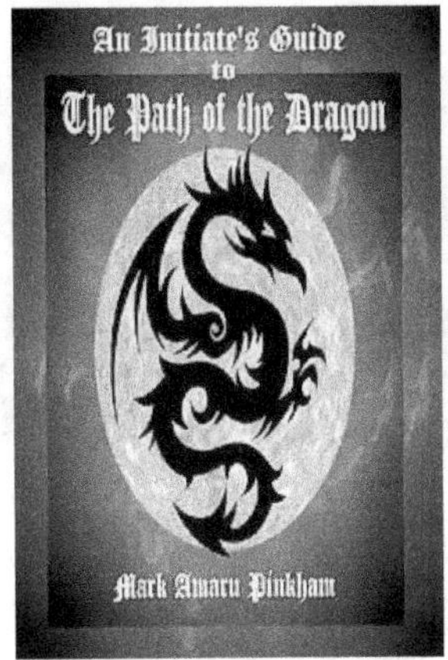

An Initiate's Guide to the Path of the Dragon presents:

1. The Dragon Orders, Lineages, and Families in Asia and Europe
2. Emperor Sigismund, Vlad Tepe III, Saint Germain and the Order of the Dragon
3. The Descent of the Dragon Tribes and Families from Middle Earth
4. Over 150 pages of Alchemical Practices of the Dragon Masters and the Siddhas
5. The Dragon Schools of the Left Hand Path and Goddess Tradition
6. The Ancient Courts and Edens of the Dragon King of the World
7. Descent of Jesus & Mary Magdalene from the Dragon Pharaoh Akhenaton
8. Ceremonial Dragon Magic
9. And Much, Much More. Fully Illustrated 460 pgs. $21.95

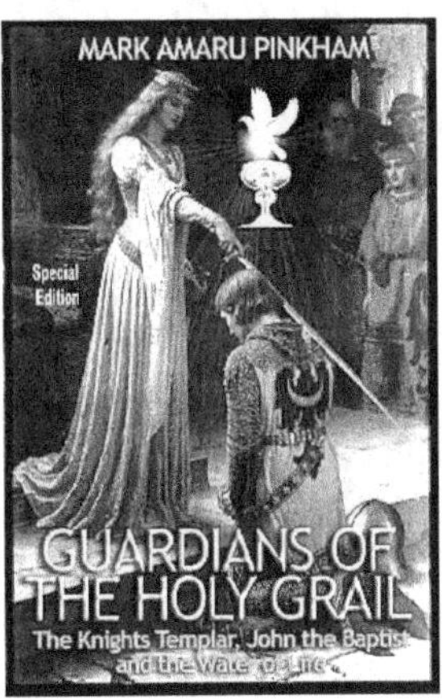

- *Guardians of the Holy Grail: The Knights Templar, John the Baptist, and the Water of Life-Special Edition.*
- 1. The ancient and current location of the Holy Grail
- 2. What the Holy Grail truly is
- 3. The Holy Grail Mysteries of the Knights Templar
- 4. The heretical Holy Grail practices of the Templars
- 5. The many Holy Chalices and their locations
- 6. The Holy Grail Relics of the Arma Christi
- 7. The origin of the Holy Grail Mysteries in the Far East
- 8. Mary Magdalene and the Grail Bloodline
- 9. The Fisher Kings and their Grail Castles
- 10. John the Baptist and the Human Holy Grails
    - Richly Illustrated 340 pgs. $16.95

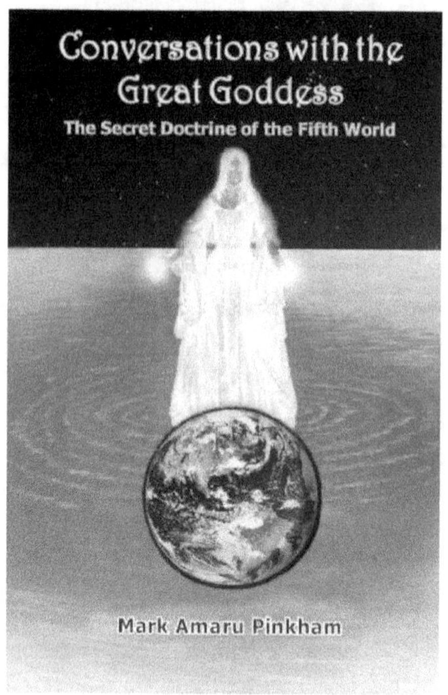

CONVERSATIONS WITH THE GREAT GODDESS
THE SECRET DOCTRINE OF THE FIFTH WORLD

A Doctrine Received Directly from the Universal Great Goddess

THE TRUE HISTORY OF AN ANCIENT BATTLE:
GOD vs GODDESS; PATRIARCHY vs MATRIARCHY

***The Kumaras: Pleiadian-Venusian founders of the Goddess Tradition**
*** The Truth about Lucifer, the Goddess's First Son & King of the World**
*** Lemuria, the Cradle of the Matriarchy, love and allowance**

*** Atlantis, the Cradle of the Patriarchy, dualism and domination**
*** The Spread of the Goddess's Worldwide Venus Culture**

*** The Evolution of the Goddess's Planetary Bull Cult**
*** The Last Stand and Defeat of Patriarchal Nazism by the Matriarchy**
*** The Coming United Civilization of the Fifth World of Venus**

Richly Illustrated 200 pgs. $14.95

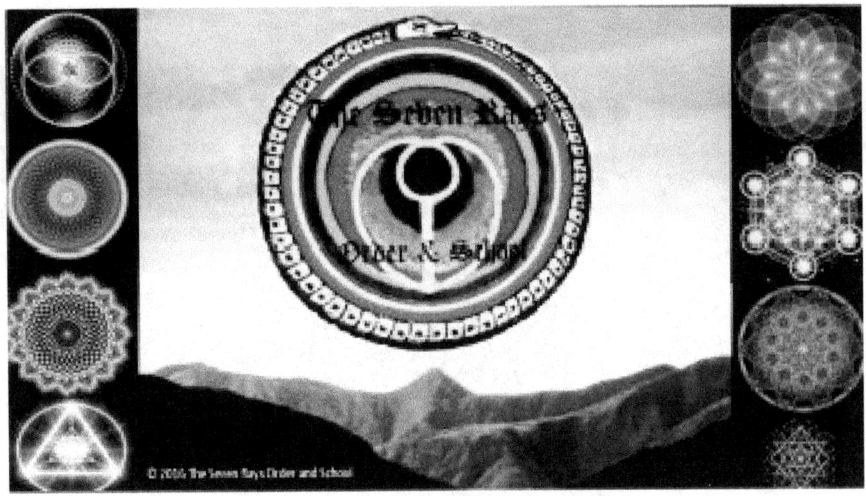

www.SevenRayOrder.com

Become a member of the World's Most Ancient Mystery School: The Order of the Seven Rays, which has also been known as the Melchizedek Priesthood and The Great White Brotherhood. This order was founded by **the Pleiadian Master Sanat Kumara or Karttikeya**, the "Son of the Pleiades," who first taught **The Path of the Dragon** and Gnostic-Alchemical Path on Earth. Over many ages this Orders' teachings have awakened many worthy spiritual seekers to the highest Self-Knowledge & intutive revelation of I AM THE CREATOR; THE INFINITE, ETERNAL SPIRIT DWELLS WITHIN ME AS ME.

The Order and Mystery School of the Seven Rays is a complete online school of esotericism that teaches: * Alchemy *Gnosticism *Yoga and Meditation *Sacred Geometry *Martial Arts *Esoteric World History Survival Skills *Shaivism *Esoteric Astrology, Healing and much more!

The Order and Mystery School of the Seven Rays includes these branches:
***The Path of the Dragon**
***The School of Seven Ray Healing**
***The School of Seven Ray Astrology**
***The Mysteries of the Knights Templar**
***The School of Shaivism**
***Spiritual Warrior Training**

The teachings of the Order and Mystery School of the Seven Rays and its branches are offered online and via Live Stream. Please visit the above website for a list of the books, DVDs, courses, spiritual tours,and upcoming seminars it is currently offering.

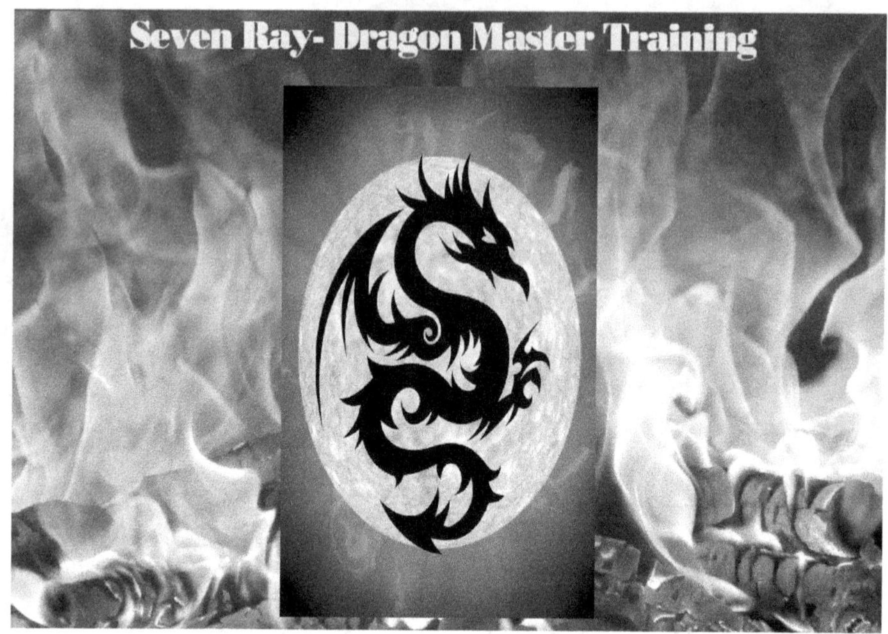

Seven Ray-Dragon Master Training is for those Dragons-in-Training who are ready to make a serious, long-term commitment to the Path of the Dragon. The curriculum of this training gives the Left Hand Path aspirant all the tools he or she needs to become a Dragon Master. Those that graduate from this training have the option of becoming administrators and teachers of the Order of the Seven Rays that was anciently created by the Pleiadian Dragon Master, Karttikeya or Sanat Kumara - the founder of the Path of the Dragon and Earth's current Dragon King. It also provides the graduate with the opportunity to become a Lord or Lady Knight of the Dragon Ways and help oversee his courts in Sedona and around the globe.

www.sevenrayorder.com/seven-ray-spiritual-warrior-trainin

Printed in the USA
CPSIA information can be obtained
at www.ICGtesting.com
LVHW080230140824
788229LV00012B/586